# A Study on Suicide

Jianjun Li

# A Study on Suicide

## Diagnosis and Solutions

SSAP

Springer

Jianjun Li
Guizhou University
Guiyang, China

ISBN 978-981-13-9497-3 ISBN 978-981-13-9499-7 (eBook)
https://doi.org/10.1007/978-981-13-9499-7

Jointly published with Social Sciences Academic Press
The print edition is not for sale in Mainland of China. Customers from Mainland of China please order the print book from: Social Sciences Academic Press.



This Springer imprint is published by the registered company Springer Nature Singapore Pte Ltd.
The registered company address is: 152 Beach Road, #21-01/04 Gateway East, Singapore 189721, Singapore

# Introduction—Suicide: A Grave Social and Public Health Issue

Suicide is a grave social and public health issue. Data released by the World Health Organization (WHO) in May 2005 shows that suicide was the leading cause of accidental death. Each year, over a million people around the globe die from suicide, while the number of those who attempt suicide may be 10–20 times that. This means that on average, a person dies from suicide every 40 s, and there is a suicide attempt every three seconds. The number of those who die by their own hands exceeds even the death toll of armed conflicts or traffic accidents around the globe. In 2001, the number of those who died from suicide was far higher than the numbers of those who died from homicide (500,000) and in armed conflicts (230,000).[1]

Suicide is among the top ten causes of death in most countries with relevant data available. It was also among the top three causes of death for youth.[2] According to statistics, in 1990, the number of people worldwide who died from suicide was 1.4 million, 1.6% of the total deaths of the year. The decline in disability-adjusted life years (DALY) caused by suicide and accidental death stood at 15.9%. The highest rates of suicide among men were reported in Lithuania, the Russian Federation, Latvia, and Estonia (annual suicide rate > 60.0 per 100,000 individuals), while the highest rates of suicide among women were seen in Sri Lanka, China, Hungary, and Estonia (annual suicide rate > 14.0 per 100,000 individuals).[3]

Suicide was a fairly grave problem in China. Data shared at the inaugural National Crisis Intervention and Suicide Prevention Seminar held in November 1992 in Nanjing showed that each year, 140,000–160,000 persons die from suicide in the Chinese mainland, approximately 400 persons per day on average, and the number of people attempting suicide is usually estimated to be ten times this figure. The death toll is far higher than the number of deaths caused by traffic accidents.

---

[1](2005, September 14). WHO data show that suicide already main cause of death in mankind. *China Youth Daily*.

[2]Liu and Li (1996).

[3]WHO releases world ranking for suicide. *Chinanews.com*. Retrieved from: http://www.chinanews.com/life/news/2009/05-22/1703440.shtml. Date of retrieval: July 10, 2011.

According to the annual World Health Statistics released by the WHO, in 1989, the suicide rate in the Chinese mainland stood at 17.07 per 100,000 individuals, with the number of those dead from suicide standing at 190,000 to 210,000. This figure accounted for 30% of the total number of suicidal deaths worldwide.[4] Generally speaking, the actual number of suicides may be three to five times the reported figure.[5] If we are to extrapolate from this, the number of deaths from suicide in the Chinese mainland may be as high as 600,000 annually. According to data from China's National Disease Surveillance System (1991–1995), the suicide rate in China was 19.58 per 100,000 individuals. In particular, those aged 15–34 accounted for 40.7% of all deaths from suicide. The Ministry of Health officially announced China's suicide rate for the first time at the WHO/Beijing High-Level Seminar on Mental Health held in 1999: 22.2 per 100,000 individuals in 1993. Oddly, in global statistics published by the WHO in 2009, the numbers for China were dated to 1999, which were 13.0/100,000 for males and 14.8/100,000 for females.[6] Clearly, the 1999 figures were the most updated data from the Chinese government.

In absolute terms, China's suicide numbers rank at the top of the world. Each year, around 42% of all deaths from suicide worldwide occur in China, which is home to 25% of the world's population.[7] According to the WHO, suicide rates among Chinese youth had been comparatively high by the end of the last century, specifically, the second highest in the world following those of Sri Lanka. In particular, suicide among those aged 15–24 accounts for 26.64% of all suicides, while suicide in the 25–34 age group accounts for 18.94% of all suicides (between 1987 and 1989).[8] It is worth noting that suicides among those in the 5–14 age group account for 1.02% of all suicides.

The higher rates of suicide among youths have a significant impact on the years of potential life lost (YPLL) in China. According to a report from the Ministry of Health to the WHO, in 1998, suicide was the top cause of death among 15–34-year-olds in China. In particular, the suicide rate in the 15–24 age group stood at 10.63 per 100,000 individuals and 22.41 per 100,000 individuals in the 25-to-34-year-old group.[9]

At the Third National Conference on Mental Health Work held in October 2001, then Deputy Health Minister Yin Dakui stated: "Each year, around 250,000 people in China die as a result of suicide. It is estimated that more than two million attempt suicide. Numbers show that of the 370 million people under 17 in China, around 30 million suffer from emotional, mental or behavioral problems… by the year 2020,

[4] WHO (1989c).

[5] Guetzloe (1991).

[6] http://www.who.int/mental_health/prevention/suicide_rates/en/print.html. Accessed: 10 August 2010.

[7] Yang et al. (1997).

[8] WHO (1989b).

[9] Li and Philip (2001).

China's mental health burden will increase to a quarter of the overall national health burden."[10]

Beijing Huilongguan Hospital released results of a seven-year study at the inaugural International Seminar on Suicide Prevention organized by the Beijing Suicide Research and Prevention Center between December 3 and December 9, 2002. The results showed China's average annual suicide rate to be 23.0 per 100,000 individuals (2.3 times the global average of 10.0 per 100,000 individuals), with an average of 287,000 deaths from suicide each year. Suicide had become the fifth cause of death for the Chinese population, and the top cause of death in the 15–34 age group, accounting for 19% of all deaths in this group.[11] Internationally, countries with suicide rates greater than 20.0 per 100,000 individuals are known as high suicide rate countries, and China is one of them.

Data on suicide attempts around China is not available for the time being. Assuming suicidal deaths to suicide attempts ratio of 1–2, that would put the number of suicide attempts in China each year in the millions.

The suicide rate among Chinese women was the highest in the world. It stood at 20.40 per 100,000 individuals in 1987 (14.90 per 100,000 individuals for men), 19.50 per 100,000 individuals in 1988 (15.00 per 100,000 individuals for men),[12] 19.60 per 100,000 individuals in 1989 (14.70 per 100,000 individuals for men),[13] and 18.40 per 100,000 individuals in 1990 (13.00 per 100,000 individuals for men).[14]

In 1994, the suicide rate among women in rural China stood at 30.54 per 100,000 individuals (compared to 23.67 per 100,000 individuals for men in rural areas) while in the cities, the suicide rate was 7.03 per 100,000 individuals (compared to 6.45 per 100,000 individuals for men in the cities).[15] In 1998, the suicide rate for rural women aged 15–24 was 15.96 per 100,000 individuals (compared to 8.67 per 100,000 individuals for men in the same age group), while for 25–34-year-old rural women, the suicide rate was 33.21 per 100,000 individuals (20.18 per 100,000 individuals for men in the same age group). For rural women aged 35–44, the suicide rate was 24.24 per 100,000 individuals (19.41 per 100,000 individuals for men in the same age group).[16]

---

[10] Yin (2002).

[11] Lin (2002a).

[12] WHO (1989a).

[13] WHO (1989b).

[14] http://www.who.int/mental_health/prevention/suicide_rates/en/print.html. Accessed: 10 July 2010.

[15] http://www.hotlife.com.cn/learning/yx-ml/information/WHO/1.htm. Date of retrieval: 20 June 2011.

[16] Lin (2002a).

Suicide rates are significantly higher among women than men in China. This is a phenomenon unique to China. Suicide among Chinese women has become a significant social problem.[17] As drastic social transformation continues, so will the increase in suicide rate, which will have significant negative impact on society.

At the WHO/Beijing High-Level Seminar on Mental Health held in Beijing in 1999, experts clearly stated that the prevention of suicide was one of the top three issues in mental health that China must tackle at that time.

Today, suicide research has yet to become a stand-alone academic discipline. It is generally believed that such research is but a small branch of social research. Few people in China are aware still less approve of "suicidology," which is already quite developed in the West. In our opinion, suicides in China have distinct features, even though they also share similarities with those in other countries. China's experience with the prevention and control of suicides also shows some distinctive features.

There should be recognition of the tremendous impact of suicide on social mentality, as well as efforts to explore the physical, psychological, and social roots of suicide through the study of the current state, nature, development, and frequency of suicide in China under social transformation. At the same time, we should also recognize that suicide rate is not an indicator of social progress or backwardness, and that on the individual level, suicide is a matter of neither shame nor pride. New values should be adopted to evaluate and control suicide.

As social changes continue in China, the irreversible modernization process will lead to major changes in the country's social structure and transform the traditional mentality of Chinese people. Further, such changes will have an unprecedented impact on people's way of thinking, emotional patterns, and values. New features will emerge for the problem of suicide in China.

We firmly believe that with unremitting efforts and effective countermeasures, China can keep its suicide rate under control.

## References


Guetzloe, E. C. (1991). *Suicide and the exceptional child. ERIC Digests.*

Li, X. & Philip, M. (2001). Causes of death for those of reproductive age and who died from suicide in China in 1998. *Chinese Journal of Public Health, 17*(7), 658.

Lin, J. (2002a). High rates of suicide in China, research and preventive institutions in short supply. *China Youth Daily*, December 11.

Li, J. (2002b). A comparative study of suicide among young females in China and Japan. *Journal of China Youth University for Political Sciences, 6*, 14–18.

Liu, H. & Li, X. (1996). The current state of research into suicide, and trends. *Guowai Yixue (Jingshenbingxue Fence), 23*(2), 125–126.

WHO. (1989a). *World Health Statistics Annual* (pp. 362–375).

WHO. (1989b). *World Health Statistics Annual* (pp. 364–369).

WHO. (1989c). *World Health Statistics Annual* (p. 367).

WHO. (1990). *World Health Statistics Annual* (pp. 364–369).


[17] Li (2002b).

Yang, G., Huang, Z., Chen, A. (1997). Levels of accidental harm among Chinese populations, and trends. *Chinese Journal of Epidemiology, 18*(3), 142–145.

Yin, D. (2002). United, with a practical mind, we promote mental health on all fronts in the new century: Report of the 3rd National Conference on Mental Health Work. *Chinese Mental Health Journal, 16*(1), 6.

# Contents

# Chapter 1
# Suicides in China: Rates, Means, and Distribution

Suicide rate refers to the number of suicidal deaths per 100,000 individual people per year. Changes in suicide rate can be used to gauge the waxing and waning of determining factors. To date, we do not yet have a comprehensive and accurate set of data for suicide in China. A good set of data is the basis of any study on suicide and key source of reference for designing effective countermeasures.

The data released by the World Health Organization (WHO) and China's National Disease Surveillance System may not be very accurate. This is due to, first of all, the sheer size of China's territory and population, which makes collection and compilation of statistics particularly challenging. A second reason is defects of the suicide recording system, the health administration system, and judicial system. The third reason is political: It is generally believed that suicide rate is a reflection of social, political, economic, and institutional problems and is thus the "dark side" that is best left unspoken of. The fourth reason has to do with historical, cultural, and psychological factors. Suicide is considered a source of dishonor (especially those that fall under "egoistic suicide" and "anomic suicide" in Émile Durkheim's classification) and among those who are superstitious, the ghosts of those who died of suicide "haunt" the living. Many are for that reason reluctant to admit to having made suicide attempts. The fifth reason is a technical one: Sometimes cases of suicide are mislabeled as accidents or homicides. Finally, there is also an economic dimension; for urban residents, death gives rise to insurance payment issues. For example, Japan's Ministry of Health and Welfare reported the country's 1988 suicide rate to the WHO as 14.3 per 100,000 individuals while the number of suicides reported by Japanese press was 23,744, which is equivalent to a suicide rate higher than 20.0 per 100,000 individuals. According to the American sociologist Erwin Stengel, the actual suicide rate is three to five times the official numbers.[1] China's National Bureau of Statistics has been releasing data in this area since 1987, while the WHO started to release such data provided by China's Ministry of Health in 1989.

[1]Stengel (1952).



J. Li, *A Study on Suicide*,
https://doi.org/10.1007/978-981-13-9499-7_1

Internationally, countries with a suicide rate higher than 20.0 per 100,000 individuals are known as high suicide rate countries.

The means and distribution of suicide vary across countries and population groups. In China, they are strongly linked to social and cultural customs. Preferred suicide methods in China include poisoning, hanging, drowning, among others, which can be linked to such traditional beliefs about the importance of preserving the physical integrity of the body of the dead so as to facilitate "reincarnation". By contrast, in the West, it is more common for people to choose more violent ways to end their lives, such as through the use of firearms, suicidal jumps, and traffic accidents. In Japan, the practice of suicide by disembowelment (seppuku) also finds deep roots in the culture. The distribution of suicide is closely related to both natural conditions (the weather and geographic conditions, etc.) and social and cultural factors.

# 1 Suicide Mortality Rate

## *1.1 Suicide Mortality Rate in China*

Of the more than 100 countries for which the WHO provides data on suicide rates, China has been ranked near the top. Furthermore, China is the only country in which the suicide rate for females is higher than that for males. In China, rural suicide rate is three times the urban rate, and the suicide rate for females aged 15–24 is the highest in the world.

The earliest statistics available on suicide in China (released by the National Bureau of Statistics in 1987) are as follows: The urban suicide mortality rate in 1979 was 10.90 per 100,000 individuals, and the rural rate was 15.30 per 100,000 individuals; in 1980, the urban suicide mortality rate was 12.50 per 100,000 individuals, while the that of rural areas was 15.40 per 100,000 individuals; in 1985, the urban suicide mortality rate was 11.20 per 100,000 individuals while the rural rate was 29.50 per 100,000 individuals.[2]

Calculations based on the 1979, 1980, and 1985 data for the urban and rural populations in *China Statistical Yearbook 1990* show that in 1979, a total of 20,159 individuals expired by suicide in the cities with another 120,941 in rural areas, making up a total of 141,100 and an overall suicide rate of 14.46 per 100,000 individuals; in 1980, the number of urban individuals who died of suicide stood at 23,925, while another 122,530 died in rural areas from the same reason, making a total of 146,455 and an overall suicide rate of 14.83 per 100,000 individuals; and in 1985, the number of urban number was 38,579, and the rural number was 196,464, making a total of 235,043 and an overall suicide rate of 23.26 per 100,000 individuals.

[2]Department of Social Statistics and National Bureau of Statistics (1987).

**Table 1** Suicide mortality rates by age groups in China, 1987–1989 (Unit: 100,000 people)

| Year | Sex | Age group | 5–14 | 15–24 | 25–34 | 35–44 | 45–54 | 55–64 | 65–74 | 75 and above |
|---|---|---|---|---|---|---|---|---|---|---|
| 1987 | Male | 14.9 | 1.1 | 16.2 | 13.0 | 15.2 | 15.4 | 26.4 | 54.1 | 79.1 |
| | Female | 20.4 | 1.1 | 32.7 | 18.1 | 17.0 | 19.8 | 30.2 | 50.1 | 73.7 |
| 1988 | Male | 15.0 | 1.0 | 15.8 | 13.8 | 15.4 | 16.0 | 27.7 | 49.9 | 90.1 |
| | Female | 19.5 | 1.0 | 30.4 | 17.7 | 18.4 | 18.6 | 26.5 | 44.3 | 71.0 |
| 1989 | Male | 14.7 | 0.5 | 14.0 | 13.3 | 15.4 | 17.1 | 27.4 | 52.5 | 93.3 |
| | Female | 19.6 | 0.8 | 29.1 | 20.3 | 19.3 | 17.8 | 25.6 | 43.4 | 69.0 |

*Sources* WHO (1989, 1990a, pp. 364–369)

According to data from the National Disease Surveillance System (1991–1995), the suicide rate in China stood at 19.85 per 100,000 individuals. Specifically, the urban rate was 6.50 per 100,000 individuals while the rural rate was 22.89 per 100,000 individuals. The male-to-female suicide ratio was 0.82:1. Individuals aged 15–34 accounted for 40.7% of deaths from suicide, while those aged above 60 made up another 29.74% of the total.[3]

Between 1987 and 1989, individuals aged 15–24 made up 26.64% of all deaths from suicide in China, while those aged 25–34 accounted for 18.94% of the total. The suicide rate among China's elderly people was also high during this period. In 1987, the suicide rate for males aged 55–64 stood at 26.40 per 100,000 individuals and the rate for females of the same age group was 30.20 per 100,000 individuals; among people aged 65–74, the suicide rate was 54.10 per 100,000 individuals for men and 50.10 per 100,000 individuals for women; and among those 75 years old and older, the suicide rate was 79.10 per 100,000 individuals for men and 73.70 per 100,000 individuals for women. In 1989, among those aged 55–64, the suicide rate for males stood at 27.40 per 100,000 individuals and 25.60 per 100,000 individuals for females; among those aged 65–74, the suicide rate was 52.50 per 100,000 individuals for men and 43.40 per 100,000 individuals for women; and among those 75 or older, the suicide rate was 93.30 per 100,000 individuals and 69.00 per 100,000 individuals for men and women, respectively (see Table 1).[4] By 1994, China's suicide rate had risen again, reaching 22.85 per 100,000 individuals, with an estimated total of 273,900 suicidal deaths (see Table 2).

In a study titled Global Burden of Diseases (GBD) jointly conducted by the World Bank, the WHO, and Harvard University, it was found that in the year 1990, the suicide mortality rate in China stood at 30.30 per 100,000 individuals (against a global average of 10.70 per 100,000 individuals) and that the suicide rate among Chinese women was 33.50 per 100,000 individuals (against a global average of 7.10 per 100,000 individuals). Of the 786,000 deaths from suicide worldwide in 1990, 43.6% or 343,000 occurred in China; and 55% of all suicide deaths among

[3]Yang et al. (1997).

[4]WHO (1989, 1990a, pp. 364–369).

**Table 2** Suicide and suicide mortality rates in China, 1994

| | | Suicide rate (per 100,000 individuals) | Estimated no. of suicidal deaths | Suicide mortality as a percentage of all suicide attempts |
|---|---|---|---|---|
| Urban | Male | 6.45 | 8010 | 2.92 |
| | Female | 7.03 | 8621 | 3.15 |
| | Overall | 6.74 | 16,631 | 6.07 |
| Rural | Male | 23.67 | 115,004 | 41.99 |
| | Female | 30.54 | 142,260 | 51.94 |
| | Overall | 27.03 | 257,264 | 93.93 |
| Overall | Male | 20.16 | 123,014 | 44.9 |
| | Female | 25.64 | 150,881 | 55.09 |
| | Overall | 22.85 | 273,895 | 100 |

*Source* WHO (1995)

**Table 3** Suicide mortality rates by age groups in China, 2015–2017 (1/100k)

| Year | Gender | Age group | 5–14 | 15–24 | 25–34 | 35–44 | 45–54 | 55–64 | 65–74 | 75+ |
|---|---|---|---|---|---|---|---|---|---|---|
| 2015 | Male | 7.715 | 0.58 | 2.74 | 4.58 | 5.07 | 8.75 | 12.13 | 22.91 | 49.96 |
| | Female | 5.715 | 0.44 | 1.62 | 3.17 | 3.45 | 6.21 | 8.57 | 17.12 | 33.74 |
| 2016 | Male | 7.465 | 0.61 | 2.34 | 5.03 | 4.77 | 8.6 | 12.35 | 21.12 | 43.72 |
| | Female | 5.51 | 0.32 | 1.68 | 3.06 | 3.06 | 6.31 | 8.74 | 15.37 | 29.23 |
| 2017 | Male | 6.975 | 0.64 | 2.44 | 4.83 | 4.57 | 8.37 | 10.74 | 20.11 | 39.24 |
| | Female | 4.96 | 0.35 | 1.52 | 2.61 | 2.57 | 5.9 | 7.88 | 14.25 | 24.32 |

*Sources* National Health Commission, *China Health Statistics Yearbook 2016–2018*

women occurred in China.[5] However, according to China's Ministry of Health, the suicide mortality rate for 1990 was only 18.80 per 100,000 individuals.

In the global statistics for suicide released by the WHO for 2009 and 2011, the 1999 data was cited for China: a suicide rate of 13.00 per 100,000 individuals for males and 14.80 per 100,000 individuals for females. Clearly, the Chinese government no longer provided data on China's suicide rate to the WHO after 1999.

Between 2015 and 2017, China witnessed a higher suicide mortality rate among the elderly. In 2015, the suicide mortality rate of those aged 65–74 was 22.91/100,000 for males, and 17.12/100,000 for females; aged over 75 was 49.96/100,000 for males and 33.74/100,000 for females. In 2016, the rate of those aged 65–74 was 21.12/100,000 for males and 15.37/100,000 for females; the rate of those aged over 75 was 39.24/100,000 for males and 24.32/100,000 for females (Table 3).

[5]Philip et al. (1999).

## 1.2 *Causes of Death for Working Age Population in Urban and Rural China*

In 1998, suicide was the number one cause of death for those aged 15–34 in China and the fourth cause of death among those aged 35–44 (see Table 5).

In 2009, suicide was the fourth cause of death for the 15–24 and 25–34 age groups and the fifth cause of death for the 35–44 age group (see Table 6).

### 1.2.1 The Statistical Approach

The statistical approach for Tables 4, 5, 6, 7, 8, and 9 is as follows.

(a) The statistical approach for various age groups. First, for men in the 15–24 age group, the population count is as follows: (total urban population × proportion of 15–19 + urban males + total urban population × proportion of 20–24 urban males) + (total town population × proportion of 15–19 + males living in towns + total town population × proportion of 20–24 males living in towns). The statistical methods for the corresponding age groups among urban women are the same as those for men. Second, the proportion of female (or male) of various age groups within the rural population = total rural population × proportion of rural female (male) within this age group to the total rural population. Third, we calculated the population of urban and rural male and female across the various age groups using the following: city males + city females + town males + town females + rural males + rural females within the age group.
In population statistics, no distinction is made between "cities" and "cities and towns." However, the corresponding mortality rate is officially expressed as a "city" rate (the *China Health Statistical Yearbook* published by the Ministry of Health does not have a corresponding mortality rate for "towns." Therefore, the author believes that the "city" statistics released by the Ministry of Health also includes "town" numbers).
(b) Calculation of the mortality rates for various causes of death in various age groups. As the mortality data from the *China Health Statistics Yearbook* is based on a five-year age cohort, for ten-year age group intervals we have employed the method of dividing the sum total by two. For instance, the mortality rate of suicide among rural women in the 15–24 group = (suicide mortality rate of rural women aged 15–19 + suicide mortality rate of rural women aged 20–24)/2. The margin of error should be negligibly small.
(c) Mortality rate from traffic accidents as shown in the tables and figures includes two types of deaths: accidents involving motor vehicles and those that do not.
(d) The numbers of suicides across the various age groups (general population, rural, urban, female, male, rural female, rural male, urban female, urban male) are calculated follows: population of age group × suicide rate (numbers for rural female, rural male, urban female, urban male can be directly calculated with the data shown in Table 6, so we can obtain the figures for the following

**Table 4** Suicide mortality rates in China's urban and rural populations by age group, 2003–2009 (Unit: Per 100,000 individuals)

| Year | Urban and rural | Total of all age groups | 5–9 | 10–14 | 15–19 | 20–24 | 25–29 | 30–34 | 35–39 | 40–44 | 45–49 | 50–54 | 55–59 | 60–64 | 65–69 | 70–74 | 75–79 | 80–84 | 85 years and above |
|---|---|---|---|---|---|---|---|---|---|---|---|---|---|---|---|---|---|---|---|
| 2003 | Urban (total) | 10.96 | 0.21 | 1.10 | 1.93 | 4.60 | 6.30 | 9.50 | 10.75 | 11.67 | 14.97 | 18.65 | 18.03 | 23.55 | 31.19 | 41.73 | 62.28 | 79.24 | 75.59 |
| | Urban (male) | 10.90 | 0.18 | 1.25 | 1.75 | 4.10 | 5.23 | 8.26 | 9.53 | 11.61 | 14.43 | 19.13 | 17.08 | 25.07 | 35.91 | 51.41 | 72.97 | 87.53 | 89.34 |
| | Urban (female) | 11.05 | 0.21 | 0.92 | 2.11 | 5.14 | 7.45 | 10.78 | 12.03 | 11.76 | 15.53 | 18.12 | 19.04 | 21.95 | 26.46 | 32.34 | 53.13 | 73.18 | 66.83 |
| | Rural (total) | 17.29 | 0.13 | 1.05 | 1.86 | 6.15 | 8.57 | 15.91 | 18.64 | 17.75 | 24.28 | 35.43 | 33.56 | 38.48 | 57.20 | 77.04 | 130.79 | 159.12 | 138.18 |
| | Rural (male) | 15.07 | 0.28 | 3.30 | 3.19 | 5.45 | 6.16 | 9.24 | 11.61 | 13.59 | 19.75 | 27.94 | 23.21 | 42.13 | 59.24 | 88.55 | 109.67 | 130.79 | 101.42 |
| | Rural (female) | 17.44 | 0.44 | 1.05 | 3.19 | 7.54 | 10.84 | 15.07 | 16.94 | 19.47 | 26.73 | 30.09 | 33.72 | 36.25 | 50.33 | 64.13 | 77.86 | 72.73 | 101.58 |
| 2005 | Urban (total) | 12.89 | 0.13 | 0.90 | 2.61 | 7.15 | 6.16 | 8.41 | 11.45 | 11.23 | 13.41 | 18.53 | 21.70 | 32.68 | 41.49 | 70.70 | 96.82 | 128.10 | 103.67 |
| | Urban (male) | 12.65 | 0.00 | 1.48 | 2.60 | 6.29 | 4.81 | 6.52 | 10.63 | 9.73 | 12.73 | 20.18 | 24.80 | 31.46 | 44.20 | 78.90 | 111.95 | 139.39 | 105.99 |
| | Urban (female) | 13.13 | 0.27 | 0.27 | 2.62 | 8.03 | 7.54 | 10.34 | 12.32 | 12.85 | 14.14 | 16.77 | 18.37 | 33.97 | 38.76 | 62.93 | 83.91 | 1119.78 | 96.72 |
| | Rural (total) | 10.08 | 0.72 | 1,52 | 2.29 | 4.62 | 2.88 | 7.24 | 8.86 | 9.89 | 7.54 | 15.41 | 17.38 | 22.87 | 39.15 | 42.89 | 65.16 | 82.98 | 97.50 |
| | Rural (male) | 9.62 | 1.03 | 1.99 | 1.87 | 3.71 | 1.89 | 5.76 | 7.61 | 8.88 | 7.21 | 15.74 | 17.23 | 25.03 | 39.82 | 46.00 | 74.23 | 96.54 | 77.12 |
| | Rural (female) | 10.64 | 0.00 | 0.96 | 2.80 | 5.65 | 4.05 | 8.98 | 10.33 | 11.12 | 7.95 | 15.02 | 17.58 | 20.13 | 38.35 | 39.33 | 56.30 | 71.93 | 111.71 |
| 2006 | Urban (total) | 5.02 | 0.00 | 0.24 | 1.80 | 2.54 | 3.42 | 3.81 | 4.42 | 6.18 | 5.55 | 6.15 | 7.67 | 9.22 | 9.62 | 14.38 | 18.59 | 27.67 | 39.22 |
| | Urban (male) | 5.39 | 0.00 | 0.31 | 1.88 | 2.42 | 2.75 | 3.88 | 4.28 | 6.78 | 6.24 | 7.24 | 8.72 | 10.11 | 11.21 | 18.16 | 21.89 | 34.75 | 57.37 |
| | Urban (female) | 4.65 | 0.00 | 0.17 | 1.71 | 2.68 | 4.13 | 3.73 | 4.56 | 5.55 | 4.84 | 5.04 | 6.60 | 8.36 | 8.08 | 10.87 | 15.72 | 22.42 | 28.84 |
| | Rural (total) | 9.26 | 0.09 | 0.97 | 3.47 | 3.83 | 4.22 | 6.55 | 7.27 | 9.94 | 8.29 | 13.65 | 16.59 | 20.89 | 26.35 | 36.11 | 48.02 | 65.82 | 74.03 |
| | Rural (male) | 9.56 | 0.08 | 1.47 | 2.63 | 4.35 | 3.87 | 5.83 | 5.97 | 10.19 | 8.42 | 14.44 | 17.83 | 24.24 | 29.67 | 45.01 | 58.04 | 87.89 | 83.46 |
| | Rural (female) | 8.95 | 0.09 | 0.42 | 4.38 | 3.30 | 4.58 | 7.28 | 8.61 | 9.68 | 8.16 | 12.81 | 15.26 | 17.20 | 22.91 | 27.82 | 40.08 | 51.59 | 69.61 |

(continued)

**Table 4** (continued)

| Year | Urban and rural | Total of all age groups | 5–9 | 10–14 | 15–19 | 20–24 | 25–29 | 30–34 | 35–39 | 40–44 | 45–49 | 50–54 | 55–59 | 60–64 | 65–69 | 70–74 | 75–79 | 80–84 | 85 years and above |
|---|---|---|---|---|---|---|---|---|---|---|---|---|---|---|---|---|---|---|---|
| 2007 | Urban (total) | 4.89 | 0.06 | 0.46 | 1.29 | 2.71 | 2.89 | 3.43 | 4.76 | 5.28 | 5.48 | 6.22 | 6.25 | 7.37 | 8.35 | 14.16 | 14.83 | 23.13 | 22.70 |
| | Urban (male) | 5.46 | 0.00 | 0.54 | 1.46 | 3.17 | 3.25 | 3.84 | 6.27 | 6.88 | 6.47 | 6.35 | 6.34 | 8.52 | 8.26 | 17.02 | 16.72 | 27.75 | 28.64 |
| | Urban (female) | 4.30 | 0.00 | 0.38 | 1.12 | 2.21 | 2.50 | 3.02 | 3.19 | 3.60 | 4.44 | 6.09 | 6.15 | 6.21 | 8.43 | 11.59 | 13.28 | 19.91 | 19.53 |
| | Rural (total) | 10.31 | 0.08 | 0.77 | 2.73 | 4.25 | 4.14 | 5.04 | 8.54 | 11.15 | 7.73 | 16.71 | 20.43 | 22.34 | 28.45 | 40.55 | 57.21 | 86.73 | 97.52 |
| | Rural (male) | 10.97 | 0.16 | 1.03 | 3.03 | 4.93 | 4.00 | 4.40 | 7.79 | 10.36 | 7.41 | 18.21 | 22.33 | 27.27 | 34.27 | 51.69 | 67.46 | 103.51 | 127.97 |
| | Rural (female) | 9.64 | 0.00 | 0.50 | 2.42 | 3.58 | 4.29 | 5.68 | 9.30 | 11.96 | 8.05 | 15.17 | 18.45 | 17.13 | 22.67 | 30.23 | 48.85 | 75.13 | 81.08 |
| 2008 | Urban (total) | 3.59 | 0.21 | 0.80 | 1.57 | 2.07 | 2.25 | 2.58 | 3.46 | 3.61 | 3.82 | 4.78 | 4.63 | 4.85 | 6.11 | 7.38 | 9.66 | 14.39 | 13.93 |
| | Urban (male) | 4.00 | 0.20 | 0.46 | 1.57 | 2.52 | 2.44 | 2.43 | 4.25 | 4.38 | 4.65 | 5.67 | 4.52 | 5.26 | 7.52 | 9.02 | 10.85 | 16.00 | 16.82 |
| | Urban (female) | 10.97 | 0.00 | 0.16 | 1.03 | 3.03 | 4.93 | 4.00 | 4.40 | 7.79 | 10.36 | 7.41 | 18.21 | 22.33 | 27.27 | 34.27 | 51.69 | 67.46 | 103.51 |
| | Rural (total) | 8.25 | 0.00 | 0.31 | 2.88 | 4.11 | 3.71 | 4.34 | 7.59 | 9.16 | 7.01 | 13.40 | 17.72 | 18.52 | 20.51 | 26.93 | 41.18 | 51.87 | 62.48 |
| | Rural (male) | 8.62 | 0.00 | 0.30 | 3.18 | 3.54 | 3.06 | 4.29 | 7.33 | 8.46 | 7.78 | 14.85 | 19.31 | 17.96 | 27.32 | 31.46 | 47.19 | 68.40 | 106.10 |
| | Rural (female) | 7.87 | 0.00 | 0.32 | 2.57 | 4.67 | 4.36 | 4.39 | 7.85 | 9.90 | 6.20 | 11.89 | 16.02 | 19.14 | 13.60 | 22.76 | 36.40 | 41.28 | 42.47 |
| 2009 | Urban (total) | 4.95 | 0.13 | 0.37 | 1.41 | 2.78 | 2.56 | 2.94 | 3.82 | 4.29 | 4.53 | 5.18 | 6.33 | 7.52 | 9.94 | 13.23 | 20.64 | 29.67 | 31.07 |
| | Urban (male) | 5.43 | 0.06 | 0.26 | 1.27 | 2.92 | 2.61 | 3.64 | 4.43 | 4.51 | 5.36 | 6.24 | 7.49 | 8.86 | 11.54 | 15.31 | 23.72 | 31.76 | 34.34 |
| | Urban (female) | 4.47 | 0.00 | 0.50 | 1.55 | 2.62 | 2.52 | 2.20 | 3.18 | 4.07 | 3.67 | 4.10 | 5.17 | 6.19 | 8.41 | 11.34 | 17.97 | 28.06 | 29.05 |
| | Rural (total) | 9.10 | 0.00 | 0.40 | 2.38 | 4.80 | 3.45 | 3.69 | 4.94 | 8.81 | 7.47 | 12.19 | 14.96 | 19.83 | 23.68 | 35.10 | 53.00 | 81.16 | 104.92 |
| | Rural (male) | 9.76 | 0.00 | 0.39 | 2.67 | 4.91 | 3.16 | 3.39 | 5.78 | 9.55 | 7.20 | 14.18 | 17.90 | 22.09 | 26.48 | 43.21 | 64.07 | 90.31 | 130.25 |
| | Rural (female) | 8.41 | 0.00 | 0.41 | 2.07 | 4.68 | 3.74 | 4.00 | 4.09 | 8.03 | 7.75 | 10.11 | 11.87 | 17.38 | 20.80 | 27.34 | 43.80 | 74.78 | 91.90 |

(continued)

**Table 4** (continued)

| Year | Urban and rural | Total of all age groups | 5–9 | 10–14 | 15–19 | 20–24 | 25–29 | 30–34 | 35–39 | 40–44 | 45–49 | 50–54 | 55–59 | 60–64 | 65–69 | 70–74 | 75–79 | 80–84 | 85 years and above |
|---|---|---|---|---|---|---|---|---|---|---|---|---|---|---|---|---|---|---|---|
| 2010 | Urban (total) | 6.86 | | 0.45 | 2.03 | 3.07 | 3.29 | 3.58 | 4.08 | 4.91 | 5.61 | 6.28 | 7.94 | 11.54 | 15.54 | 24.88 | 32.77 | 57.37 | 89.46 |
| | Urban (male) | 7.37 | | 0.43 | 1.97 | 3.25 | 2.95 | 3.57 | 4.20 | 5.19 | 6.27 | 7.64 | 8.86 | 13.02 | 17.27 | 29.25 | 39.88 | 68.88 | 117.48 |
| | Urban (female) | 6.32 | | 0.47 | 2.09 | 2.87 | 3.66 | 3.59 | 3.95 | 4.62 | 4.92 | 4.88 | 7.02 | 10.05 | 13.88 | 20.98 | 26.65 | 48.47 | 71.95 |
| | Rural (total) | 10.01 | | 0.26 | 2.32 | 4.04 | 4.90 | 4.71 | 5.88 | 6.18 | 7.58 | 9.06 | 13.71 | 17.67 | 27.02 | 44.25 | 68.78 | 108.13 | 191.74 |
| | Rural (male) | 10.61 | | 0.33 | 2.10 | 4.67 | 5.02 | 4.61 | 5.11 | 6.08 | 8.87 | 9.51 | 15.87 | 18.57 | 29.19 | 51.44 | 88.71 | 151.03 | 256.81 |
| | Rural (female) | 9.39 | | 0.19 | 2.58 | 3.34 | 4.78 | 4.81 | 6.67 | 6.30 | 6.26 | 8.60 | 11.52 | 16.73 | 24.81 | 37.31 | 52.30 | 79.49 | 159.70 |
| 2011 | Urban (total) | 5.28 | 0.08 | 0.63 | 1.45 | 2.43 | 2.55 | 2.54 | 3.68 | 4.67 | 4.73 | 5.61 | 6.62 | 8.34 | 9.85 | 13.97 | 24.10 | 37.13 | 38.91 |
| | Urban (male) | 5.78 | 0.00 | 0.94 | 1.91 | 2.80 | 3.07 | 2.87 | 4.60 | 5.53 | 5.65 | 6.41 | 7.49 | 9.35 | 9.86 | 15.97 | 24.14 | 42.83 | 45.08 |
| | Urban (female) | 4.77 | 0.16 | 0.29 | 0.98 | 2.05 | 2.01 | 2.20 | 2.74 | 3.81 | 3.80 | 4.79 | 5.75 | 7.33 | 9.85 | 12.19 | 24.07 | 32.57 | 34.94 |
| | Rural (total) | 9.28 | 0.19 | 0.85 | 2.44 | 4.59 | 4.15 | 3.43 | 5.43 | 7.62 | 8.91 | 9.66 | 17.39 | 17.82 | 25.59 | 35.23 | 46.36 | 78.50 | 93.46 |
| | Rural (male) | 9.95 | 0.21 | 0.88 | 2.90 | 5.54 | 4.16 | 3.47 | 5.38 | 7.25 | 9.11 | 10.30 | 19.18 | 19.48 | 29.57 | 41.69 | 50.99 | 104.13 | 148.44 |
| | Rural (female) | 8.58 | 0.16 | 0.81 | 1.92 | 3.60 | 4.15 | 3.39 | 5.48 | 7.99 | 8.71 | 8.97 | 15.52 | 16.04 | 21.47 | 28.87 | 42.39 | 60.52 | 63.76 |
| 2012 | Urban (total) | 4.82 | 0.24 | 0.72 | 1.41 | 2.46 | 2.28 | 2.17 | 3.01 | 3.95 | 4.72 | 4.95 | 5.34 | 7.50 | 10.51 | 14.88 | 22.06 | 28.63 | 32.36 |
| | Urban (male) | 5.30 | 0.23 | 0.61 | 1.61 | 2.92 | 2.59 | 2.19 | 3.03 | 4.93 | 5.43 | 5.46 | 6.07 | 8.61 | 11.83 | 17.35 | 25.83 | 32.92 | 35.19 |
| | Urban (female) | 4.33 | 0.25 | 0.84 | 1.20 | 1.98 | 1.96 | 2.16 | 3.00 | 2.96 | 3.99 | 4.43 | 4.62 | 6.38 | 9.19 | 12.56 | 18.79 | 25.18 | 30.50 |
| | Rural (total) | 8.58 | 0.14 | 0.67 | 2.50 | 3.91 | 4.72 | 4.25 | 5.51 | 7.31 | 8.95 | 9.07 | 13.23 | 15.49 | 19.79 | 26.58 | 43.47 | 53.08 | 71.17 |
| | Rural (male) | 9.09 | 0.13 | 0.83 | 2.64 | 3.90 | 4.94 | 4.44 | 6.11 | 7.36 | 9.64 | 9.77 | 14.33 | 16.71 | 21.64 | 29.90 | 47.50 | 64.93 | 92.21 |
| | Rural (female) | 8.05 | 0.15 | 0.49 | 2.35 | 3.91 | 4.49 | 4.07 | 4.93 | 7.26 | 8.25 | 8.32 | 12.10 | 14.18 | 17.83 | 23.20 | 39.79 | 43.79 | 58.72 |

(continued)

**Table 4** (continued)

| Year | Urban and rural | Total of all age groups | 5–9 | 10–14 | 15–19 | 20–24 | 25–29 | 30–34 | 35–39 | 40–44 | 45–49 | 50–54 | 55–59 | 60–64 | 65–69 | 70–74 | 75–79 | 80–84 | 85 years and above |
|---|---|---|---|---|---|---|---|---|---|---|---|---|---|---|---|---|---|---|---|
| 2013 | Urban (total) | 5.29 | 0.09 | 0.46 | 1.83 | 2.87 | 3.33 | 3.59 | 3.57 | 4.84 | 4.02 | 5.88 | 7.25 | 9.04 | 11.67 | 14.69 | 18.98 | 29.52 | 29.23 |
| | Urban (male) | 6.02 | 0.06 | 0.52 | 1.79 | 3.21 | 3.61 | 4.02 | 4.03 | 5.41 | 4.83 | 7.02 | 8.94 | 10.60 | 13.79 | 17.15 | 23.39 | 34.90 | 40.02 |
| | Urban (female) | 4.54 | 0.13 | 0.38 | 1.87 | 2.52 | 3.06 | 3.15 | 3.10 | 4.26 | 3.18 | 4.68 | 5.55 | 7.47 | 9.58 | 12.41 | 15.12 | 25.10 | 22.28 |
| | Rural (total) | 8.77 | 0.13 | 1.09 | 3.03 | 3.45 | 4.78 | 5.63 | 5.24 | 6.44 | 6.97 | 10.84 | 11.83 | 15.56 | 22.06 | 30.96 | 43.95 | 59.18 | 72.40 |
| | Rural (male) | 9.82 | 0.13 | 1.09 | 3.34 | 3.61 | 5.04 | 6.30 | 5.96 | 7.40 | 8.10 | 12.62 | 13.84 | 17.62 | 25.47 | 37.05 | 53.66 | 73.17 | 95.03 |
| | Rural (female) | 7.66 | 0.13 | 1.08 | 2.68 | 3.30 | 4.51 | 4.94 | 4.48 | 5.45 | 5.85 | 8.96 | 9.77 | 13.40 | 18.59 | 24.79 | 35.27 | 48.38 | 58.92 |
| 2014 | Urban (total) | 5.01 | 0.05 | 0.96 | 1.92 | 1.83 | 3.33 | 3.05 | 2.83 | 3.67 | 4.13 | 6.26 | 5.53 | 9.81 | 12.86 | 15.85 | 19.48 | 25.69 | 41.19 |
| | Urban (male) | 5.71 | 0.05 | 1.06 | 2.21 | 2.09 | 3.60 | 3.33 | 2.93 | 4.46 | 5.09 | 7.74 | 6.46 | 10.84 | 15.06 | 19.37 | 24.08 | 28.56 | 57.34 |
| | Urban (female) | 4.29 | 0.05 | 0.84 | 1.60 | 1.57 | 3.06 | 2.75 | 2.74 | 2.86 | 3.14 | 4.69 | 4.60 | 8.77 | 10.65 | 12.56 | 15.42 | 23.29 | 30.61 |
| | Rural (total) | 8.61 | 0.04 | 0.90 | 2.60 | 2.89 | 5.16 | 5.36 | 4.78 | 6.19 | 6.88 | 10.08 | 11.24 | 15.16 | 21.44 | 30.99 | 42.02 | 55.83 | 70.29 |
| | Rural (male) | 9.65 | 0.03 | 0.93 | 2.89 | 3.57 | 5.83 | 5.77 | 5.51 | 7.47 | 8.13 | 11.46 | 13.24 | 16.80 | 25.31 | 35.46 | 49.16 | 67.51 | 93.54 |
| | Rural (female) | 7.51 | 0.04 | 0.85 | 2.26 | 2.21 | 4.47 | 4.95 | 4.01 | 4.87 | 5.63 | 8.63 | 9.18 | 13.44 | 17.52 | 26.50 | 35.53 | 46.62 | 56.19 |
| 2015 | Urban (total) | 5.07 | 0.08 | 1.08 | 1.30 | 1.77 | 3.29 | 2.84 | 2.52 | 4.20 | 4.11 | 7.26 | 6.09 | 9.70 | 13.17 | 15.32 | 18.16 | 26.81 | 41.09 |
| | Urban (male) | 5.85 | 0.05 | 1.14 | 1.62 | 2.26 | 4.02 | 3.33 | 2.96 | 5.16 | 4.88 | 8.56 | 7.52 | 11.25 | 15.67 | 16.88 | 21.62 | 33.17 | 49.91 |
| | Urban (female) | 4.27 | 0.11 | 1.00 | 0.97 | 1.27 | 2.58 | 2.32 | 2.08 | 3.23 | 3.33 | 5.89 | 4.68 | 8.13 | 10.69 | 13.86 | 15.11 | 21.53 | 35.35 |
| | Rural (total) | 8.39 | 0.03 | 0.88 | 2.81 | 2.88 | 4.63 | 4.77 | 4.45 | 5.89 | 7.06 | 11.53 | 10.71 | 14.94 | 21.99 | 29.58 | 39.85 | 52.48 | 65.60 |
| | Rural (male) | 9.58 | 0.03 | 1.10 | 3.44 | 3.63 | 5.70 | 5.28 | 5.24 | 6.91 | 8.93 | 12.63 | 13.11 | 16.63 | 26.14 | 32.95 | 46.40 | 66.90 | 81.78 |
| | Rural (female) | 7.16 | 0.02 | 0.63 | 2.10 | 2.12 | 3.53 | 4.25 | 3.63 | 4.85 | 5.22 | 10.39 | 8.27 | 13.20 | 17.77 | 26.14 | 33.81 | 40.92 | 55.71 |

(continued)

**Table 4** (continued)

| Year | Urban and rural | Total of all age groups | 5–9 | 10–14 | 15–19 | 20–24 | 25–29 | 30–34 | 35–39 | 40–44 | 45–49 | 50–54 | 55–59 | 60–64 | 65–69 | 70–74 | 75–79 | 80–84 | 85 years and above |
|---|---|---|---|---|---|---|---|---|---|---|---|---|---|---|---|---|---|---|---|
| 2016 | Urban (total) | 4.90 | 0.02 | 0.98 | 1.56 | 1.56 | 2.79 | 3.38 | 2.45 | 3.72 | 3.87 | 7.36 | 5.83 | 10.67 | 11.91 | 13.62 | 16.96 | 24.26 | 37.05 |
| | Urban (male) | 5.62 | 0.05 | 1.25 | 1.58 | 1.90 | 3.27 | 4.24 | 2.88 | 4.49 | 4.57 | 8.15 | 7.00 | 12.53 | 13.76 | 17.32 | 21.05 | 26.29 | 46.18 |
| | Urban (female) | 4.15 | | 0.66 | 1.54 | 1.20 | 2.32 | 2.49 | 2.00 | 2.94 | 3.17 | 6.52 | 4.65 | 8.78 | 10.08 | 10.18 | 13.39 | 22.57 | 30.98 |
| | Rural (total) | 8.09 | 0.06 | 0.86 | 2.52 | 2.41 | 4.77 | 5.24 | 4.37 | 5.13 | 6.71 | 11.9 | 9.65 | 16.05 | 19.77 | 25.30 | 34.15 | 45.16 | 59.31 |
| | Rural (male) | 9.31 | | 1.13 | 2.73 | 3.13 | 5.88 | 6.71 | 5.45 | 6.24 | 7.81 | 13.87 | 11.28 | 18.60 | 23.35 | 30.04 | 38.63 | 53.93 | 76.23 |
| | Rural (female) | 6.87 | 0.06 | 0.56 | 2.31 | 1.68 | 3.66 | 3.76 | 3.29 | 4.02 | 5.60 | 9.93 | 8.02 | 13.49 | 16.19 | 20.55 | 29.66 | 36.39 | 42.39 |
| 2017 | Urban (total) | 4.31 | 0.09 | 0.96 | 1.40 | 1.59 | 2.67 | 2.87 | 2.35 | 2.92 | 3.57 | 7.17 | 4.55 | 9.11 | 10.58 | 13.07 | 14.03 | 21.60 | 25.31 |
| | Urban (male) | 5.04 | 0.17 | 1.39 | 1.81 | 1.87 | 3.66 | 3.38 | 2.92 | 3.59 | 4.12 | 8.81 | 5.52 | 9.78 | 12.09 | 14.78 | 17.38 | 27.80 | 33.04 |
| | Urban (female) | 3.56 | | 0.46 | 0.96 | 1.29 | 1.71 | 2.32 | 1.77 | 2.23 | 3.00 | 5.42 | 3.58 | 8.43 | 9.08 | 11.49 | 11.10 | 16.40 | 20.15 |
| | Rural (total) | 7.66 | 0.02 | 0.94 | 2.49 | 2.47 | 4.47 | 4.91 | 3.94 | 4.33 | 6.11 | 11.76 | 8.12 | 15.52 | 20.51 | 24.50 | 31.57 | 42.73 | 48.56 |
| | Rural (male) | 8.91 | 0.03 | 0.96 | 2.73 | 3.33 | 5.82 | 6.47 | 4.65 | 5.55 | 7.38 | 13.15 | 9.37 | 18.30 | 24.47 | 29.11 | 37.17 | 54.52 | 65.52 |
| | Rural (female) | 6.36 | | 0.92 | 2.21 | 1.60 | 3.08 | 3.34 | 3.20 | 3.08 | 4.86 | 10.31 | 6.85 | 12.65 | 16.54 | 19.90 | 26.51 | 33.47 | 38.30 |

*Source* Ministry of Health, *China Health Statistics Yearbook* (2004–2010)

**Table 5** List of main causes of death for Chinese males and females at working age in urban and rural areas, 1998

| Age group | 15–24 | | 25–34 | | 35–44 | |
|---|---|---|---|---|---|---|
| Rural female | Pop. 79,635,412 | | Pop. 92,590,396 | | Pop. 66,451,134 | |
| | Cause of death | Mortality rate (Per 100,000 individuals) | Cause of death | Mortality rate (Per 100,000 individuals) | Cause of death | Mortality rate (Per 100,000 individuals) |
| | 1 Suicide | 15.96 | 1 Suicide | 33.21 | 1 Malignant tumors | 47.90 |
| | 2 Traffic accidents | 5.33 | 2 Malignant tumors | 17.68 | 2 Suicide | 24.24 |
| | 3 Malignant tumors | 4.43 | 3 Diseases of the circulatory system | 12.58 | 3 Diseases of the circulatory system | 22.28 |
| | 4 Diseases of the circulatory system | 3.08 | 4 Traffic accidents | 9.54 | 4 Diseases of the respiratory system | 10.97 |
| | 5 Drowning | 2.58 | 5 Infectious diseases | 5.65 | 5 Traffic accidents | 10.83 |
| Rural male | Pop. 81,480,977 | | Pop. 92,266,233 | | Pop. 69,182,291 | |
| | Cause of death | Mortality rate (Per 100,000 individuals) | Cause of death | Mortality rate (Per 100,000 individuals) | Cause of death | Mortality rate (Per 100,000 individuals) |
| | 1 Traffic accidents | 13.95 | 1 Traffic accidents | 31.43 | 1 Malignant tumors | 81.49 |
| | 2 Suicide | 8.67 | 2 Malignant tumors | 25.76 | 2 Diseases of the circulatory system | 41.37 |
| | 3 Drowning | 7.11 | 3 Suicide | 20.18 | 3 Traffic accidents | 32.28 |
| | 4 Malignant tumors | 6.31 | 4 Diseases of the circulatory system | 13.23 | 4 Diseases of the digestive system | 20.89 |
| | 5 Diseases of the circulatory system | 3.82 | 5 Infectious diseases | 9.23 | 5 Suicide | 19.41 |
| Urban female | Pop. 20,096,543 | | Pop. 26,074,066 | | Pop. 21,564,760 | |
| | Cause of death | Mortality rate (Per 100,000 individuals) | Cause of death | Mortality rate (Per 100,000 individuals) | Cause of death | Mortality rate (Per 100,000 individuals) |
| | 1 Suicide | 4.60 | 1 Malignant tumors | 11.93 | 1 Malignant tumors | 44.35 |

(continued)

**Table 5** (continued)

| Age group | 15–24 | | 25–34 | | 35–44 | |
|---|---|---|---|---|---|---|
| | 2 Malignant tumors | 4.18 | 2 Suicide | 7.77 | 2 Diseases of the circulatory system | 21.31 |
| | 3 Traffic accidents | 3.81 | 3 Traffic accidents | 5.55 | 3 Traffic accidents | 7.52 |
| | 4 Diseases of the circulatory system | 1.94 | 4 Diseases of the circulatory system | 5.40 | 4 Suicide | 5.88 |
| | 5 Accidental poisoning | 1.73 | 5 Accidental poisoning | 2.51 | 5 Diseases of the digestive system | 4.64 |
| Urban male | Pop. 19,960,096 | | Pop. 26,103,939 | | Pop. 22,069,573 | |
| | Cause of death | Mortality rate (Per 100,000 individuals) | Cause of death | Mortality rate (Per 100,000 individuals) | Cause of death | Mortality rate (Per 100,000 individuals) |
| | 1 Traffic accidents | 8.10 | 1 Traffic accidents | 16.53 | 1 Malignant tumors | 63.58 |
| | 2 Malignant tumors | 5.47 | 2 Malignant tumors | 15.23 | 2 Suicide | 28.40 |
| | 3 Diseases of the circulatory system | 3.86 | 3 Diseases of the circulatory system | 10.21 | 3 Diseases of the circulatory system | 21.68 |
| | 4 Drowning | 2.54 | 4 Suicide | 6.62 | 4 Diseases of the respiratory system | 16.53 |
| | 5 Leukemia | 2.17 | 5 Homicide | 4.65 | 5 Traffic accidents | 9.53 |
| | 6 Suicide | 2.10 | | | 6 Suicide | 8.16 |
| Urban and rural male and female | Pop. 201,173,029 | | Pop. 237,034,634 | | Pop. 179,267,758 | |
| | Cause of death | Mortality rate (Per 100,000 individuals) | Cause of death | Mortality rate (Per 100,000 individuals) | Cause of death | Mortality rate (Per 100,000 individuals) |
| | 1 Suicide | 10.63 | 1 Suicide | 22.41 | 1 Malignant tumors | 62.37 |
| | 2 Traffic accidents | 8.94 | 2 Traffic accidents | 19.92 | 2 Diseases of the circulatory system | 30.28 |
| | 3 Malignant tumors | 5.27 | 3 Malignant tumors | 18.39 | 3 Traffic accidents | 20.04 |
| | 4 Drowning | 4.53 | 4 Diseases of the circulatory system | 11.78 | 4 Suicide | 18.19 |

(continued)

**Table 5** (continued)

| Age group | 15–24 | | 25–34 | | 35–44 | |
|---|---|---|---|---|---|---|
| | 5 Diseases of the circulatory system | 3.24 | 5 Infectious diseases | 6.29 | 5 Diseases of the digestive system | 13.79 |
| | 6 Various infectious diseases | 2.49 | 6 Diseases of the digestive system | 5.40 | 6 Diseases of the respiratory system | 10.59 |
| | 7 Homicide | 1.93 | 7 Drowning | 4.37 | 7 Infectious diseases | 10.21 |
| | 8 Accidental falls from height | 1.78 | 8 Diseases of the respiratory system | 3.91 | 8 Diseases relating to the endocrinological system, nutrition, and metabolism | 4.37 |
| | 9 Diseases of the respiratory system | 1.57 | 9 Accidental falls from height | 3.47 | 8 Accidental falls from height | 4.22 |
| | 10 Accidental poisoning | 1.40 | 10 Homicide | 3.31 | 10 Diseases of the urinary and reproductive systems | 4.02 |

*Note* Mortality rates for different causes of death and population figures for the three age groups are calculated based on the mortality rates for various five-year age group intervals as contained in the 1998 *National Health Statistics Annual Report* of the Ministry of Health and the corresponding population by age group for 1998 as provided in *China Demographic Yearbook* 1999

items: number of rural suicides, urban suicides, male suicides, and female suicides. After obtaining these figures, we calculated the suicide rate for rural areas, urban areas, males, and females in various age groups based on age group population numbers). Although this is a reverse calculation, i.e., we first determined the number of suicides and then calculated the suicide rate (official figures are available for suicide rates but not the actual number of suicides), the premise of this solution is that the number of suicides and the population size is constant. Thus, it should be relatively accurate.

### 1.2.2 Discussions

Compared to the 1998 and 2009 figures, we see that there have been some changes in the rankings of various causes of death for the three age groups in 2017. The suicide rate has dipped significantly. However, the data also tells us that suicide remains the leading cause of death for all age groups. In particular, it is the fourth cause of death for both rural and urban women in all three age groups, i.e., 15–24, 25–34 and 35–44.

**Table 6** List of main causes of death for Chinese males and females of working age in urban and rural areas, 2009

| Age group | 15–24 | | 25–34 | | 35–44 | |
|---|---|---|---|---|---|---|
| Rural female | Pop. 44,398,825 | | Pop. 35,877,215 | | Pop. 56,069,726 | |
| | Cause of death | Mortality rate (Per 100,000 individuals) | Cause of death | Mortality rate (Per 100,000 individuals) | Cause of death | Mortality rate (Per 100,000 individuals) |
| | 1 Traffic accidents | 7.69 | 1 Malignant tumors | 10.14 | 1 Malignant tumors | 46.53 |
| | 2 Malignant tumors | 6.03 | 2 Traffic accidents | 6.50 | 2 Diseases of the circulatory system | 21.69 |
| | 3 Suicide | 3.38 | 3 Diseases of the circulatory system | 4.69 | 3 Traffic accidents | 13.49 |
| | 4 Diseases of the circulatory system | 2.45 | 4 Suicide | 3.87 | 4 Suicide | 6.06 |
| Rural male | Pop. 47,486,365 | | Pop. 36,679,975 | | Pop. 54,958,212 | |
| | Cause of death | Mortality rate (Per 100,000 individuals) | Cause of death | Mortality rate (Per 100,000 individuals) | Cause of death | Mortality rate (Per 100,000 individuals) |
| | 1 Traffic accidents | 20.88 | 1 Traffic accidents | 21.22 | 1 Malignant tumors | 74.13 |
| | 2 Malignant tumors | 7,54 | 2 Malignant tumors | 14.71 | 2 Diseases of the circulatory system | 47.00 |
| | 3 Drowning | 4.76 | 3 Diseases of the circulatory system | 8.67 | 3 Traffic accidents | 44.66 |
| | 4 Diseases of the circulatory system | 4.12 | 4 Accidental falls from height | 3.45 | 4 Diseases of the digestive system | 11.06 |
| | 5 Suicide | 3.79 | 3 Suicide | 3.28 | 5 Accidental falls from height | 10.19 |
| | | | | | 6 Infectious diseases | 8.01 |
| | | | | | 7 Suicide | 7.76 |
| Urban female | Pop. 38,640,986 | | Pop. 41,828,062 | | Pop. 53,896,954 | |
| | Cause of death | Mortality rate (Per 100,000 individuals) | Cause of death | Mortality rate (Per 100,000 individuals) | Cause of death | Mortality rate (Per 100,000 individuals) |
| | 1 Malignant tumors | 4.03 | 1 Malignant tumors | 9.6 | 1 Malignant tumors | 32.95 |

(continued)

**Table 6** (continued)

| Age group | 15–24 | | 25–34 | | 35–44 | |
|---|---|---|---|---|---|---|
| | 2 Traffic accidents | 3.75 | 2 Diseases of the circulatory system | 3.53 | 2 Diseases of the circulatory system | 14.20 |
| | 3 Suicide | 2.08 | 3 Traffic accidents | 3.41 | 3 Traffic accidents | 6.41 |
| | 4 Diseases of the circulatory system | 1.96 | 4 Suicide | 2.36 | 4 Suicide | 3.63 |
| Urban male | Pop. 40,682,753 | | Pop. 39,852,632 | | Pop. 50,168,269 | |
| | Cause of death | Mortality rate (Per 100,000 individuals) | Cause of death | Mortality rate (Per 100,000 individuals) | Cause of death | Mortality rate (Per 100,000 individuals) |
| | 1 Traffic accidents | 9.75 | 1 Traffic accidents | 12.71 | 1 Malignant tumors | 45.46 |
| | 2 Malignant tumors | 5.92 | 2 Malignant tumors | 11.12 | 2 Diseases of the circulatory system | 40.11 |
| | 3 Diseases of the circulatory system | 3.86 | 3 Diseases of the circulatory system | 8.36 | 3 Traffic accidents | 21.10 |
| | 4 Drowning | 3.62 | 4 Suicide | 3.13 | 4 Diseases of the digestive system | 8.43 |
| | 5 Suicide | 2.10 | | | 5 Infectious diseases | 5.69 |
| | | | | | 6 Suicide | 4.47 |
| Urban and rural male and female | Pop. 171,208,929 | | Pop. 154,237,884 | | Pop. 215,093,161 | |
| | Cause of death | Mortality rate (Per 100,000 individuals) | Cause of death | Mortality rate (Per 100,000 individuals) | Cause of death | Mortality rate (Per 100,000 individuals) |
| | 1 Traffic accidents | 10.62 | 1 Malignant tumors | 11.41 | 1 Malignant tumors | 49.92 |
| | 2 Malignant tumors | 5.90 | 2 Motor vehicle traffic accident | 11.09 | 2 Diseases of the circulatory system | 30.95 |
| | 3 Diseases of the circulatory system | 3.12 | 3 Diseases of the circulatory system | 6.35 | 3 Traffic accidents | 21.57 |
| | 4 Suicide | 2.84 | 4 Suicide | 3.16 | 4 Diseases of the digestive system | 6.03 |

(continued)

**Table 6** (continued)

| Age group | 15–24 | | 25–34 | | 35–44 | |
|---|---|---|---|---|---|---|
| | 5 Drowning | 2.36 | 4 Accidental falls from height | 1.75 | 5 Suicide | 5.46 |
| | 6 Accidental falls from height | 1.45 | 6 Drowning | 1.35 | 6 Infectious diseases | 4.28 |
| | 7 Congenital physical deformities and chromosomal abnormalities | 1.12 | 7 Other accidental occurrences and harmful effects | 1.33 | 7 Accidental falls from height | 4.19 |
| | 8 Other accidental occurrences and harmful effects | 1.11 | 8 Accidental poisoning | 1.28 | 8 Diseases of the respiratory system | 3.96 |
| | 9 Homicide | 0.94 | 9 Infectious diseases | 1.27 | 9 Diseases of the urinary and reproductive systems | 2.98 |
| | 10 Accidental poisoning | 0.93 | 8 Diseases of the respiratory system | 1.17 | 10 Other accidental occurrences and harmful effects | 2.93 |

*Note* Mortality rates of different causes of death and population of the three age groups are calculated based on the crude mortality rate, injury rate, and crude mortality rate for specific causes of death in major disease groups among various five-year age group intervals in the population as provided in the Ministry of Health's *2010 China Health Statistics Yearbook* as well as the corresponding age group population figures for 2009 provided in the *China Population and Employment Statistics Yearbook 2010*

The suicide rate and number of suicides in different population groups in rural and urban areas of China are shown in Table 8. From this, we see the following:

First, in the 15–44 age group, the rural suicide rate is 1.6 times the urban rate and the number of rural suicides is 1.7 times the urban number.

Second, women account for 46.46% of all suicides and men, 53.54%. The suicide rate among women is lower than among men. This is a marked difference from the situation in 1998. However, quite a few scholars and practitioners questioned this change after working on a significant number of suicide cases (after summarizing sporadic cases or suicide statistics specific to each region and industry, they found that not much had changed in the sex ratio of suicide rate). Of course, this may also have something to do with the growing gender imbalance in China in recent years.

Third, the number of suicides in the 35–44 age group is 1.2 times the total of the 15–24 and 25–34 age groups. Clearly, this age group remains a high-risk group for suicide.

The suicide rates in different population groups in 2017 are shown in Table 9. From the table, we can see the following characteristics:

**Table 7** List of main causes of death for Chinese males and females at working age in urban and rural areas, 2017[a]

| Age group | 15–24 | | 25–34 | | 35–44 | |
|---|---|---|---|---|---|---|
| | Cause of death | Mortality rate (1/100,000) | Cause of death | Mortality rate (1/100,000) | Cause of death | Mortality rate (1/100,000) |
| Rural female | 1 Malignant tumors | 3.25 | 1 Malignant tumors 4 | 11.9 | 1 Malignant tumors | 26.50 |
| | 2 Traffic | 2.95 | 2 Diseases of the circulatory system | 6.72 | 2 Diseases of the circulatory system | 14.22 |
| | 3 Diseases of the circulatory system | 1.92 | 3 Traffic | 6.13 | 3 Traffic | 6.49 |
| | 4 Suicide | 1.91 | 4 Suicide | 3.21 | 4 Suicide | 3.14 |
| | 5 Drowning | 0.87 | 5 Diseases of the digestive system | 1.74 | 5 Diseases of the respiratory system | 1.81 |
| | 6 Accidental poisoning | 0.61 | 6 Drowning | 1.2 | 6 Infectious diseases | 1.36 |
| | 7 Accidental falls from height | 0.60 | 7 Infectious diseases | 1.16 | 7 Diseases of the digestive system | 1.33 |
| | 8 Diseases of the respiratory system | 0.43 | 8 Accidental poisoning | 1.04 | 8 Internal secretion, malnutrition | 1.19 |
| | 9 Infectious diseases | 0.39 | 9 Accidental falls from height | 1.01 | 9 Accidental falls from height | 1.14 |
| | 10 Murder | 0.30 | 10 Diseases of the respiratory system | 0.93 | 10 Accidental poisoning | 1.01 |
| Rural male | 1 Traffic | 11.29 | 1 Traffic | 6.43 | 1 Diseases of the circulatory system | 47.25 |
| | 2 Malignant tumors | 5.33 | 2 Diseases of the circulatory system | 18. 99 | 2 Malignant tumors | 42.79 |
| | 3 Drowning | 4.27 | 3 Malignant tumors | 17.39 | 3 Traffic | 23.42 |
| | 4 Internal secretion | 4.19 | 4 Suicide | 6.15 | 4 Diseases of the digestive system | 8.21 |
| | 5 Diseases of the circulatory system | 4.19 | 5 Accidental falls from height | 5.52 | 5 Accidental falls from height | 6.95 |
| | 6 Suicide | 3.03 | 6 Drowning | 3.78 | 6 Infectious diseases | 6.45 |
| | 7 Accidental falls from height | 1.74 | 7 Accidental poisoning | 3.55 | 7 Suicide | 5.10 |
| | 8 Accidental poisoning | 1.27 | 8 Infectious diseases | 3.28 | 8 Accidental poisoning | 4.57 |
| | 9 Infectious diseases | 0.89 | 9 Diseases of the digestive system | 2.79 | 9 Diseases of the respiratory system | 4.24 |
| | 10 Diseases of the respiratory system | 0.74 | 10 Diseases of the respiratory system | 1.96 | 10 Drowning | 2.64 |

(continued)

**Table 7** (continued)

| Age group | 15–24 | | 25–34 | | 35–44 | |
|---|---|---|---|---|---|---|
| | Cause of death | Mortality rate (1/100,000) | Cause of death | Mortality rate (1/100,000) | Cause of death | Mortality rate (1/100,000) |
| Rural female | 1 Malignant tumors | 2.14 | 1 Malignant tumors | 8.68 | 1 Malignant tumors | 23.93 |
| | 2 Traffic | 1.94 | 2 Diseases of the circulatory system | 4.24 | 2 Diseases of the circulatory system | 10.56 |
| | 3 Diseases of the circulatory system | 1.41 | 3 Traffic | 3.58 | 3 Traffic | 4.2 |
| | 4 Suicide | 1.13 | 4 Suicide | 2.02 | 4 Suicide | 2.00 |
| | 5 Drowning | 0.61 | 5 Diseases of the respiratory system | 0.86 | 5 Diseases of the respiratory system | 1.38 |
| | 6 Accidental falls from height | 0.56 | 6 Accidental falls from height | 0.69 | 6Internal secretion | 1.19 |
| | 7 Accidental poisoning | 0.44 | 7 Infectious diseases | 0.68 | 7 Diseases of the digestive system | 1.16 |
| | 8 Diseases of the respiratory system | 0.41 | 8 Drowning | 0.66 | 8 Infectious diseases | 1.04 |
| | 9 Infectious diseases | 0.18 | 9 Internal secretion | 0.56 | 9 Accidental falls from height | 1.00 |
| | 10 Diseases of the digestive system | 0.18 | 10 Diseases of the digestive system | 0.50 | 10 Drowning | 0.71 |
| Urban male | 1 Traffic | 6.57 | 1 Traffic | 13.93 | 1 Diseases of the circulatory system | 37.17 |
| | 2 Malignant tumors | 3.49 | 2 Malignant tumors | 11.31 | 2 Malignant tumors | 32.12 |
| | 3 Diseases of the circulatory system | 2.68 | 3 Diseases of the circulatory system | 12.50 | 3 Traffic | 13.78 |
| | 4 Drowning | 2.47 | 4 Suicide | 3.52 | 4 Diseases of the digestive system | 6.14 |
| | 5 Suicide | 1.84 | 5 Accidental falls from height | 3.47 | 5 Infectious diseases | 4.56 |
| | 6 Accidental falls from height | 1.30 | 6 Drowning | 2.37 | 6 Accidental falls from height | 4.56 |
| | 7 Accidental poisoning | 0.80 | 7 Infectious diseases | 2.04 | 7 Suicide | 3.26 |
| | 8 Diseases of the respiratory system | 0.52 | 8 Accidental poisoning | 1.99 | 8 Diseases of the respiratory system | 2.84 |
| | 9 Infectious diseases | 0.43 | 9 Diseases of the digestive system | 1.90 | 9 Accidental poisoning | 2.77 |
| | 10 Murder | 0.40 | 10 Diseases of the respiratory system | 1.44 | 10 Internal secretion, malnutrition and metabolism | 2.34 |

(continued)

**Table 7** (continued)

| Age group | 15–24 | | 25–34 | | 35–44 | |
|---|---|---|---|---|---|---|
| | Cause of death | Mortality rate (1/100,000) | Cause of death | Mortality rate (1/100,000) | Cause of death | Mortality rate (1/100,000) |
| Urban and rural male and female | 1 Traffic | 5.79 | 1 Traffic | 12.57 | 1 Malignant tumors | 31.41 |
| | 2 Malignant tumors | 3.58 | 2 Malignant tumors | 12.33 | 2 Diseases of the circulatory system | 27.49 |
| | 3 Diseases of the circulatory system | 2.57 | 3 Diseases of the circulatory system | 10.66 | 3 Traffic | 12.06 |
| | 4 Drowning | 2.11 | 4 Suicide | 3.73 | 4 Diseases of the digestive system | 4.25 |
| | 5 Suicide | 1.99 | 5 Accidental falls from height | 2.68 | 5 Suicide | 3.39 |
| | 6Accidental falls from height | 1.06 | 6Drowning | 2.00 | 6 Infectious diseases | 3.38 |
| | 7 Accidental poisoning | 0.78 | 7 Infectious diseases | 1.79 | 7 Accidental falls from height | 3.44 |
| | 8 Diseases of the respiratory system | 0.53 | 8 Accidental poisoning | 1.76 | 8 Diseases of the respiratory system | 2.58 |
| | 9 Infectious diseases | 0.47 | 9 Diseases of the digestive system | 1.52 | 9 Accidental poisoning | 2.25 |
| | 10 urogenital system diseases | 0.39 | 10 Diseases of the respiratory system | 1.30 | 10 urogenital system diseases | 1.91 |

*Note* The table above has been made according to *China Population & Employment Statistics Yearbook 2018*. The population grouped by age adopted cluster sampling method. However, it is based on three levels as cities, towns and rural areas and the proportions of population is hard to calculate. Statistics by other methods indicated enormous errors and thus abandoned.

[a] Suicide rates and suicide numbers for the above three groups are calculated based on the suicide rate for various five-year age group intervals as provided in the National Health Commission's *China Health Statistics Yearbook 2018*.

First, for the 15–44 age group, the rural suicide rate is 1.6 times that of the urban rate.

Second, for the 15–44 age group, the suicide rate of men is 1.7 times that of women. In fact, statistics show that from 2006, regardless of urban or rural areas, male suicide rates rapidly exceed those of female.

Third, the 2017 statistics show that age and suicide rate are basically positively correlated. The older the age, the higher the suicide rate. In particular, the suicide rate rises sharply after the elderly entering sixties.

According to statistics from China's Ministry of Health, in recent years the suicide rate for people of all ages has generally declined significantly. This is the result of the attention paid to the issue by Chinese officials as well as the theoretical study on the issue and the preventive measures proposed by the Chinese academic circles.

**Table 8** Suicide rate and numbers among Chinese men and women of working age in rural and urban areas, 2009

| Age group | 15–24 | | 25–34 | | 35–44 | | 15–44 | |
|---|---|---|---|---|---|---|---|---|
| | Suicide rate (per 100,000 individuals) | Suicidal deaths | Suicide rate (per 100,000 individuals) | Suicidal deaths | Suicide rate (per 100,000 individuals) | Suicidal deaths | Suicide rate (per 100,000 individuals) | Suicidal deaths |
| Overall | 2.84 | 4959 | 3.16 | 4825 | 5.46 | 11,812 | 3.99 | 21,596 |
| Rural | 3.58 | 3301 | 3.57 | 2591 | 6.86 | 7613 | 4.90 | 13,505 |
| Urban | 2.09 | 1658 | 2.75 | 2234 | 4.05 | 4199 | 3.05 | 8091 |
| Female | 2.77 | 2305 | 3.12 | 2375 | 4.85 | 5354 | 3.71 | 10,034 |
| Male | 3.01 | 2654 | 3.20 | 2450 | 6.07 | 6458 | 4.28 | 11,562 |
| Rural female | 3.38 | 1501 | 3.87 | 1388 | 6.06 | 3398 | 4.61 | 6287 |
| Rural male | 3.79 | 1800 | 3.28 | 1203 | 7.67 | 4215 | 5.19 | 7218 |
| Urban female | 2.08 | 804 | 2.36 | 987 | 3.63 | 1956 | 2.79 | 3747 |
| Urban male | 2.10 | 854 | 3.13 | 1247 | 4.47 | 2243 | 3.32 | 4344 |

*Note* Suicide rates and suicide numbers for the above three groups are calculated based on the suicide rate for various five-year age group intervals as provided in the Ministry of Health's *2010 China Health Statistics Yearbook* and the corresponding age group population figures for 2009 carried in the *China Population and Employment Statistics Yearbook 2010*

**Table 9** Suicide rates and numbers among Chinese men and women of working age in rural and urban areas, 2017 (1/100,000)[a]

| Age group | 15-24 | 25-34 | 35-44 | 15-44 |
|---|---|---|---|---|
| | Suicide rate (per 100,000 individuals) | Suicide rate (per 100,000 individuals) | Suicide rate (per 100,000 individuals) | Suicide rate (per 100,000 individuals) |
| All | 1.98 | 3.72 | 3.37 | 3.02 |
| Rural | 2.47 | 4.68 | 4.12 | 3.75 |
| Urban | 1.48 | 2.77 | 2.63 | 2.29 |
| All females | 1.52 | 2.61 | 2.57 | 2.23 |
| All males | 2.44 | 4.83 | 4.18 | 3.82 |
| Rural female | 1.91 | 3.21 | 3.14 | 2.75 |
| Rural male | 3.03 | 6.15 | 5.1 | 4.76 |
| Rural female | 1.13 | 2.02 | 2.0 | 1.71 |
| Urban male | 1.84 | 3.52 | 3.26 | 2.88 |

*Note* The table above has been made according to *China Population & Employment Statistics Yearbook 2018*. The population grouped by age adopted cluster sampling method. However, it is based on three levels as cities, towns and rural areas and the proportions of population is hard to calculate. Statistics by other methods indicated enormous errors and thus abandoned.
[a] Suicide rates and suicide numbers for the above three groups are calculated based on the suicide rate for various five-year age group intervals as provided in the Ministry of Health's *2010 China Health Statistics Yearbook* and the corresponding age-group population figures for 2009 carried in the *China Population and Employment Statistics Yearbook 2010*

In a speech given on May 14, 2011, at the 9th annual National Conference on Crisis Intervention and Suicide Prevention held in Hangzhou, professor Xiao Shuiyuan, Dean of the Xiangya School of Public Health, Central South University, said that: "Based on our preliminary studies, the rapid decline in China's suicide rate, especially in rural areas, can be explained by a number of factors: socioeconomic development, the development of mental health services, the government's efforts to prevent suicide, and the improvement of the educational attainment of the population."[6]

However, as China's social transformation continues apace and new social problems emerge, our research and prevention efforts must keep in both in complexity and sustainability. At the same time, as the population ages, suicide among the elderly will also become a key topic in suicide studies. China's status as the no. 1 country in the world in terms of suicide rate will likely remain unchanged for some time to come.

[6]Zhang (2012).

## 1.3 Key Feature of Suicides on the Mainland of China

The following features are distinctive to suicide in the Chinese mainland:

First, the suicide rates are high among the young and the old;
Second, the suicide rate is higher among women than among men;
Third, the suicide rate is higher in rural areas than in cities;
Fourth, the age of those who commit suicide is both decreasing on one end and increasing on the other;
Fifth, high death-to-attempt ratio;
Sixth, the chief methods of choice are poisoning and hanging; and
Seventh, high incidence of group or copycat suicide is significant.

New features have shown up in suicides in China since 2006, which are: 1. Suicide rate has dropped apparently, especially the rate for females. 2. Male suicide rate has been higher than female suicide rate. 3. There has seen a prominent suicide rate among the older age. 4. Higher suicide rates in rural areas than urban areas.

## 1.4 Suicide Rate in Hong Kong

Though the suicide rate in Hong Kong is not as high as in the Chinese mainland, it has also been on the rise in recent years. According to The Samaritan Befrienders Hong Kong, the average suicide rate in Hong Kong stood at 11.60 per 100,000 individuals between 1989 and 1993, with the rate of the 10–24 age group at 4.90 per 100,000 individuals.[7] The suicide rate in Hong Kong was a decade high in 2000, at 13.50 per 100,000 individuals. According to the findings of a study conducted by the Faculty of Social Sciences, Hong Kong University, announced on September 21, 2001, Hong Kong's 2001 suicide rate is 16.00 per 100,000 individuals.[8] Suicide is in the seventh place in a list of top causes of death among Hong Kong residents, with the highest suicide rate seen in the 40–49 age group and the above 60 age group. Hong Kong's 2004 suicide rate is 15.30 per 100,000 individuals.[9] Suicide rate figures released by Hong Kong Jockey Club Centre for Suicide Research and Prevention for the 2005–2009 period are shown in Fig. 1, Tables 10 and 11.

In recent years, due to the impact of the Asian financial crisis and the global economic downturn, Hong Kong's economy has been in a continued slump. Unemployment rates have been high, and many local residents have been affected mentally. A 1999–2000 report from Hong Kong Coroner's Court shows

[7]Xu (1995).

[8]http://hk.news.yahoo.com/030130/12/pqe8.html. Accessed: 20 July 20 2010.

[9]http://news.china.com/zh_cn/news100/11038989/20060428/13282080.html. Accessed: 21 June 2010.

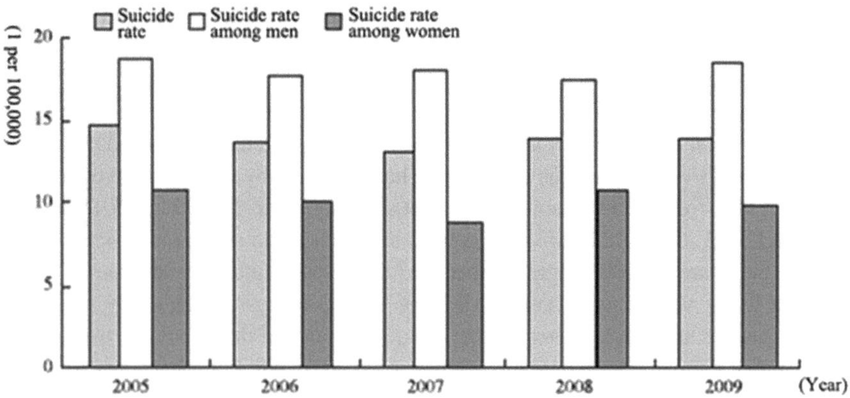


**Fig. 1** Suicide rate in Hong Kong by gender, 2005–2009

**Table 10** Suicide rate by gender in Hong Kong, 2005–2009 (Unit: Per 100,000 individuals)

| Year | Suicide rate | Suicide rate male | Suicide rate female |
|---|---|---|---|
| 2005 | 14.6 | 18.8 | 10.8 |
| 2006 | 13.6 | 17.6 | 10.0 |
| 2007 | 13.1 | 17.9 | 8.8 |
| 2008 | 14.0 | 17.5 | 10.9 |
| 2009 | 13.8 | 18.4 | 9.8 |

*Source* http://csrp.hku.hk/WEB/gh/statistics.asp

**Table 11** Suicide rate by age in Hong Kong, 2005–2009 (Unit: Per 100,000 individuals)

| Year | Under 15 | 15–24 | 25–34 | 35–44 | 45–54 | 55–64 | 65 and above | Overall suicide rate |
|---|---|---|---|---|---|---|---|---|
| 2005 | 0.2 | 7.1 | 14.6 | 16.7 | 16.2 | 19.6 | 30.4 | 14.6 |
| 2006 | 0.2 | 8.3 | 13.3 | 14.8 | 14.1 | 14.3 | 30.3 | 13.6 |
| 2007 | 0.5 | 7.3 | 13.9 | 12.9 | 13.2 | 16.0 | 28.5 | 13.1 |
| 2008 | 0.6 | 9.2 | 13.8 | 14.7 | 13.1 | 17.4 | 30.4 | 14.0 |
| 2009 | 0.3 | 8.4 | 13.0 | 13.6 | 15.2 | 17.2 | 28.9 | 13.8 |

that 60% of all deaths from suicide were related to financial issues.[10] The poor economic performance has had a direct impact on the family and interpersonal relations of Hong Kong residents.

According to Paul Yip Siu-fai, head of the Hong Kong Jockey Club Centre for Suicide Research and Prevention, structural changes in the Hong Kong population have also had an impact on the suicide rate in Hong Kong. Statistics from Hong Kong's

[10]http://www.phoenixtv.com.cn/home/phonenixweekly/75/26hk.html. Accessed: 21 June 2010.

Census and Statistics Department reveal the following issues: First, Hong Kong's population is aging. Up to 14% of the population is above 60 years old, and this figure is expected to rise steeply to 28% by 2020. Suicide among the elderly, at 27.0 per 100,000 individuals, has become a salient issue. Second, the divorce rate is going up, and it is now very common for singles to live alone. In particular, 5% of those above 50 are single and living alone. The divorce rate has increased by more than fivefold in the past 20 years, from 2000 persons in the 1980s to more than 13,000 in 2001. Between 1991 and 2001, the number of single parents has risen by an average of 5.4% per year. Today, there are 45,000 single mothers, 13,000 single fathers, and around 80,000 children living with single parents. Marriage has been regarded as a key prevention against suicide and suicide rates among single parents and divorcees are two to three times higher than among individuals who are married. In addition, the issues associated with marriages between mainland Chinese and Hong Kong residents are also becoming increasingly salient. Children born in the mainland have shown poor adaptation after moving to Hong Kong, and this had resulted in a group of marginalized youth. Third, the birth rate in Hong Kong has been on a constant decline, with the total fertility rate falling from 1.93‰ in the 1980s to 0.927‰ in 2001, far lower than the replacement level of 2.1% and one of the lowest in the world. The decline in birth rate and the increase in the number of childless women have on one hand led to less cohesion in marriages and on the other, played a role in the increased suicide rate among women.

The Coroner's Court of Hong Kong documents show that there were 916 suicides in 2017 and the sucide rate was 12.36 (with a rate of 12.36 per 100,000 individuals). The number dropped 0.58 to 2.51 compared to 2016.[11][12] For a better comparisom, it is an international practice to standardize these statistics according to different ages. In 2017, the standardized suicide rate in Hong Kong, where there is a big number of aged population, is an estimate of 9.5, lower than the national level of 10.5 (WHO 2018).[13]

The main features are as follows:

First, the suicide rate in Hong Kong has generally declined in recent years. Although there is no significant drop in suicide for the elderly over the age of 70, the number of suicide for other age groups has basically shown a downward trend.

Second, the number for men is higher than that for women. By gender, among the 916 suicides in Hong Kong in 2017, 569 were males, accounting for 62.12%, while 347 were females, accounting for 37.88%.

Third, means of suicide is mainly falls from height. According to suicide means, falls from height is the main suicide means in Hong Kong, accounting for 21.07%; followed by hanging, accounting for 21.07%; the third is carbon monoxide poisoning (burning charcoal), accounting for 12.12%.

[11]Census and Statistics Department Hong Kong Special Administrative Region People's Republic of China 2017.

[12]The Samaritan Befrienders Hong Kong 2017 Annual Report.

[13]"Working Together to Prevent Suicide" The HKU Centre for Suicide Research and Prevention releases the latest figures and prevention recommendations on suicide. https://www.hku.hk/press/c_news_detail_18364.html Accessed: 10 September 2018.

Fourth, the suicide rate of the elderly is higher than that of the young. According to different age groups, the suicide rate was the highest in the age of 70 years old, accounting for 26.74%; the suicide rate in the 60–69 age group comes to the second place, accounting for 14.86%.

Studies show that the suicide rate among the elderly has been higher than that of other age groups and it sees a drop from 27.1 in 2008 to 20.83 in 2017, which is a good sign. Meanwhile, the suicide rate among 0–14 age group has remained at a low of 0.3–0.8.

Hong Kong's suicide rate in 2017 (1/100,000)[a]

| Suicide type | Gender | 0-9 | 10-19 | 20-29 | 30-39 | 40-49 | 50-59 | 60-69 | 70 + | 不详 | Subtotal | Total |
|---|---|---|---|---|---|---|---|---|---|---|---|---|
| Fire | Male | 0 | 0 | 1 | 0 | 0 | 1 | 0 | 0 | 0 | 2 | 2 |
| | Female | 0 | 0 | 0 | 0 | 0 | 0 | 0 | 0 | 0 | 0 | |
| Drug | Male | 0 | 0 | 2 | 3 | 0 | 1 | 2 | 3 | 0 | 11 | 29 |
| | Female | 0 | 1 | 1 | 4 | 2 | 4 | 3 | 3 | 0 | 18 | |
| Poison | Male | 0 | 0 | 0 | 1 | 3 | 0 | 0 | 4 | 0 | 8 | 10 |
| | Female | 0 | 0 | 0 | 1 | 0 | 0 | 0 | 1 | 0 | 2 | |
| Hanging | Male | 0 | 2 | 8 | 14 | 8 | 22 | 25 | 37 | 0 | 116 | 193 |
| | Female | 0 | 0 | 6 | 11 | 5 | 15 | 7 | 33 | 0 | 77 | |
| Fall from height | Male | 0 | 24 | 46 | 37 | 31 | 37 | 51 | 76 | 2 | 304 | 495 |
| | Female | 0 | 6 | 25 | 27 | 27 | 36 | 30 | 40 | 0 | 191 | |
| Carbon monoxide | Male | 0 | 0 | 6 | 23 | 13 | 19 | 8 | 5 | 0 | 74 | 111 |
| | Female | 0 | 1 | 2 | 15 | 8 | 7 | 4 | 0 | 0 | 37 | |
| Drowning | Male | 0 | 1 | 3 | 6 | 3 | 4 | 1 | 12 | 1 | 31 | 40 |
| | Female | 0 | 0 | 0 | 1 | 1 | 0 | 5 | 2 | 0 | 9 | |
| Pointed objects | Male | 0 | 1 | 0 | 0 | 5 | 0 | 1 | 1 | 0 | 8 | 9 |
| | Female | 0 | 0 | 0 | 0 | 0 | 1 | 0 | 0 | 0 | 1 | |
| Others | Male | 0 | 0 | 2 | 2 | 1 | 4 | 4 | 1 | 1 | 15 | 27 |
| | Female | 0 | 0 | 4 | 1 | 1 | 2 | 1 | 3 | 0 | 12 | |
| Subtotal | Male | 0 | 28 | 68 | 86 | 64 | 88 | 92 | 139 | 4 | 569 | 916 |
| | Female | 0 | 8 | 38 | 60 | 44 | 65 | 50 | 82 | 0 | 347 | |
| Total | | 0 | 36 | 106 | 146 | 108 | 153 | 142 | 221 | 4 | | 916 |

[a] The Samaritan Befrienders Hong Kong 2017 Annual Report

Number of suicides among different age groups in Hong Kong in 2015–2017[a]

| | Gender | 0-9 | 10-19 | 20-29 | 30-39 | 40-49 | 50-59 | 60-69 | 70+ | unclear | Total |
|---|---|---|---|---|---|---|---|---|---|---|---|
| 2017 | Male | 0 | 28 | 68 | 86 | 64 | 88 | 92 | 139 | 4 | 569 |
| | Female | 0 | 8 | 38 | 60 | 44 | 65 | 50 | 82 | 0 | 347 |
| | Total | 0 | 36 | 106 | 146 | 108 | 153 | 142 | 221 | 4 | 916 |
| 2016 | Male | 0 | 17 | 76 | 83 | 83 | 126 | 117 | 132 | 4 | 638 |
| | Female | 0 | 7 | 29 | 42 | 58 | 61 | 45 | 74 | 0 | 316 |
| | Total | 0 | 24 | 105 | 125 | 141 | 187 | 162 | 206 | 4 | 954 |
| 2015 | Male | 0 | 15 | 76 | 92 | 104 | 126 | 102 | 125 | 3 | 643 |
| | Female | 0 | 8 | 37 | 60 | 61 | 73 | 57 | 82 | 1 | 379 |
| | Total | 0 | 23 | 113 | 152 | 165 | 199 | 159 | 207 | 4 | 1022 |

[a] The Samaritan Befrienders Hong Kong 2017 Annual Report

Different suicide types in Hong Kong in 2015-2017[a]

| | | 2017 | | 2016 | | 2015 | |
|---|---|---|---|---|---|---|---|
| Suicide type | Gender | Subtotal | Total | Subtotal | Total | Subtotal | Total |
| Fire | Male | 2 | 2 | 2 | 2 | 1 | 1 |
| | Female | 0 | | 0 | | 0 | |
| Drug | Male | 11 | 29 | 14 | 20 | 22 | 42 |
| | Female | 18 | | 6 | | 20 | |
| Poison | Male | 8 | 10 | 4 | 8 | 4 | 10 |
| | Female | 2 | | 4 | | 6 | |
| Hanging | Male | 116 | 193 | 140 | 206 | 134 | 219 |
| | Female | 77 | | 66 | | 85 | |
| Fall from height | Male | 304 | 495 | 334 | 514 | 343 | 536 |
| | Female | 191 | | 180 | | 193 | |
| Carbon monoxide | Male | 74 | 111 | 86 | 117 | 96 | 142 |
| | Female | 37 | | 31 | | 46 | |
| Drowning | Male | 31 | 40 | 31 | 50 | 20 | 38 |
| | Female | 9 | | 19 | | 18 | |
| Pointed objects | Male | 8 | 9 | 11 | 16.00 | 5 | 8.00 |
| | Female | 1 | | 5.00 | | 3 | |
| Others | Male | 15 | 27 | 16 | 21 | 18.00 | 26 |
| | Female | 12 | | 5 | | 8 | |

[a] The Samaritan Befrienders Hong Kong 2017 Annual Report

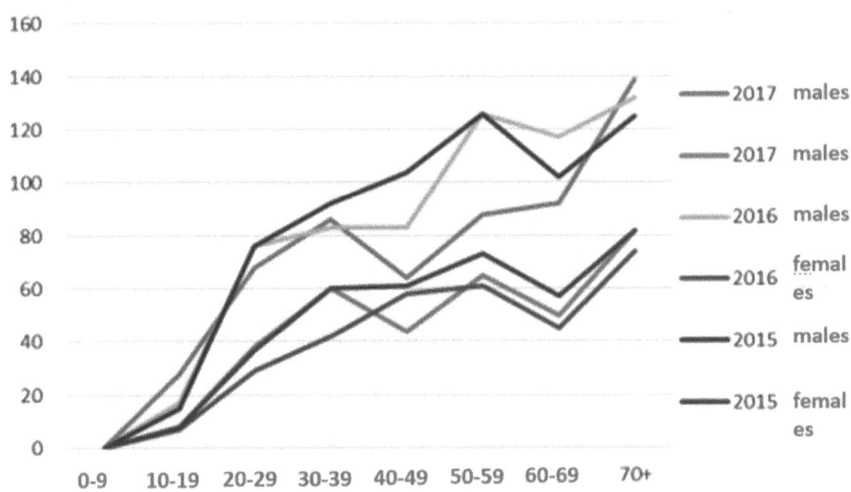


Number of suicides of males and females in Hong Kong in 2015–2017. *Note* The Samaritan Befrienders Hongkong 2017 Annual Report

## 1.5 Suicide Rate in Taiwan

The suicide rate of Taiwan is lower than that of the Chinese mainland. In 2001, according to Taiwan's "National Fire Agency" and "Ministry of Health and Welfare," suicide was one of the top three causes of death in Taiwan for three consecutive years.[14] The number deaths from suicide was 2172 in 1997, 2177 in 1998, 2281 in 1999, 2360 in 2000, 2781 in 2001, and more than 4000 in 2004 (refer to Fig. 2).[15] The suicide mortality rate of Taiwan in 1993 was 6.20 per 100,000 individuals. In 1998, the suicide mortality rate was 7.60 per 100,000 individuals (specifically, 8.50 per 100,000 individuals for males and 5.60 per 100,000 individuals for females. The rate for those aged 15–24 was 3.90 per 100,000 individuals, specifically, 5.10 per 100,000 individuals for males and 2.70 per 100,000 individuals for females). In the same year, the suicide mortality rate for those aged above 65 was the highest at 25.60 per 100,000 individuals. The rate for males in this age group was 31.60 per 100,000 individuals and 18.30 per 100,000 individuals for females.[16] In 1999, the suicide mortality rate in Taiwan rose to 12.45 per 100,000 individuals and then further to 15.31 per 100,000 individuals in 2004 and 18.80 per 100,000 individuals in 2005. The rate has been rising at growing increments.[17] Between 1984 and 2005, the suicide mortality rate and the number of those dead from suicides in Taiwan first fell slightly, then stayed around the same level for a while, and then rose rapidly.[18] In 2010, the suicide mortality rate in Taiwan was 13.60 per 100,000 individuals.[19]

In Taiwan, the suicide rate is higher for men than for women. This is in line with international norms though diametrically opposed to the Chinese mainland's situation. In 2001, 68.4% of those dead from suicide were male, and 31.6% female. The number of males dead from suicide was up 15.6% from the previous year while the increase for females was 6.5%. In terms of both the absolute number of deaths and the growth rate, the figures for males were more than twice those for females.

By age groups, in 2001, 6.8% of those dead from suicide were under 24, significantly lower than that of the Chinese mainland; 36.1% of suicidal deaths were from the 25–44 age group, and 57.2% from the above 45 age group. Clearly, the suicide rate in Taiwan is positively correlated with age. As for the absolute number of deaths, the figure of the under 24 age group increased by 14.6% over the previous year, while the number of those aged between 25 and 44 rose by 10.7%. In

[14]Dang (2001).

[15]Data for 2002 and 2003 not found despite extensive searches by the author.

[16]*World Health Statistics Annual*. http://www.sinorama.com.tw/jp/9704/704112j4.htm. Accessed: 15 June 2011.

[17]Media criticized for encouraging suicide, Min Health to bring together monitoring capacity. *Lihpao*. http://www.lihpao.com/?action-viewnews-itemid-90086. Accessed: 15 July 2010.

[18]Yang and Yang (2007).

[19]Media reports worsen suicide rate in China. *Chinanews.com*. http://www.chinanews.com/tw/2011/09-09/3319222.shtml. Accessed: 15 July 2012.

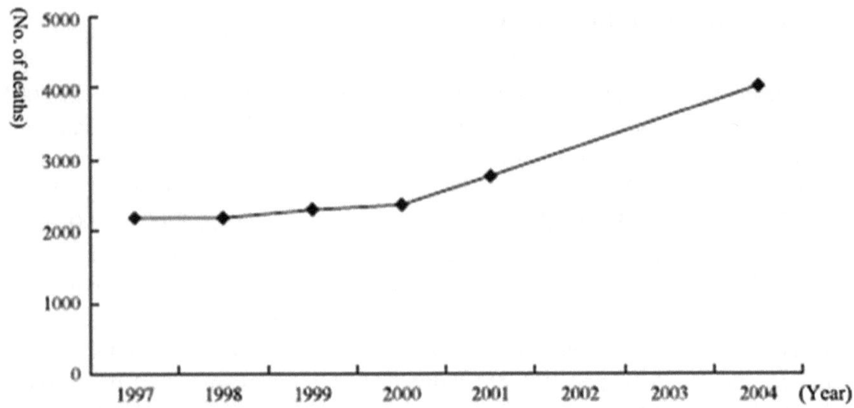


**Fig. 2** Number of suicidal deaths in Taiwan, 1997–2004

the same period, the number for the 45–64 age group increased by 17.6% and for the above 65 age group, it rose by 9.1%.[20]

This is the ranking of Taiwanese counties and cities by suicide rate, from the highest to the lowest, for the period 2000–2002: Nantou County, Keelung City, Hualien County, Taitung County, Tainan County, Yunlin County, Miaoli County, Pingtung County, Chiayi County, Kaohsiung County, Yilan County, Hsinchu County, Tainan City, Kaohsiung City, Changhua County, Taoyuan County, Hsinchu City, Chiayi City, Taipei City, Taichung County, Penghu County, Taipei County, and Taichung City.[21]

Taiwan's "Ministry of Health and Welfare" found in an analysis that among men who died from suicide, 58% were unemployed; among the females, 50% were housewives and another 15% were unemployed. Obviously, the continued economic downturn, high unemployment rate, and the rash of suicides following the 1999 Jiji, Nantou earthquake are key reasons for the increase in the suicide rate in Taiwan in recent years.[22]

According to the statistics from the Taiwan Suicide Prevention Center, Taiwan's suicides in recent years has the following characteristics:

First, the overall suicide rate in Taiwan has remained rather stable in recent years. In 2017, the number of suicides in Taiwan was 3,871, ranking suicide as the 11th cause of death. Among them, male death was ranked 11th and female death was ranked 12th. The number of suicides inTaiwan in 2017 increased by 106 from 3,765 in 2016, an increase of 2.8%, and by 196 from 3,675 in 2015, an increase of

[20]Key socioeconomic indicators for "governance": government should pay more attention to rising suicide rate. http://www.npf.org.tw/symposium/morm.2002-08-09. Accessed: 15 September 2010.

[21]Kuo et al. (2010).

[22]Suicide rate in Taiwan last year highest in nine years. *Chinanews.com*. http://www.chinanews.com/2001-03-30/26/82157.html. Accessed: 15 September 2010.

5.3%. At the same time, the rough death rate in Taiwan in 2017 was 16.4 per 100,000 individuals, an increase of 2.5% from 16 per 100,000 individuals in 2016 and 4.5% from 15.7 in 2015. In terms of standardized suicide mortality for Taiwan in 2017, it was 12.5 per 100,000 individuals, an increase of 1.6% from 12.3 in 2016 and an increase of 3.3% from 12.1 in 2015.

Second, male suicide rates continue to be higher than that of female. In 2017, the male suicide rate in Taiwan was 20.7 per 100,000 individuals, and the female suicide rate was 9.9 per 100,000 individuals. In 2016, the male suicide rate in Taiwan was 21.1 per 100,000 individuals, and the female suicide rate was 9.5 per 100,000 individuals. In 2015, the male suicide rate in Taiwan was 20.1 per 100,000 individuals, and the female suicide rate was 9.7 per 100,000 individuals.

Third, the suicide rate of the elderly is much higher than that of other age groups. In 2017, the suicide rate of over 65 years old in Taiwan was 31.1 per 100,000 individuals. while the age of 45–64 years old was 21.1 per 100,000 individuals, and the age of 25–44 years old was 16.6 per 100,000 individuals, age of 15- 24 years old group was 6.4 per 100,000 individuals, and the suicide rate of those below 14 years old was 0.1 per 100,000 individuals.

Number of suicides in Taiwan in 2017–2017[a]

| Year | Suicides | Standardizes suicide rate (1/100,000) | Rough suicide rate (1/100,000) |
|---|---|---|---|
| 2017 | 3871 | 12.5 | 16.4 |
| 2016 | 3765 | 12.3 | 16.0 |
| 2015 | 3675 | 12.1 | 15.7 |
| 2014 | 3542 | 11.8 | 16.1 |
| 2013 | 3565 | 12.0 | 15.3 |
| 2012 | 3766 | 13.1 | 16.2 |

[a] Taiwan Suicide Prevention Center: http://tspc.tw/tspc/portal/know/know_content.jsp?type=2&sno=65

Suicide mortality rate among different age groups in 2013–2017 (1/100,000)[a]

| Year | Gender | ≤ 14 | 15-24 | 25-44 | 45-64 | ≥ 65 |
|---|---|---|---|---|---|---|
| 2017 | Male | 0.1 | 8.1 | 21.4 | 29.9 | 43.8 |
| | Female | 0.1 | 4.6 | 11.8 | 12.7 | 20.3 |
| | Total | 0.1 | 6.4 | 16.6 | 21.1 | 31.1 |
| 2016 | Male | 0.4 | 8.6 | 22.0 | 28.2 | 46.2 |
| | Female | 0.0 | 4.8 | 10.2 | 12.2 | 20.3 |
| | Total | 0.2 | 6.8 | 16.1 | 20.1 | 32.3 |
| 2015 | Male | 0.3 | 8.2 | 20.4 | 28.2 | 43.6 |
| | Female | 0.1 | 3.3 | 11.5 | 13.2 | 20.5 |
| | Total | 0.2 | 5.9 | 15.9 | 20.6 | 31.2 |
| 2014 | Male | 0.0 | 6.8 | 20.5 | 28.0 | 43.2 |
| | Female | 0.1 | 3.2 | 11.0 | 12.0 | 20.9 |
| | Total | 0.1 | 5.1 | 15.7 | 19.9 | 31.3 |
| 2013 | Male | 0.2 | 6.0 | 21.6 | 28.4 | 43.9 |
| | Female | 0.0 | 4.3 | 10.5 | 12.3 | 21.7 |
| | Total | 0.1 | 5.2 | 16.0 | 20.1 | 32.1 |

[a] Taiwan Suicide Prevention Center: http://tspc.tw/tspc/portal/know/know_content.jsp?type=2&sno=65

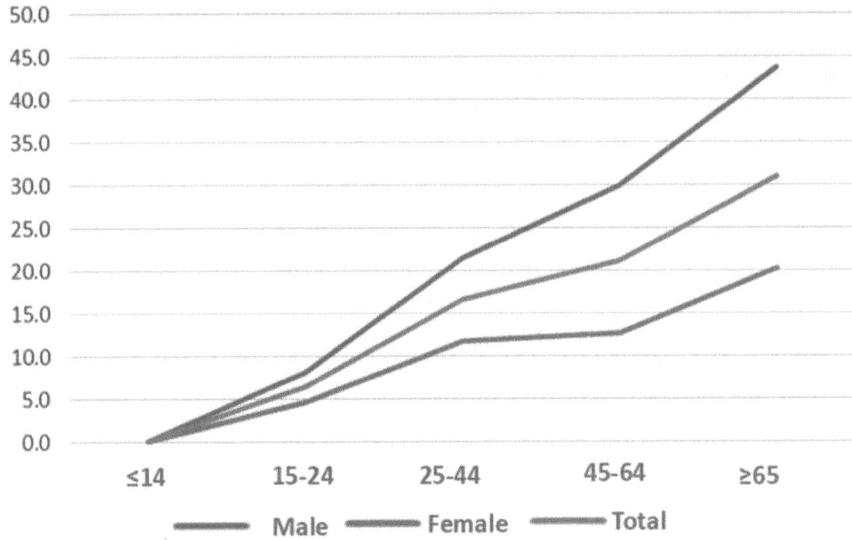


Taiwan's suicide mortality rate of different age groups in 2017. *Note* Taiwan Suicide Prevention Center: http://tspc.tw/tspc/portal/know/know_content.jsp?type=2&sno=65

## 2 Attempted Suicide and Suicidal Ideation Rates

### *2.1 Over Two Million Failed Attempts in China Each Year*

Attempted suicide refers to a suicidal action taken by a person who has had suicidal thoughts. While he or she may not have "succeeded" in this attempt for various reasons, such an attempt may still cause physical injury or disability.

There are no nationwide data on attempted suicide in China. In October 2001, then-Vice Health Minister Yin Dakui observed at the 3rd National Mental Health Work Conference that the number of attempted suicides in China was estimated to be more than two million per year.[23] Assuming a 10:1 ratio of attempted suicides to suicidal deaths, then in 1998, the rate of attempted suicides among young people aged 15–24 in China would be 106.3 per 100,000 individuals, 224.10 per 100,000 individuals for those aged 25–34, and 181.99 per 100,000 individuals for those aged 35–44.

A survey of 2466 high school students in Hefei, Anhui, showed that the rate of attempted suicide was as high as 3%.[24] According to a 2002 survey of the Suigang'ao Research Institute of Guangzhou, in the city's primary and secondary schools, 5.2% of students admitted to having used a blade or other sharp objects to cut themselves (deliberate self-harm) during the year, 1.9% of students admitted to

[23] Yin (2002).

[24] Zhang et al. (1999).

having attempted suicide, and 69.5% agreed with the statement that they were facing "serious pressure" in their studies and at work.[25] Speaking of attempted suicide rate, we should also consider regional disparity in terms of emergency services, medical care, and basic knowledge among residents about first-aid, which are typically less adequate in rural areas than in urban areas. This means suicide attempts are more likely to result in deaths in rural than in urban areas, where timely intervention or emergency response may help prevent deaths. For example, in one district in the city of Shanghai, in 1980–1985, of 1134 attempted suicides 857 individuals survived thanks to emergency treatment.[26]

According to data released by WHO, from 2000 to 2012, the global age-standardized suicide rate was reduced by 26%. But at the same time, WHO estimated that 788,000 people worldwide committed suicide in 2015, and the number of people attempting to commit suicide was 25 times that number.[27]

An investigation was conducted based on the sample of a mental disorder epidemic survey conducted in Tianjin in 2011. Altogether 4438 individuals who were over 18 years old and stayed in the local place in Tianjin for over 3 months participated in the investigation. It found that 76 of them have attempted suicide[28], of which the rate was 1.71%

## 2.2 *High Risk of Repeat Attempts*

Those who have attempted suicide before are of the highest risk of trying again. A number of studies have shown that around 10% of this group eventually die of suicide and 25% would repeat the attempt.[29] Therefore, it is important for us to keep track of the rate of attempted suicide.

Adolescents aged 15–24 account for up to 70% of those who attempt "quasi-suicide" and "deliberate self-harm," and the deliberate self-harm rate among Chinese teenagers is 49.33 per 100,000 individuals. Japan has the highest rate of deliberate self-harm among its teenagers, with 80% of those who commit deliberate self-harm being teenagers.[30] The attempted suicide rate in Japan is ten times the suicide mortality rate. In 1998, the attempted suicide rate was 347.00 per 100,000 individuals with approximately 310,000 attempts.[31]

---

[25] Tan (2002).

[26] Bu et al. (1987).

[27] Suicide Prevention Day: More elderly people in China committed suicide than other countries. http://datanews.caixin.com/2017-09-10/101143112.html

[28] Zhang et al. (2018).

[29] Liu and Xiao (2002).

[30] He (1997a, p. 379).

[31] Retrieved from: http://www.mhlw.go.jp/houdou/2002/12/h1218-3b. Date of retrieval: June 10, 2011.

## 2.3 *Suicidal Ideation Rate*

Suicidal ideation is the thought of suicide experienced by the subject on an incidental basis. It is an imaginary attempt at, or intention to commit, suicide, with no explicit action in this direction. Suicidal ideation is an important part of suicidal behavior. The study on suicidal ideation rate is important for us to better understand the roots of suicide and is of great significance to our efforts to prevent suicide. Only with the survey and determination of suicidal ideation and targeted education and intervention can we nip suicide behavior in the bud and effectively intervene and prevent suicide.

Suicidal ideation is hidden, universal, and sporadic, occurs in groups, and can vary from one individual to another.

### 2.3.1 High Rates of Suicidal Ideation in China

He Zhaoxiong investigated 4239 people between March and August 1991 using the Eysenck Personality Questionnaire (EPQ) and found out that 31.16% of the respondents showed positive signs of suicidal ideation. In particular, the positive rate was as high as 41.21% among those aged 15–24, 36.78% among those aged 25–34, and 37.95% among 35–44-year-olds.[32] Xu Yong, et al. tested 1600 15-year-old high school students in Hefei, Anhui, with the Family Environmental Scale (Chinese version) (FES-CV). The results were that 27.63% of males and 38.18% of females tested positive for suicidal ideation.[33]

The positive rate for suicidal ideation is also high among China's college students. In a mass survey of college students (1994–1995) conducted by Jin Shenghua, 34.3% of those surveyed were found to "have thought of suicide before" (with the rate higher among women than men at a ratio of 38.6:30.0), while 4.4% of those surveyed had "had experience in committing suicide" (higher among males than females at a ratio of 5.5:3.2). Comparison with a survey of US college students on suicidal ideation conducted around the same time shows no big difference in the suicidal ideation rates between Chinese and US students.[34]

Chen Changhui et al. tested 2366 college students (freshmen to seniors) in Guizhou University, Guizhou University of Technology, Guizhou Normal University, Guizhou Minzu University, and Guiyang College of Traditional Chinese Medicine using the Symptom Checklist (SCL-90),[35] 1397 or 59% male and 969 or 41% female. The respondents were from a variety of departments: humanities, history, law, economics, management, science, engineering, agriculture, and medicine. The results show that 22.12% of the students tested positive for

[32]He (1997b, pp. 265–266).

[33]Xu and Gao (1999).

[34]Jin (1996).

[35]Chen and Wang (1993).

suicidal ideation. In particular, a higher proportion of females tested positive for suicidal ideation than males, with a rate of 28.41%; the suicidal ideation rate was generally higher among science majors than humanities majors, despite that the suicidal ideation rate was also comparatively high among foreign language majors (28.71% for males and 33.10% for females); and female students from minority ethnic groups showed the highest suicidal ideation rate with 36.06% testing positive. There was no significant correlation between the positive rate and the student's seniority at school (i.e., freshman or senior).[36]

### 2.3.2 Suicidal Ideation Rate in Hong Kong and Taiwan

The suicidal ideation rate has been on the rise in Hong Kong in recent years. According to the results of a study by the Chinese University of Hong Kong (CUHK) Faculty of Medicine, 26% of the 7000 secondary school students surveyed had felt sadness and despair, 36% had had thoughts of suicide, and some 15% had even thought seriously about committing suicide.[37] A 1997 study by the Hong Kong Baptist University showed that 10.7% of secondary school students had thought about committing suicide before. Another 2002 CUHK study on secondary school students in Hong Kong found 14.9% of secondary school students to have had thoughts of suicide.[38]

Although the suicide mortality rate in Taiwan is not as high as in the Chinese mainland, the suicidal ideation rate is also fairly high. In 2000, Eden Social Welfare Foundation conducted an island-wide survey among students aged 12–22 with the help of TVBS Poll Center. The results show that 26.4% of the students surveyed had thoughts of suicide. Only 1% of youth entertaining thoughts of suicide would approach professional crisis counselors or helplines such as Taiwan Life International or the Teacher Chang Foundation for help; 8% of the students would tell their family or friends; and 17.5% of those surveyed would keep quiet about their thoughts of suicide. The results of the survey also show that 25% of those surveyed felt their lives to be "very empty" and "joyless and painful"; and that 3.4% of them "often" felt this way; 19.3% of the students were unhappy with how their lives had turned out, and 1.7% of them "often" or "always" felt this way; 7.4% of students felt that "there is no meaning and joy in life" and 1% of the students "often" felt this way, meaning that they are at a high risk of committing suicide. According to the results of the survey, the top cause of suicide among Taiwanese students is schooling pressure (18.6% of the total), followed by parent–child conflicts at home (7.3%).

---

[36]Test conducted in October 2003.

[37]Wang (2002).

[38]*Ming Pao*, June 19, 2004.

## 3 Gender Ratio of Suicide

### *3.1 Higher Suicide Rates Among Women*

Generally, around the world, suicide rates are higher among men than women. In the USA, ratio of males to females in the 15–24 age group committing suicide is 291.9:100, and that in the 25–34 age group is 438:100. Or simply put, there are four male suicides for every female suicide.[39] The situation in China is the opposite: In China, the number of women committing suicide is far higher than that of men (especially in rural areas). In particular, among 15–24-year-olds, almost twice as many women committing suicide. This is absolutely unique in the world (refer to Tables 12, 13, and 14). According to data from the WHO, between 1987 and 1989 the ratio of men to women in the 15–24 age group committing suicide was 52.9:100, and that in the 25–34 age group was 75.6:100 (refer to Table 15).

In 1998, the suicide rate among Chinese youth aged 15–24 was 10.63 per 100,000 individuals, that among rural females in this age group was 15.96 per 100,000 individuals compared to 8.67 per 100,000 individuals for rural males in the same age group. To a large extent, the high suicide rate among rural women in China is caused by the high suicide rate among rural women in this age group.

According to a study by Michael R. Philips, Liu Huaqing, Zhang Yanping et al, between 1990 and 1994, on average, 99,266 rural women aged 15–39 committed suicide each year, accounting for 31% of all suicidal deaths in China for the period and 57.3% of all suicidal deaths among rural women. The suicide mortality rate for women in this age group was 29.40 per 100,000 individuals, which was 4.9 times the suicide mortality rate for men in urban areas and nearly twice the rate of rural men.[40]

The suicidal ideation rate is also higher among Chinese women. Of the 4329 individuals surveyed by He Zhaoxiong, 41.52% of the females had thoughts of suicide compared to 32.07% of the males.[41] Undoubtedly, the high suicide rate among China's young women, in particularly those in rural areas, has become a significant social problem.

In the opinion of He Zhaoxiong and David Lester of the Center for the Study of Suicide in the USA, the causes of this gender anomaly in China are as follows: first, the skewing of China's general gender ratio; second, marriage and family planning; third, poverty; fourth, family conflicts and interpersonal issues; and fifth, the lack of gender equality.[42]

In Hong Kong and Taiwan, the gender ratio for suicides is in line with world-wide patterns (i.e., higher for men than for women). According to David Lester,[43]

---

[39]WHO (1990b, p. 117).

[40]Xie (1999).

[41]He (1997c, p. 334).

[42]He and Lester (1997).

[43]Lester (1994).

**Table 12** Gender ratio in suicides among the Chinese population, 1987–1989 (Female = 100)

| Year | Age | | | | | | | | |
|---|---|---|---|---|---|---|---|---|---|
| | 5–14 | 15–24 | 25–34 | 35–44 | 45–54 | 55–64 | 65–74 | 75 and above | Overall |
| 1987 (male) | 110.2 | 51.9 | 76.8 | 93.9 | 90.5 | 97.0 | 107.0 | 78.8 | 77.44 |
| 1988 (male) | 114.0 | 55.6 | 82.3 | 89.8 | 90.4 | 103.2 | 103.0 | 85.6 | 80.51 |
| 1989 (male) | 65.2 | 51.6 | 69.8 | 85.9 | 101.3 | 111.3 | 109.0 | 86.2 | 78.13 |
| Average (male) | 97.9 | 52.9 | 75.6 | 89.4 | 94.3 | 104.0 | 106.6 | 83.6 | 80.20 |

*Sources* WHO (1989, 1990c, p. 117)

**Table 13** Gender ratio in suicides in certain Chinese cities, 1987–1989 (Female = 100)

| Year | Age | | | | | | | | |
|---|---|---|---|---|---|---|---|---|---|
| | 5–14 | 15–24 | 25–34 | 35–44 | 45–54 | 55–64 | 65–74 | 75 and above | Overall |
| 1987 (male) | 107.1 | 54.2 | 84.2 | 107.8 | 93.6 | 92.6 | 97.3 | 76.7 | 81.65 |
| 1988 (male) | 109.0 | 62.8 | 94.3 | 81.3 | 87.7 | 100.3 | 102.0 | 75.3 | 83.84 |
| 1989 (male) | 57.7 | 56.8 | 81.0 | 99.3 | 91.5 | 99.5 | 106.0 | 83.1 | 85.56 |
| Average (male) | 90.8 | 57.4 | 85.5 | 96.6 | 91.1 | 97.3 | 102.0 | 83.9 | 83.73 |

*Sources* WHO (1989, 1990c, p. 117)

**Table 14** Gender ratio in suicides in some rural areas of China, 1987–1989 (Female = 100)

| Year | Age | | | | | | | | |
|---|---|---|---|---|---|---|---|---|---|
| | 5–14 | 15–24 | 25–34 | 35–44 | 45–54 | 55–64 | 65–74 | 75 and above | Overall |
| 1987 (male) | 111.7 | 51.1 | 73.24 | 87.5 | 88.6 | 99.4 | 112.2 | 80.1 | 75.47 |
| 1988 (male) | 116.7 | 53.8 | 77.7 | 93.2 | 91.7 | 104.5 | 103.4 | 91.9 | 79.25 |
| 1989 (male) | 69.6 | 48.2 | 64.7 | 80.1 | 106.3 | 114.7 | 111.5 | 88.2 | 82.64 |
| Average (male) | 101.2 | 51.6 | 71.7 | 86.3 | 96.0 | 107.3 | 109.0 | 86.8 | 77.05 |

*Sources* WHO (1989, 1990c, p. 117)

**Table 15** Suicide rate in China by age group, 1988–1989 (Unit: Per 100,000 individuals)

| Year | Sex | Age | | | | | | | |
|---|---|---|---|---|---|---|---|---|---|
| | | 5–14 | 15–24 | 25–34 | 35–44 | 45–54 | 55–64 | 65–74 | 75 and above |
| 1988 | Male | 1.0 | 15.8 | 13.8 | 15.4 | 16.8 | 27.7 | 49.9 | 90.1 |
| | Female | 1.0 | 30.4 | 17.7 | 18.4 | 18.6 | 26.5 | 44.4 | 71.0 |
| 1989 | Male | 0.5 | 14.0 | 13.3 | 15.4 | 17.1 | 27.4 | 52.5 | 93.3 |
| | Female | 0.8 | 29.1 | 20.3 | 19.4 | 17.8 | 25.6 | 43.4 | 69.0 |

*Source* WHO (1990b)

the ratio is 121:100 for Hong Kong and 124:100 for Taiwan. The 1996 male-to-female ratio for suicides in Hong Kong is 150:100.[44] The 2001 male-to-female ratio for individuals aged under 19 committing suicide is 113:100 (53.1–46.9%).[45]

---

[44]Suen (1996).

[45]Retrieved from: http://www.sps.org.hk/sps-stat.htm. Date of retrieval: May 20, 2008.

### *3.2 More Male Suicides: Suicide Sex Ratio Among Populations in the Mainland of China*

In 2006, male suicide rate started to rapidly overtake female either in urban or rural areas in the mainland of China.

Chinese (mainland) suicide rate sex ratio among different ages (female = 100)

| Age / Year | 5–14 | 15–24 | 25–34 | 35–44 | 45–54 | 55–64 | 65–74 | 75+ | Total |
|---|---|---|---|---|---|---|---|---|---|
| 2002 (male) | 76.49 | 62.97 | 77.40 | 97.52 | 99.27 | 134.89 | 161.02 | 159.26 | 102.16 |
| 2003 (male) | 191.22 | 80.59 | 65.45 | 76.98 | 89.81 | 96.87 | 135.70 | 132.88 | 91.15 |
| 2004 (male) | 107.02 | 80.93 | 65.12 | 79.52 | 84.81 | 112.56 | 125.88 | 112.06 | 88.10 |
| 2005 (male) | 300.00 | 75.76 | 61.40 | 79.04 | 103.67 | 109.41 | 116.47 | 112.01 | 93.69 |
| 2006 (male) | 273.53 | 93.45 | 82.81 | 95.85 | 117.80 | 128.43 | 149.33 | 150.44 | 109.93 |
| 2007 (male) | 196.59 | 134.94 | 100.00 | 111.59 | 113.90 | 134.46 | 152.55 | 144.33 | 117.86 |
| 2008 (male) | 64.86 | 103.84 | 90.32 | 105.30 | 132.22 | 106.09 | 160.15 | 172.20 | 114.21 |
| 2009 (male) | 78.02 | 107.78 | 102.73 | 125.30 | 128.68 | 138.73 | 142.20 | 131.13 | 117.93 |
| 2010 (male) | 115.15 | 110.20 | 95.90 | 95.54 | 130.94 | 124.27 | 131.11 | 164.81 | 114.45 |
| 2011 (male) | 142.96 | 153.80 | 115.49 | 113.69 | 119.79 | 124.33 | 134.14 | 160.93 | 117.83 |
| 2012 (male) | 104.05 | 117.27 | 111.67 | 118.07 | 121.25 | 122.64 | 128.58 | 137.74 | 116.24 |
| 2013 (male) | 104.65 | 115.24 | 121.14 | 131.87 | 143.67 | 140.92 | 142.97 | 156.13 | 129.84 |
| 2014 (male) | 116.29 | 140.84 | 121.67 | 140.68 | 146.76 | 131.54 | 141.60 | 154.19 | 130.17 |
| 2015 (male) | 131.82 | 169.50 | 144.56 | 146.99 | 140.96 | 141.51 | 133.86 | 148.09 | 135.00 |
| 2016 (male) | 189.84 | 138.78 | 164.35 | 155.59 | 136.40 | 141.41 | 148.19 | 149.57 | 135.48 |
| 2017 (male) | 184.78 | 160.73 | 184.98 | 162.55 | 141.84 | 136.37 | 141.12 | 161.33 | 140.63 |
| Average (male) | 148.58 | 115.41 | 106.56 | 114.75 | 121.99 | 126.53 | 140.30 | 146.69 | 115.92 |

It is clear that from 2006, Chinese (mainland) male suicide rate began to be higher than female, and the gap still widened. In 2017, the figure is 1.4 times the size of female suicides.

## 4 China Falls Under the "East Asian Model" of Suicide Age Distribution[46]

Generally speaking, the suicide rate rises with age, with a steep increase when it comes to the elderly segment of the population. In Émile Durkheim's view, the positive correlation between suicide rate and age is a general principle.[47]

Kaoru Oohashi of Japan put countries around the world into three different groups based on the relationship between suicide rate and age.[48]

[46]The model is also known as the "Japan model".

[47]Durkheim (1998a, p. 216).

[48]Inamura (1977).

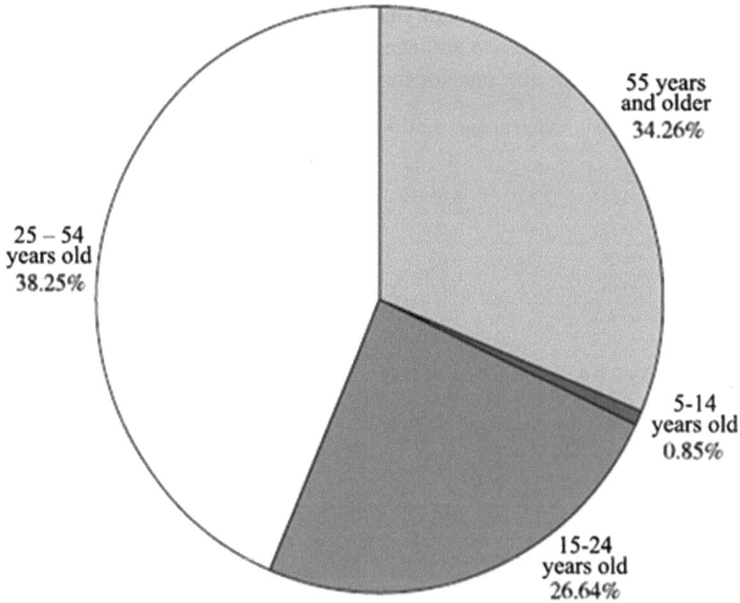


**Fig. 3** Age distribution of suicide in China

The Hungarian model: The suicide rate increases with age and rises sharply for those over 60. Countries in this category include Hungary, the former Soviet Union, Bulgaria, Czechoslovakia, Austria, Belgium, France, Germany, Ireland, and the former Yugoslavia, mostly in eastern and central Europe.

The Finnish model: The suicide rate curve is in the inverted V shape, peaking at the age of 45. Before the age of 45, the suicide rate increases with age and after that it decreases with age. Examples of countries in this category are "welfare states" such as Sweden, Norway, Finland, Denmark, the Netherlands, the UK, Australia, New Zealand, Canada, and the USA.

The Japanese model: There are two peaks in the suicide rate curve: for youth (under 25 years old) and at an old age (over 60 years old).[49] This model is manifested largely in East Asia, including Japan and China (Hong Kong SAR included), and other examples are Sri Lanka, Singapore, Thailand, Mexico, Brazil, and Chile.

According to statistics released by the WHO in 1990, the suicide rate in China reaches its first peak in the 15–24 group and then declines slightly or stays around the same level until it passes the 55-year-old mark where a second peak appears (see Table 15). Between 1987 and 1989, among those who have committed suicide in China, young people aged 15–24 accounted for 26.64% of the total, another 38.25% were 25–54, 34.26% were 55 and older, and 0.85% were children aged 5–14 (see Fig. 3).[50]

[49]Inamura (1978).

[50]WHO (1989).

In Taiwan, the age distribution of suicide is different. There is a simple positive correlation between suicide rate and age. In 1995, the suicide rate of those over 65 in Taiwan was six times the rate for those aged 15–24.[51]

China suicide rate among different ages (2016–2017, 1/100,000)

| Year | Gender | 5～14 | 15～24 | 25～34 | 35～44 | 45～54 | 55～64 | 65～74 | 75⁺ |
|---|---|---|---|---|---|---|---|---|---|
| 2016 | Male | 0.61 | 2.34 | 5.03 | 4.77 | 8.60 | 12.35 | 21.12 | 43.72 |
| | Female | 0.32 | 1.68 | 3.06 | 3.06 | 6.31 | 8.74 | 15.37 | 29.23 |
| 2017 | Male | 0.64 | 2.44 | 4.83 | 4.57 | 8.37 | 10.74 | 20.11 | 39.24 |
| | Female | 0.35 | 1.52 | 2.61 | 2.57 | 5.90 | 7.88 | 14.25 | 24.32 |

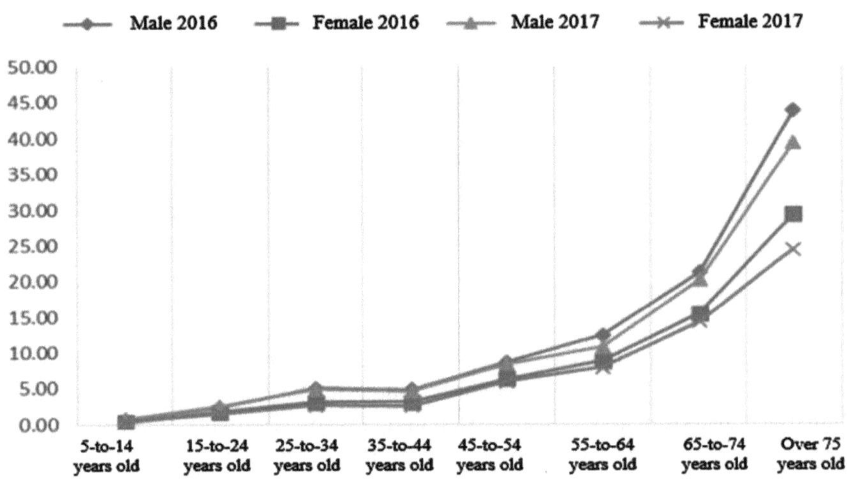


Age distribution of suicide rate in China (2016–2017, 1/100,000)

According to *China Health Statistics Yearbook*, the suicide rate in China reached the first peak at 25-to-34 years old (both male and female), and then declined slightly or basically maintained flat. But after 45 years old, it continued to rise to the peak.

## 5 A Comparative Study on the Means of Suicide

### *5.1 Primary Means of Suicide in the Chinese Mainland*

The primary means of suicide in China are poisoning and hanging, which together account for 80–90% of all cases.[52] The primary means of suicide for Chinese youth

[51]http://www.sinorama.com.tw/jp/9704/704112j2.htm. Accessed: 10 February 2012.
[52]He (1997d, p. 505).

are poisoning, hanging, drowning, fall (jump), knife cut, gas poisoning, and traffic accident (railway and road). The primary means of suicide for Chinese college students in recent years are fall (jump), hanging, drowning, and knife cut.

It is worth noting that with rapid economic and social development in recent years, the means of suicide in China have also taken on characteristics commonly seen in industrialized nations. For example, there has been an increase in jumps from height due to the increase in the number of urban high-rise buildings, viaducts, and bridges; the increase in subways and light rails has led to an increase in rail-related suicides; the widespread use of cooking gas in urban areas has led to an increase in suicide by gas poisoning; the increase in migrant worker population has led to an increase in suicides on railways and highways; the spread of drugs has led to an increase in drug abuse and suicide; the widespread use of explosives in civil construction has led to an increase in suicides by explosion; and the use of hazardous chemicals and highly toxic pesticides has increased the incidence of suicide by poisoning.

### 5.1.1 Suicide by Poisoning and Hanging

Following the implementation of the household responsibility system in rural China, the rate of suicide by agricultural chemical poisoning increased sharply as pesticides were stored in households. The term "drinking pesticide" has even become a synonym for "rural suicide." In rural areas, suicide by poisoning is usually performed with agricultural chemicals, mainly organophosphorus pesticides and rat poison. In urban areas, suicide by poisoning is mainly performed using sedatives and medications for insomnia, mainly barbiturates, diazepam, antipsychotics, antidepressants, and chemical agents.

According to an official of the Ministry of Agriculture's Institute for the Control of Agrochemicals, 62% of those who commit suicide use agricultural chemicals or rat poison, while 75% of what is used are stored in homes; if we could effectively manage the distribution of rat poison and organophosphorus pesticides, we would be able to dramatically reduce the incidence of suicide in rural areas.[53]

As for quasi-suicide cases, the use of poison is even more prevalent, accounting for more than 90% of all cases.

Hanging as a means of suicide is a straightforward operation that requires only a rope, belt, or some object that can be fashioned into a similar form, like a tie, a piece of clothing, or a towel. The mortality rate from hanging is high, and this method is widely used by many individuals with strong suicidal tendencies. The selection or making of tools, the choice of position, the choice of heights, etc., can all be done in many possible ways, and an individual falls unconscious soon without much suffering. This is a suicide method that is widely used and difficult to prevent.

---

[53]Pesticide regulation in China at a time of high suicide rates. http://www.21cbh.com/HTML/2003-1-2/7621.html. Accessed: 20 May 2008.

The choice of suicide method is directly related to one's cultural background. According to a survey, among Chinese men and women living in the USA who commit suicide, 25 and 11%, respectively, opt to use firearms. These rates are far lower than their US-born counterparts (60% for men and 39% for women). At the same time, the rates of suicide by hanging are much higher compared to the local population.[54]

### 5.1.2 Falls (Jumps): From High-Rises and Bridges

It is worth noting that in recent years, the number of suicide cases in China involving jumps from buildings has increased significantly and that this method has become the main means of suicide for college students. For example, in 2001, among seven students from Guangdong universities who committed suicide, five jumped from buildings and one from a bridge, one used poison.[55] Suicide by jumping off a building accounted for 71.43% of all suicides. Between May 1989 and October 1991, a total of eight college students from Fujian Normal University committed suicide, four jumped from a building, two drowned themselves, one took poison, and one committed suicide on the railroad. In other words, half of these cases involved jumping from a building.[56] Between 1991 and 1995, there were 28 suicides among college students from seven key universities and one general university in Beijing. Of these, 13 (46.43%) jumped, five (7.666%) hung themselves, four (14.9%) consumed poison, four (14.9%) drowned, one (3.57%) killed himself on the railway, and one (3.57%) used cooking gas. The jumpers included more women than men, and the majority of them jumped from schools or dormitory buildings. In some schools, the same building is chosen. Suicide by consuming poison mostly took place in the dormitory or at home. Up to 75% of deaths by drowning occurred in the same location.[57] According to available statistics, in the year 2005 alone, a total of 19 Beijing college students leapt to their deaths.

In February 2006, four persons killed themselves within the space of ten days at one agricultural university in southern China, jumping off the university's laboratory, teaching, and dormitory buildings.[58] On June 19, the same year, a student surnamed Bai at a university in Beijing jumped off a building, killing himself and a passerby surnamed Ouyang.

From these incidents of suicide by high-rise jumps and the existence of "popular" drowning sites, we can conclude that there is a contagious effect with regard to college students' choice of suicide means and location.

---

[54]Guo et al. (1993).

[55]*China Youth Daily*, March 2, 2002. *Southern Metropolis Daily*, March 8, 2002.

[56]Su et al. (1993).

[57]Cui and Fang (1998).

[58]*Beijing Youth Daily,* March 7, 2006.

The number of suicides by jumping off buildings has increased significantly. On the one hand, it is due to the increase of high-rise buildings in China; and on the other hand, it is because the housing conditions of urban residents have significantly improved. It is now very common for one to occupy a single room, which makes it more convenient to commit suicide.

The growing number of viaducts and overpasses in cities has also made things easier for those contemplating suicide.

Bridges along the Yangtze River are quite popular among people attempting suicide. Nearly 2000 persons have ended their lives jumping off the bridge since the bridge over the Yangtze River in Nanjing opened to motor traffic in 1968.[59] Hundreds have also killed themselves by jumping off the Yangtze River Bridge in Wuhan and the bridge over the Qiantang River. In recent years, jumps from Yangtze River bridges have declined due to increased patrol and rescue efforts. However, suicides sometimes still occur despite best efforts at prevention. In 2001 alone, the Nanjing Traffic Police Team No. 9 rescued a total 38 people seeking to commit suicide on the Yangtze River Bridge.[60] A total of 215 people jumped from Nanjing's Yangtze River Bridge between January 2003 and September 2004, 110 were under the age of 30, 74 were between 30 and 50 years old, and 31 were over the age of 50, with the oldest being 85 years old.[61] In 2006, nearly 700 persons were rescued from suicide attempts on the bridge.[62] Those who commit suicide jumping off bridges often do so in an instant and disappear quickly without a trace, leaving no chance for anyone to bear witness. Therefore, many such cases may not have been included in statistics.

In modern cities, people often experience this: They feel dizzy when they are on top of a skyscraper, and then are tempted by danger as they imagine themselves jumping. This psychological drive is named desire to fall by US psychologist Scott Herdman. A person who had been saved after jumping off the Nanjing Yangtze River Bridge reported feeling as light as a leaf when falling from the bridge.

Falling from a high altitude, especially a skyscraper, is undoubtedly an overwhelming experience for a living person. However, for those committing suicide, jumping offers little room for return in comparison with other means. Once one is off, gravity will do the rest. Research shows that the huge fear caused by falling from a high altitude can cause a person's adrenaline level to spike, which in turn pushes up the heart rate till the heart stops entirely. The person thus dies in the air rather than upon reaching the ground.

---

[59] *Jiangnan Times,* January 22, 2007.

[60] Han (2002).

[61] Zhang (2005).

[62] Wang (2007).

### 5.1.3 Railway Suicides: Railroads and Subway Rails

The International Classification of Diseases (ICD-10) published by the WHO defines suicides by railway (including subway systems) as "deliberate self-harm through intentional jumps or lying down in front of a moving object."

Suicide by lying on railroad tracks has been rare in China in recent years. Those who kill themselves in this way are mostly youths between the ages of 20 and 30 (more than 60% of the total).[63] There are fewer victims aged under 18 or over 55. More than 65% of the victims are male. Suicide locations are, in most cases, not far from inhabited areas for this makes it easier for other to find and claim the dead body. Death by running into (under) a train usually occurs along slow track sections or at stations, while cases of suicide by lying on railroad tracks, crashing into trains, and jumping onto tracks occur mostly along fast track sections. The most common way to commit suicide on a railway is to lie across the railway track. This, which accounts for more than half of the cases, is followed by crashes and running under trains. Jumping onto tracks is rare. More than 80% of these cases occur at night.[64] The ratio of males to females choosing to commit suicide by lying on railway tracks is 2.1:1. This appears to be because of the gory nature of the method. Most victims lay their upper body across the track. A majority of such cases (73.33%) occur between May and October.[65] A sensation was caused when in March 1989 the young poet Hai Zi (Zha Haisheng) committed suicide by lying on the railway track in Shanhaiguan. On April 10, 2001, in the train station of Lechang City, Guangdong Province, a young woman committed suicide with her 8-year-old son and 5-year-old daughter by doing the same.

Ratnayake et al. defined suicide behavior in the subway as: (1) "suicide" or intentional self-harming behavior on subway property leading to death; (2) "suicide attempt" or intentional self-harming behavior on subway property that does not result in death; and (3) "suicide incident" which is either a death by suicide attempted suicide on subway property.[66]

Subway suicide is a new phenomenon that recently emerged in China. Cases have been reported in Beijing, Shanghai, Guangzhou, and Nanjing. Until now, the number is far lower than in Japan. Between the completion of the Shanghai Metro in July 1995 and the end of 2003, there were 65 cases of suicide, causing 48 deaths while 17 were rescued. Most of the individuals in these cases were women, particularly young women.[67] On June 8 and 9, 2005, Shanghai Metro Lines 1 and 2 saw a number of suicide attempts where the individuals lay on the rails. During the Spring Festival of 2012, two people (one male and one female) killed themselves by lying on the tracks at Lujiazui Station of Shanghai Metro Line 2 within the space of nine days.

---

[63]Zhong (2000a, p. 130).

[64]Zhong (2000a, p. 130).

[65]Xiao and Wang (1997).

[66]Ratnayake et al. (2007).

[67]Ouyang (2004).

### 5.1.4 Suicide During the Spring Festival Travel Crush

The Spring Festival travel crush is a phenomenon unique to China. In addition to the 150 million rural migrant workers in cities, there are also hundreds of millions of Chinese who work and live away from their hometowns. This creates a massive flow of people heading home for the Spring Festival each year. People are willing to traverse hundreds of miles to be with their families. The tradition of going home for the Spring Festival goes back to ancient times. In 2004, a total of 1.9 billion trips were made during the Spring Festival travel crush, and in 2005, the number rose to almost 1.95 billion. In 2006, the figure passed the two billion mark. In particular, in 2003, 134.7 million passenger trips were made by train during the crush (with an addition of 1.667 billion by road and 9 million by air). In 2003, the figure was 137 million, 140 million in 2004, 149 million in 2006, 159 million in 2007, 210 million in 2010, peaked at 230 million in 2011, and dropped slightly to 220 million in 2012. The figure surged to 357 million in 2017, with an addition of 2.52 billion by road, 58.3 million by air, and 43.5 million by water. Such figures far exceed the carrying capacity of China's railway system. As such, trains are severely overcrowded and signs of mental illness are frequently seen among passengers. Acts of violence and suicide attempts have occurred on numerous occasions. Each year, during the Spring Festival travel crush, there have been reports of passengers killing themselves by jumping off moving trains. For many, especially those with a history of mental illness are under stress, or already nervous because they are carrying large amounts of cash, traveling long distances in crowded and poorly ventilated spaces while sleep-deprived can trigger panic or other negative psychological responses. A number of passengers have jumped from heights at Beijing West Station after long-distance travel in a less-than-clear state of mind. The incidence of mental illness spikes each year during the Spring Festival travel crush. In fact, there have been trains serving migrant workers on which multiple cases of suicide and harm to others have been reported. According to statistics from the Guangzhou Railway Police, the number of suicides by passengers while traveling in trains has increased in recent years. Ten acts of suicide were committed on-board trains departing from Guangzhou Station during the Spring Festival travel crush in 2001. Another 12 occurred during the same period in 2002. Data shows that sudden onset of mental illness on trains most frequently occur on those heading west from coastal areas, with more than 95% of those afflicted being migrant workers. These overcrowded "special" trains travel for many hours with poor ventilation. Thus, passengers are prone to developing anxiety and hallucinations as well as exhibit symptoms of mental illness suddenly.[68]

There are reports of suicides on passenger aircraft in China. On July 20, 2000, on China Eastern Airlines' flight MU5368 from Shenzhen to Shanghai, a young woman committed suicide by taking poison due to emotional issues. She was in deep coma when found and was finally saved through emergency treatment. On

[68]Guo (2003).

April 11, 2006, China Southern Airlines' flight CZ6403 flew from Shenyang to Kunming via Chongqing. On the flight, a young man committed suicide using a razor blade in the lavatory. A week later, on CZ628 from Tokyo to Shenyang, a woman committed suicide by cutting her wrist.[69] On November 13, 2010, on a flight from Madrid to Beijing, a 40-year-old individual tried to commit suicide by means of arson and was subsequently sentenced to four years in prison.[70]

### 5.1.5 Suicide by Explosion

Suicide by explosion has also been occurring in China in recent years. This appears to have something to do with the influence of media. In recent years, Palestinians in the Palestinian–Israeli conflict have frequently carried out suicide bombings against the Israelis, and suicidal car bombings have also been on the rise in Iraq. International media outlets also carry countless reports on terrorist attacks perpetrated by suicide bombers. This is known internationally as the "CNN effect."[71] In China, explosives are used extensively for mining and construction and can be easily obtained, making it an easy option as a method of suicide. But explosions can also kill innocent bystanders or passersby. Most such cases have occurred in rural areas and tend to be caused by interpersonal conflicts and emotional difficulties. Suicides by explosion that occur in urban areas are mostly of the "anomic" type (using Durkheim's definition). On the night of December 3, 2000, Chen Maoqin, a 30-year-old female, deputy mayor of Yeping Town of Ankang, Shaanxi Province, committed suicide using more than 10 kg of explosives and 30 detonators to blow up the office building due to problems in her marriage. The explosion also killed her 8-year-old twin daughters who were sleeping, harmed a number of innocent people, and destroyed the entire office building. On December 3, 2006, at a road construction site in Panxian, Guizhou Province, a 33-year-old man (someone who had previously worked with explosives) detonated explosives tied to his body. This resulted in the killing of six people and serious injury to another two. Suicide bombings required would-be bombers to have access to explosives as well as the knowledge of how to use these explosives. This is more common with men. Of the 207 suicide cases recorded by Zhong Jirong et al. 12%, or 25 cases, involved the use of explosives. There have also been cases in which the detonators were inserted in anal passages or held in the victims' mouths.[72]

---

[69]Yang (2006).

[70]Liu (2011).

[71]The term "CNN effect" usually refers to the influence of the news media on political and government decisions in political conflicts or disputes. The emergence of this term reflects the pioneering position of CNN in the journalism industry.

[72]Zhong (2000b, p. 118).

### 5.1.6 Self-immolation

Self-immolation has also been a common means of suicide. In general, those who choose to self-immolate mostly do so outdoors. They pour substances such as gasoline or kerosene on themselves, and then ignite the fuel, making it easy to identify where the case occurs. The motives behind such suicides are primarily emotional issues (with self-immolation being a dramatic way of conveying certain messages), or cult influence (such as Falungong), protests and political issues. With the growing use of piped household gas and liquefied petroleum gas in China, reports of suicide by the ignition of indoor gas supply are also growing in number. According to Weng Xinhui et al., 20-to-29-year-old self-immolators made up 2.43% of total suicides in Quanzhou, Fujian Province, in 1989.[73] A number of individuals obsessed with Falungong had also killed themselves in this manner at the turn of the century. One such case that shocked the world happened on January 23, 2001, on the Tiananmen Square, during which a group of Falungong followers performed collective self-immolation, resulting in multiple deaths. On January 5, 2000, a 27-year-old man suddenly jumped into a furnace containing molten steel at a temperature of up to 1500 °C at the Guiyang Steel Plant in Guizhou and turned into ash in an instant. This is probably the only case of its kind in the world.

### 5.1.7 Suicide by Disembowelment

Suicide by disembowelment ("seppuku" in Japanese) has long been regarded as unique to Japan because the mortality rate from this method is low and because this method is exceptionally painful. In general, suicide by this method is of the "anomic" kind, that is, an attempt to reveal certain thoughts and feelings. Suicide by disembowelment has also become more common in recent years. On September 8, 2000, Luo Shugui, a resident of Baizhao Village, Duyun City, Guizhou Province, cut his abdomen open with a pair of scissors after failing to be elected as village chief; on July 20 of the same year, a young man from Huqiu Road in Nanjing, cut open his abdomen with a kitchen knife in front of his wife and children; on June 5, 2001, a young individual died at home of self-inflicted disembowelment in Nanjing's Qinhuai District; on August 21 of the same year, the bankrupt boss of a company in Taipei City cut open his abdomen in front of his 3-year-old daughter; on March 24, 2002, a young woman from Xuanwu District, Nanjing, cut open her abdomen with a pair of scissors after an argument with her husband; on January 7, 2003, a young man from Tianzhu County, Guizhou Province, stabbed his wife and then committed suicide with a dagger; on February 19, 2006, a resident of Longquan Town, Danzhai County, Guizhou Province, committed suicide this way with a dagger; and on April 9, 2007, a 74-year-old resident of Xianlin New Village in Hangzhou, committed suicide by disembowelment using a kitchen knife.

[73]He (1997e, p. 514).

### 5.1.8 "Online" Suicides

"Online" suicides are a new phenomenon that has emerged with the growing use of computers and the Internet in recent years. In addition to a large number of websites containing information on suicide and online help (some individuals help others commit suicide for profit), many Internet users also go online to search for suicide partners and learn more about how to commit suicide. In recent years, there have even been cases of "live streaming of suicide."

At midnight on January 25, 2003, a young woman in Yichang, Hubei Province, turned on her computer webcam and then took sleeping pills and turned on the gas in front of multiple online viewers. A number of Internet users who witnessed the unfolding of this scene in a Yahoo! chatroom called the Yichang Public Security Bureau from all over the country, launching an offline bid to save the girl's life. The girl was saved a few hours later. This has been the most successful case of crisis intervention for a "live streaming of suicide."

On the afternoon of September 14, 2004, a 24-year-old Sichuan woman broadcast her suicide by wrist cut in an online chatroom, triggering a joint rescue operation between the police, hospital workers, and netizens from Changsha and Pingjiang. The young woman was eventually saved.[74]

## 5.2 *Primary Means of Suicide in Hong Kong*

Falling from a height is the major suicide method in Hong Kong. According to different suicide methods, the first suicide method in Hong Kong is falling from a height, accounting for 21.07%; the second one is hanging by the neck, accounting for 21.07%; and the third one is carbon monoxide poisoning (by burning charcoal), accounting for 12.12%.

Suicide rate of Hong Kong in 2017 (1/100,000)[a]

| Suicide methods | gender | 0-9 | 10-19 | 20-29 | 30-39 | 40-49 | 50-59 | 60-69 | 70+ | unspecified | subtotal | total |
|---|---|---|---|---|---|---|---|---|---|---|---|---|
| firearm | male | 0 | 0 | 1 | 0 | 0 | 1 | 0 | 0 | 0 | 2 | 2 |
| | female | 0 | 0 | 0 | 0 | 0 | 0 | 0 | 0 | 0 | 0 | |
| drugs | male | 0 | 0 | 2 | 3 | 0 | 1 | 2 | 3 | 0 | 11 | 29 |
| | female | 0 | 1 | 1 | 4 | 2 | 4 | 3 | 3 | 0 | 18 | |
| poison | male | 0 | 0 | 0 | 1 | 3 | 0 | 0 | 4 | 0 | 8 | 10 |
| | female | 0 | 0 | 0 | 1 | 0 | 0 | 0 | 1 | 0 | 2 | |
| hanging by the neck | male | 0 | 2 | 8 | 14 | 8 | 22 | 25 | 37 | 0 | 116 | 193 |
| | female | 0 | 0 | 6 | 11 | 5 | 15 | 7 | 33 | 0 | 77 | |
| falling from a height | male | 0 | 24 | 46 | 37 | 31 | 37 | 51 | 76 | 2 | 304 | 495 |
| | female | 0 | 6 | 25 | 27 | 27 | 36 | 30 | 40 | 0 | 191 | |

(continued)

[74] *Jiangnan Times*, September 18, 2004, 13.

(continued)

| Suicide methods | gender | 0-9 | 10-19 | 20-29 | 30-39 | 40-49 | 50-59 | 60-69 | 70+ | unspecified | subtotal | total |
|---|---|---|---|---|---|---|---|---|---|---|---|---|
| carbon monoxide | male | 0 | 0 | 6 | 23 | 13 | 19 | 8 | 5 | 0 | 74 | 111 |
| | female | 0 | 1 | 2 | 15 | 8 | 7 | 4 | 0 | 0 | 37 | |
| get drowned | male | 0 | 1 | 3 | 6 | 3 | 4 | 1 | 12 | 1 | 31 | 40 |
| | female | 0 | 0 | 0 | 1 | 1 | 0 | 5 | 2 | 0 | 9 | |
| sharp weapon | male | 0 | 1 | 0 | 0 | 5 | 0 | 1 | 1 | 0 | 8 | 9 |
| | female | 0 | 0 | 0 | 0 | 0 | 1 | 0 | 0 | 0 | 1 | |
| others | male | 0 | 0 | 2 | 2 | 1 | 4 | 4 | 1 | 1 | 15 | 27 |
| | female | 0 | 0 | 4 | 1 | 1 | 2 | 1 | 3 | 0 | 12 | |
| subtotal | male | 0 | 28 | 68 | 86 | 64 | 88 | 92 | 139 | 4 | 569 | 916 |
| | female | 0 | 8 | 38 | 60 | 44 | 65 | 50 | 82 | 0 | 347 | |
| total | | 0 | 36 | 106 | 146 | 108 | 153 | 142 | 221 | 4 | | 916 |

[a] 2017 Annual Report of the Samaritan Befrienders Hong Kong

# 6 Temporal Distribution of Suicide

## *6.1 Seasonal Distribution*

In Western countries, the "peak" season for suicides is in the spring. In Durkheim's view, the number of suicides in European countries increases between January and May and declines the rest of the year.[75]

According to various domestic sources, China's peak season for suicide is in the summer, with the peak occurring in July in southern China and the trough, just before and after the Spring Festival. According to He Zhaoxiong, the number of suicides peaks in June, July, and August, the total of which accounts for 41.7% annual total. The lowest numbers are reported for the month of February.[76] Survey results from Li Wenshi et al. show that the number of suicides is the highest from May to August, with the total accounting for 48.7% of the annual total.[77] According to Zhao Mei and Ji Jianlin, the suicide rate is higher in spring, summer, and autumn, especially in summer, and the lowest in winter. Data from Yangcheng, Shanxi (1989–1991) shows that the largest number of suicides (29.96% of the total) occurs in summer. Winter witnesses 13.07% of all suicides. According to data from Kunming (1990–1992), spring sees 29.96% of all suicide cases of a year (there is little difference in temperature between the daytime and nighttime in spring), while summer sees 28.27% of the total and winter, 16.03%. According to data provided by Anhui Disease Surveillance Station (for 1990–1995), the highest proportion of suicides occurred in August and September, at 12.66 and 18.38% of the total,

[75]Durkheim (1998b, p. 79).

[76]He (1996).

[77]Li et al. (2001a, p. 236).

respectively.[78] In the case of junior and senior high school students, there are relatively more suicides in July and August, when the results of the senior high school entrance examination and the college entrance examination are released. The number of suicides is also higher among young people at the beginning of a school year or a semester (August–September, February–March). The phenomenon of "Black July"—where a number of students commit suicide following the release of the results of the senior high school and college entrance examinations—has been significant enough to draw public attention. Gao Wei et al. have found through a survey that the number of suicides peaks in mid- and late July, especially on July 23.[79]

The number of suicides by poisoning, the most common means of suicide in China, also peaks in the summer. In part of Sichuan province, a peak of 553 cases of suicide by poisoning was seen in June. Xu Chunsheng et al. discovered from a study of 414 cases where patients were hospitalized at the Affiliated Hospital of Binzhou Medical College following attempts at suicide by poisoning (1982–1988) and found that suicides occurring between June and August accounted for 41.1% of the total, while those occurring from April to June accounted for 31.6%. June 27 was determined to be the "peak day" for suicide following statistical analysis by circular distribution.[80] Hu Yan et al. examined 1756 cases of suicide by poisoning (81.44% women and 18.56% men) between 1981 and 1990 and found May 24 to September 14 to be the peak time for these suicides.[81]

This may be explained by the longer and more packed schedule in summer due to longer daytime hours and the fact that rising temperatures can lead the nervous system to produce a confused state of mind. Tempers can flare more easily in warmer weather, thus leading to more conflicts at home and with others, which are prime causes of suicide. Further, summer is a critical time for students seeking further education and for youth seeking employment. So, at this time of the year, young people are more likely to suffer setbacks in their academic or employment pursuits, thereby increasing the probability of suicide. In addition, China is a big agricultural nation and summer is the most hectic season for Chinese farmers. During this period, there may be more disputes. Another thing to note is that agrochemicals are used widely in summer and easier to obtain by those who want to use it for suicide purpose.

[78]Zhao and Ji (2000).

[79]Gao (1998).

[80]Xu et al. (1993).

[81]Hu et al. (1994).

## 6.2 Suicides by the Hours of the Day

Suicides in China occur largely in the daytime and early evenings and rarely at night. According to two sets of data from He Zhaoxiong (1980–1990), suicides occur primarily in the daytime (0600–1900 h). The first set of data shows that daytime suicides make up 72% of the total, while the second set of data reveals a proportion of 62%. This makes for a marked difference from overseas data, which show suicides to occur mostly after nightfall.[82] Li Wenshi et al. report that the number of suicides was the highest between 0600 h and 2100 h, which add up to 86.6% of the total.[83] Gao Wei et al. found in their examination of 878 cases of suicide among youths aged between 13 and 19 that 21.18% or 186 of these suicides occurred in the early morning or morning, with the peak time at 1015 h; 692 or 78.82% of the suicides occurred in the afternoons or the evening with the peak time at 1930 h.[84] Hu Yan et al. found after an examination of 1756 cases of suicide that 80% of suicides by poisoning occurred in the afternoon with the peak period between 1730 h and 2130 h.[85] This time of day is when people come home to spend time with family or to be alone after a long day of work or school. Interaction with family members increases the likelihood of conflicts, a leading cause of suicide. When individuals are alone, they are prone to anxiety and fear, and can easily feel helpless and even world-weary. There is no one around to help allay their low spirits and distress, thus the possibility of suicide increases. Furthermore, the pesticides used for suicide in rural areas and the medications used for suicide in urban areas in China are generally stored at home and are thus easily accessible.

## 6.3 Post-disaster Suicides

A strong earthquake occurred in Nantou County and its surrounding areas in Taiwan on September 21, 1999. Within the disaster area, 440,000 individuals were affected, and a rash of suicides subsequently developed. In 2000, victims who had suffered the loss of loved ones and the destruction of family businesses, etc., were reminded of their losses and took to committing suicide on major festival days such as the Spring Festival, the Ching Ming (or Tomb-sweeping) Festival, the Dragon Boat Festival, the Hungry Ghost Festival in July, and the Mid-Autumn Festival, as well as on the anniversary of the disaster. As such, the number of suicides peaked on these dates.[86] According to investigations by the Taiwan authorities concerned,

[82]He (1997f, p. 241).

[83]Li et al. (2001b, p. 237).

[84]Gao (1998).

[85]Hu et al. (1994).

[86]He (2000).

4% of the victims who lost their loved ones in the disaster described their suicidal tendencies to be "hardly suppressible."

A study conducted by scholars from Taiwan concluded that earthquakes have a significant impact on the suicide rate of earthquake victims. The group collected and examined data from the six months following the 1999 Nantou earthquake, and after controlling for factors such as the victims' place of residence, pre-disaster physical disabilities, pre-disaster socioeconomic status, and the level of urbanization, they found that earthquake victims were 1.46 times more likely to commit suicide than the general population. The team recommended targeting post-disaster psychological intervention and preventive measures at those individuals who are most seriously affected, instead of covering all those living in the area where the disaster took place.[87]

A massive earthquake occurred in Wenchuan, Sichuan Province, on May 12, 2008, causing 69,197 deaths and injuring another 374,176 persons, with 18,289 persons missing. A mini-peak in the suicide rate occurred in the disaster zone in about half a year following the disaster. On October 3, 2008, Dong Yufei, director of the Beichuan County Agricultural Office and a disaster-relief hero who lost his son to the earthquake, committed suicide; on October 8, a 59-year-old disaster victim, from Dujiangyan, jumped from his 12th-floor ward at a hospital in Chengdu and perished; on the evening of November 15, a Beichuan man committed suicide after killing his wife; on November 19, He Zonghua, director of the Personnel and Education Department of Mianyang Municipal People's Government, committed suicide jumping off a building; in the early morning of April 20, 2009, disaster-relief hero Feng Xiang (aged 33), deputy director of the Publicity Department of the Beichuan County CPC Committee who had lost his son, hung himself at home.

On November 9, 2009, a health check-up was conducted for the 36 members of the first Sichuan Model Course for Earthquake Relief Training at Sichuan Provincial People's Hospital. The results were shocking: among these disaster-relief heroes. 41.66% had anxiety, and 33.3% had depression, with some have both. In the self-assessment for anxiety, 31 persons, or 86% of the total, reported "feeling weak all over and prone to fatigue," while 27 persons (75% of the total) reported feeling "nervous and anxious." In the self-assessment for depression, 26 persons reported feeling "prone to anger and agitation," and 25 persons reported "poor quality of sleep." One statement in the self-assessment for depression is "I do not bear any hope for the future," For this, six persons chose the option "Most of the time" in response.[88]

According to Zhang Wei of the Psychological Counseling Center of East China Normal University, the emotions that people experience after a disaster are usually divided into several stages: The first stage or emotion experienced is shock as the victim has yet to come around after the sudden disaster. The second stage or

[87]Tao and Gong (2008)

[88]Song (2008).

emotion experienced occurs around two months later, when aid and concern pour in from the rest of society. This can also be termed the "honeymoon period." In the following months, individuals start to try and put their lives back to normal. However, as their homes have been destroyed and in some cases, loved ones have been lost, this is a difficult process. However, most rescue and aid resources are also leaving around this time, and there is less intense attention from the rest of society. This can cause local victims to feel neglected. This is the third period, the period of frustration. In addition, once victims settle down, it is common for them to recall the scenes when they are with their deceased loved ones. These symptoms of "flash-back"—scenes of being with loved ones, tragic scenes from the earthquake itself—occur over and over, like in a movie. Such flashbacks, when experienced over a long period of time, will lead to a strong emotional response, with insomnia being a very common symptom. If an individual is unable to find meaning in life, which is a painful experience, then he or she will seek to escape from reality. Some will resort to an extreme method like suicide in order to find relief. Generally, the six-month-mark is when such pressures can no longer be bottled up if no appropriate guidance and counseling is provided.[89] Major natural disasters are an important factor leading to suicidal behavior. The loss of life and property caused by major earthquakes, strong typhoons, floods, fires, volcanic eruptions, etc., have caused some victims to commit suicide due to pessimism or dejection, or due to mental illness. In addition, during famines caused by severe flood, drought, or pest disasters, despair and the lack of food can also lead to suicide by individuals or entire families.[90]

## 7 Places of Suicide

### 7.1 *Suicide by Poisoning and Hanging Largely Occur Indoors*

Suicide by poisoning and hanging, the primary means of suicide in China, mostly occurs indoors (at home). Statistics show that of the 360 cases of suicidal deaths in urban areas in Guiyang City from 1995 to 1999, 59.10% occurred in residential buildings.[91] With the improvement of living standards in urban and rural areas in China, it is now common for young people to have a room to themselves. In recent years, suicide among youth in their own homes has grown significantly.

[89]Xiao et al. (2008).
[90]He (1997g, p. 537).
[91]Yu et al. (2002).

## 7.2 *Jumps Mainly Occur on High-Rises and Bridges*

As the number of high-rise buildings in China's cities increases, young people have generally chosen high-rise buildings such as residential buildings and campus buildings (teaching buildings, office buildings, dormitory buildings) to jump off from. As for bridge suicides, bridges that span rivers and viaducts/overhead passes are also popular venues for suicide. As mentioned above, nearly 2000 people have jumped to death from the Nanjing Yangtze River Bridge over the nearly 40 years since the bridge was opened to traffic. Between January 2003 and September 2004, 215 individuals were recorded to have jumped from the bridge. Each year, dozens of people commit suicide by jumping from the Wuhan Yangtze River Bridge too and the same is true for the Qiantang River Bridge. Between 1937 and 1991, 918 persons committed suicide by jumping from the Golden Gate Bridge in San Francisco, 153 died jumping off the Aurora Bridge in Seattle as of 1981, and 121 people had died jumping off the harbor bridge of San Francisco by 1979.[92] The iconic Tokyo Tower (333 m high) and Eiffel Tower (324 m high) have also seen a number of suicides. On May 10, 2011, just over a year after the world's highest building, the Burj Khalifa in Dubai (888 m) had been completed, a man committed suicide jumping from the 147th floor.

## 7.3 *Committing Suicide at Famous Natural Attractions*

What is striking is that in China and Japan, scenic spots are favored as suicide locations. Many people choose beautiful mountains and rivers as their final destination.

At Mount Huangshan in China, the bodies of some 110 persons who had committed suicide were found between 1980 and 1991 (with more not yet discovered). The majority of these individuals had jumped from the "Carp's Back" ridge on top of the Tiandu Peak. More than 200 suicide cases occurred in Lushan Mountain between 1979 and 1989. Other places with frequent suicide occurrences include the Golden Peak of Mount Emei, Luoyan Peak of Mount Huashan, the Sheshen Cliff of Mount Tai, the Langshan Mountain in Nantong, the Jinshan Mountain and Beigu Mountain in Zhenjiang, and the Swallow Rock in Nanjing. Duan Xueming, director of the Mt. Emei Golden Peak Police Station, has single-handedly saved 96 individuals from suicide in just a few years (as of October 2005). The Jiulao Cave of Mt. Emei is another hotspot, with dozens of corpses found in its deep and complex interior. Those who seek to commit suicide here seem to believe that they, too, can become "immortal" by committing suicide in a place said to be "where the immortals gather" and where the body of Monk Tai'an of Xianfeng Temple stayed incorrupt for over 200 years.

[92]Zhai (1997).

## 7.4 Geographic Distribution of Suicides

According to Durkheim, the higher suicide rates in urban areas can be attributed to the high population density, as well as the accumulation and extension of basic emotional patterns over time in these areas.[93] Within the field of social psychology, it is believed that high population density results in complex interpersonal relationships and more conflicts. There is a higher probability of individuals becoming frustrated with their interpersonal relationships and emotions. However, the Chinese situation is a special one: The suicide rate is much higher in rural areas than in cities.

According to data from the National Bureau of Statistics, in the three years from 1984 to 1986, the average annual suicide rate in urban China was 11.20 per 100,000 individuals while the rural rate was 2.63 times this figure at 29.50 per 100,000 individuals.[94] Data from the National Disease Surveillance System for the period 1991–2000 shows the rural suicide mortality rate to be four times the urban rate.[95]

The suicide rate in rural China has risen sharply since the 1980s, from 15.40 per 100,000 individuals in 1980 to 29.10 per 100,000 individuals in 1991,[96] during which period, China's rural economy seen unprecedented development, indisputably pushing up rural living standard. Thus, the non-economic factors behind the rising rural suicide rate are worth noting.

The geographic distribution of suicide mortality among the vast rural areas in China shows some special features. Studying data from the National Disease Surveillance System on the causes of death for the period of 1990–2000, Yang Gonghuan et al. found that the suicide mortality rate within China's rural population is the highest in the central region, followed by the eastern region, while the rate was relatively low in rural western China.[97]

At present, the suicide rate is generally high in the rural areas of eastern and central China, especially where the boundaries of several provinces meet. This seems to be related to traditional cultural practices, the level of local economic development, and the degree of social integration. In addition, the widespread use of highly lethal pesticides is also an important cause of suicidal deaths in these areas.

[93]Durkheim (1998c, p. 16).

[94]Department of Social Statistics and National Bureau of Statistics (1987).

[95]Yang et al. (2004).

[96]He (1997h, p. 182).

[97]Yang et al. (2004).

## References


Bu, J., et al. (1987). An analysis of the types of poisons used in suicides in a certain region. *Journal of Forensic Medicine, 3*(1), 9–12.

Chen, C., & Wang, Z. (1993). Symptom checklist. In Wang, X (Ed.), *Mental health rating scale handbook (Supplement to the Chinese mental health journal*) (pp. 31–46).

Cui, Y., & Fang, M. (1998). The social and psychological factors and clinical characteristics of college students who have attempted suicide. *Chinese Journal of Clinical Psychology, 6*(3), 177.

Dang, C. (2001). *Year in review for Taiwanese society*. http://big5.china.com.cn/chinese/TCC/97547.htm. Accessed January 23, 2009.

Department of Social Statistics, & National Bureau of Statistics. (1987). *China's social statistics* (p. 273). Beijing: China Statistics Press.

Durkheim, É. (1998a). *Suicide: A study in sociology* (p. 216) (X. Zhong, L. Ma & Q. Lin, Trans.). Hangzhou: Zhejiang People's Press.

Durkheim, É. (1998b). *Suicide: A study in sociology* (p. 79) (X. Zhong, L. Ma, & Q. Lin, Trans.). Hangzhou: Zhejiang People's Press.

Durkheim, É. (1998c). *Suicide: A study in sociology* (p. 16) (X. Zhong, L. Ma, & Q. Lin, Trans.). Hangzhou: Zhejiang People's Press.

Gao, W. (1998). A study on when youth suicides occur, and interventional measures. *Chinese Journal of School Health, 19*(4), 306.

Guo, A. (2003). 20% rise in suicide rate during Spring Festival rush period, suicide prevention new task for railway police. *Information Times*, January 4.

Guo, Q., Wang, Z., & Tatsumi, T. (1993). A comparative study of suicide in nine Asian countries and regions. *Foreign Medicine (Psychiatry Volume), 4*, 206.

Han, D. (2002). A battle for life on Nanjing's Changjiang Bridge. *Jiangnan Times*, March 11.

He, Z. (1996). *Suicide and life* (p. 201). Guangzhou: Guangzhou Publishing House.

He, Z. (1997a). *The pathology of suicide* (p. 379). Beijing: China Traditional Chinese Medicine Press.

He, Z. (1997b). *The pathology of suicide* (pp. 265–266). Beijing: China Traditional Chinese Medicine Press.

He, Z. (1997c). *The pathology of suicide* (p. 334). Beijing: China Traditional Chinese Medicine Press.

He, Z. (1997d). *The pathology of suicide* (p. 505). Beijing: China Traditional Chinese Medicine Press.

He, Z. (1997e). *The pathology of suicide* (p. 514). Beijing: China Traditional Chinese Medicine Press.

He, Z. (1997f). *The pathology of suicide* (p. 241). Beijing: China Traditional Chinese Medicine Press.

He, Z. (1997g). *The pathology of suicide* (p. 537). Beijing: China Traditional Chinese Medicine Press.

He, Z. (1997h). *The pathology of suicide* (p. 182). Beijing: China Traditional Chinese Medicine Press.

He, J. (2000). Rash of suicides comes quietly upon Taiwan earthquake zone. *Chinanews.com.* http://www.chinanews.com/2000-09-23/26/47953.html. Accessed September 23, 2012.

He, Z., & Lester, D. (1997). The gender difference in Chinese suicide rates. *Medicine and Society, 10*(4), 35–36.

Hu, Y., et al. (1994). The hours and seasonality of suicide by poisoning. *Panzhihua Journal of Medicine and Pharmacy, 16*(1), 19.

Inamura, H. (1977). *Suicide studies: For the treatment and prevention of suicide* (p. 29). Tokyo: University of Tokyo Press.

Inamura, H. (1978). *Suicide among the young* (pp. 73–74). Seishin Shobo.

Jin, S. (1996). Predicting suicidal ideation in youth. *Youth Studies, 5*, 42.

Kuo, C., Chen, I., Chen, T., & Hwang, C. (2010). *A preliminary look at suicide in Taiwan*. http://www.nhu.edu.tw/~society/nsc/review/review.files/suicide.ppt. Accessed September 15, 2010.

Lester, D. (1994). The epidemiology of suicide in chinese population in six regions of the world [*sic.*]. *Chinese Mental Health Journal*, *7*, 25–36.

Li, W., et al. (2001a). Issues related to suicide. *Hebei Mental Health, 14*(4), 236.

Li, W., et al. (2001b). Issues related to suicide. *Hebei Mental Health, 14*(4), 237.

Liu, D. (2011). Attempt at self-immolation on international flight results in four years' jail. *Beijing Youth Daily*, January 6.

Liu, L., & Xiao, S. (2002). A follow-up study of individuals who have attempted suicide. *Chinese Mental Health Journal, 16*(4), 253.
Ouyang, Z. (2004). Bid to save lives by the Shanghai Metro. *Prosecutorial View, 9,* 58.
Philip, M., Liu, H., & Zhang, Y. (1999). The state of suicide in China and the relationship between suicide and society. In L. Xie (Ed.), *Report on suicides among rural women in China* (pp. 211–212). Guiyang: Guizhou People's Press.
Ratnayake, R., Links, P. S., & Eynan, R. (2007). Suicidal behaviour on subway systems: A review of the epidemiology. *Journal of Urban Health, 84*(6), 766–781.
Song, J. (2008). Free health check for 36 earthquake heroes, 75% feel anxious. *Tianfu Morning News*, November 18.
Stengel, E. (1952). Attempted suicide. *British Medical Journal, 1952*(1), 1130.
Su, X., et al. (1993). A study and analysis of the suicide case involving eight studies at Fujian Normal University. *Chinese Journal of School Health, 14*(6), 345.
Suen, K. J. (1996). *Statistics for suicide in Hong Kong*. Retrieved from: http://www.sbhk.org.hk/statistic/suicide1996.htm.
Tan, Y. (2002). 1.9% of students have attempted suicide. *Southern Metropolis Daily*, November 29.
Tao, C., & Gong, Z. (2008). Expert analysis: How to prevent a rash of suicides three months after a disaster. *The Beijing News,* June 11.
Wang, Y. (2002). Why secondary students in Hong Kong commit suicide. *Global Times*, April 11.
Wang, Y. (2007). 2000 lives lost to the river; has the Changjiang Bridge in Nanjing become a suicide "mecca"? *Jiangnan Times*, January 21.
WHO. (1989). *World health statistics annual* (pp. 364–375).
WHO. (1990a). *World health statistics annual* (pp. 364–369).
WHO. (1990b). *World health statistics annual* (p. 117).
WHO. (1990c). *World health statistics annual* (pp. 346–369).
WHO. (1995). *World health statistics annual* (pp. 709–713).
Xiao, B., et al. (2008, December). Mini peak in suicide rate half a year after Wenchuan quake. *Shanghai Evening News.*
Xiao, F., & Wang, S. (1997). An analysis of 30 cases of railway suicides. *Chinese Journal of Forensic Medicine, 12*(1), 39.
Xie, L. (Ed.). (1999). *Report on suicides among rural women in China* (p. 8). Guiyang: Guizhou People's Press.
Xu, Z. (1995). Suicide among Hong Kong youth, and prevention. *Journal of Clinical Neurology, 5*(2), 76.
Xu, Y., & Gao, H. (1999). A study of youth suicide and home environment factors. *Chinese Journal of Public Health, 15*(12), 111.
Xu, C., et al. (1993). The relationship between suicide by poisoning and the seasons. *Journal of Binzhou Medical University, 16*(3), 47–48.
Yang, F. (2006). Efforts on land and in air to save China Southern passenger committing suicide. *China Business News,* April 20.
Yang, C.-f., & Yang, C. (2007). *Preliminary analysis of regional differences for suicide rates in Taiwan.* http://faculty.nccu.edu.tw/pop/0428/2-2-1.pdf. Accessed July 16, 2012.
Yang, G., Huang, Z., & Chen, A. (1997). Levels of accidental harm among Chinese populations, and trends. *Chinese Journal of Epidemiology, 18*(3), 142–145.
Yang, G., Zhou, L., Huang, Z., & Chen, A. (2004). Trends and geographical distribution of suicide in the Chinese population. *Chinese Journal of Epidemiology, 25*(4), 282.
Yin, D. (2002). United, with a practical mind, we promote mental health on all fronts in the new century: Report of the 3rd National Conference on Mental Health Work. *Chinese Mental Health Journal, 16*(1), 6.
Yu, M., et al. (2002). A study of 360 cases of suicide in Guiyang City. *Journal of Clinical Psychological Medicine, 12*(2), 105.
Zhai, S. (1997). Bridge suicides. *Journal of Clinical Psychological Medicine, 7*(2), 100.
Zhang, X. (2005). Treasure life! *Reportage, 11.*

Zhang, Y. (2012). *Amplitude of decline in China's suicide rate rare in world.* http://news.xinhuanet.com/society/2011-05/14/c_121416339.htm. Accessed April 10, 2012.

Zhang, H., Zeng, G., et al. (1999). A study on suicide in youth and the influencing factors. *Chinese Journal of Public Health, 15*(3), 247–248.

Zhang, H., et al. (2018). Epidemiological investigation on attempted suicide among the 18 and over age group in Tianjin City. *32*(11), 889–894.

Zhao, M., & Ji, J. (2000). The current state of domestic and overseas research on suicide. *Shanghai Archives of Psychiatry, 12*(4), 225.

Zhong, J. (2000a). *Unveiling the mystery behind suicidal behavior* (p. 130). Beijing: China Procuratorial Press.

Zhong, J. (2000b). *Unveiling the mystery behind suicidal behavior* (p. 118). Beijing: China Procuratorial Press.

# Chapter 2
# Suicide Among Chinese Women

Chinese Academy of Social Sciences released the *Report on Women Development in China* in 2006.[1] In the chapter titled "Women and Health," it is revealed that China is currently the only country in the world where the suicide rate among women is much higher than that among men and that nearly 160,000 Chinese rural women commit suicide each year, half of all suicides by women in the world.

In recent years, the suicide rate in China has generally declined, which is mainly because of the declining suicide rate in rural areas of China during the past 20 years, especially the continuously declining suicide rate of women in rural areas.[2]

Among countries that provide relevant data to the WHO, China is the only country where the suicide rate is higher among women than among men. In the Chinese mainland, the suicide rate of women in the 15–24 age group is almost twice that of men in the same age group. This phenomenon is unique to China. According to the WHO, between 1987 and 1989, in China, the ratio of suicide by men and women in the 15–24 age group was 52.9:100 and the ratio for the 25–34 age group was 75.6:100.[3] In comparison, in 1988 in the USA, the male-to-female ratio of suicide in the 15–24 age group was 291.9:100 and that in the 25–43 age group was 438:100, roughly four to one.[4]

The number of suicides among urban girls aged 15–24 accounts for 12% of all deaths and 39.1% of accidental deaths. In rural areas, suicides of girls in the same age group account for 28.3% of all deaths and 63.4% of total accidental deaths.[5] Suicide is a grave issue among Chinese women and this is especially true in rural areas.

According to Dr. Bertolotti, a WHO expert of brain disorders and psychiatric diseases, suicide has become the leading cause of death among Chinese women aged 20–

---

[1]Wang (2006).
[2]Jing et al. (2010).
[3]WHO (1989, 1990a, pp. 346–369).
[4]WHO (1990b, p. 117).
[5]Liu (1995).



J. Li, *A Study on Suicide*,
https://doi.org/10.1007/978-981-13-9499-7_2

34, and that this can be attributed to two factors: First, many Asian women often have suicidal thoughts because of temporary emotional impulses. These suicides are impulse suicides. On the contrary, Western women are more likely to commit suicide because of chronic depression and alcohol dependence. Second, Chinese women in rural areas have easy access to highly toxic pesticides such as DDVP when suicidal thoughts occur to them. In addition, the lack of healthcare transport services in rural areas also contributes to the high mortality rate of suicide by poisoning. This is why the suicide rate among young Chinese women has risen sharply.[6]

Currently, suicide among Chinese women is both a major public health issue and a significant social problem.

# 1 Suicides Among Women: A Significant Social Issue

There are two distinct characteristics in the distribution of suicide rates in China: that among women is higher than that among men, and the rural rate is higher than the rural rate. The relatively high suicide rate and highest-in-the-world absolute number of suicidal deaths in China are, to a large extent, due to the high suicide rate and the large absolute number of suicidal deaths in rural areas. According to a 2004 study, the rural suicide rate was three times the urban rate and the suicide mortality rate among rural women was significantly higher than among urban women and urban men.[7] Therefore, in this section, we will focus on suicides among rural women in China.

## *1.1 Suicide Among Rural Women Is a Severe Problem*

The high suicide rate among rural women in China is mainly caused by the high suicide rate among younger women aged 15–34 in rural China. Michael R. Philips, Liu Huaqing, Zhang Yanping, et al. have made calculations based on population data provided by the 1990 population census (the Chinese mainland only), Chinese Academy of Preventive Medicine's disease surveillance statistics for the period 1990–1994, and a report by the World Bank and other international organizations on global burden of disease. As shown in Fig. 1, between 1990 and 1994, the average number of suicides each year in the Chinese mainland was 324,711, of which 21,664 (or 7%) occurred in urban areas and 303,047, in rural areas. Up to 173,230 (53%), suicidal deaths occurred to women and 129,817 (40%) to men. On average, 99,266 rural women aged 15–39 die from suicide in rural China, which is 30.57% of the total suicidal deaths in the country and 57.30% of the total suicidal deaths of rural women. The suicide mortality rate of rural women in this age group

[6]China Population Information Research Center (2002).

[7]Yang et al. (2004).

is 29.40 per 100,000 individuals. That is, in every 100,000 rural women, an average of 29.40 rural women aged 15–39 die from suicide each year. This rate is 4.7 times that of urban women of the same age group, 4.9 times that of urban men of the same age group, and nearly twice that of rural men in the same age group.[8]

An epidemiological study carried out by He Jingyi, Jiang Yonghua, Xia Bilei, et al. on suicide in some rural areas in Shandong in 1989 and 1999 shows that young people, women, and less-educated people were at a higher risk of suicide; that family disputes, conflicts with neighbors, economic difficulties, mental illnesses, and legal disputes were common causes of suicide; and that poisoning (with pesticides) was the primary means of suicide in rural areas.[9]

Zheng Rongchang, et al. studied 260 cases of suicidal deaths among rural women (in 1995–1996) and found that 238 (or 91.5% of the total) were aged between 15 and 34, and only six (2.3%) were aged above 60; 178 (68.5%) were married and "family" was, overwhelmingly, most commonly cited as their reason for suicide; 213 (81.9%) had committed suicide by poisoning.[10] Each year, 173,200 rural women die of suicide (1990–1994), and this is in itself a tremendous loss. Further, these suicides in turn also have an impact on some 510,000 surviving family members (assuming each rural woman who died of suicide leaves behind three family members).

As Lu Xun once noted: the dead are the misfortune of the living. Suicide among the marginalized in rural China can also be considered as the misfortune of those in the so-called "mainstream." If the number of rural women who die from suicide each year remains the same, then there will be 5.1 million left-behinds ten years later. The shock that suicide brings to families and society is a tremendous one, and the negative impact of suicidal deaths on surviving family members (especially children) can last a lifetime.

According to statistics from the report on the global burden of disease by the World Bank and other organizations, the number of suicidal deaths in China accounts for about 43.6% of the total suicidal deaths in the world and the number of suicidal deaths among Chinese women accounts for as much as 55% of the total suicidal deaths among females worldwide.[11]

There is no doubt that the high suicide rate of rural women in our country has serious consequences. Suicide is a denial of the meaning of life and so is a homicide. Both are disastrous for the parents, children, husbands, and lovers of the deceased and cause harm to society. Further, those who commit suicide are generally at child bearing age, and thus suicide also leads to the loss of rural labor and lower life expectancy of the general population.

Michael R. Philips, Liu Huaqing, et al. studied accidental deaths and suicidal deaths in China using two key concepts: period expected years of life lost (PEYLL) and working years of life lost (WYLL). PEYLL refers to the years of life lost to illness, accident, suicide, etc., when compared to the common life expectancy. For

[8]Xie (1999a, pp. 6–8).

[9]He et al. (2002).

[10]Zheng (1998).

[11]Kang (2002).

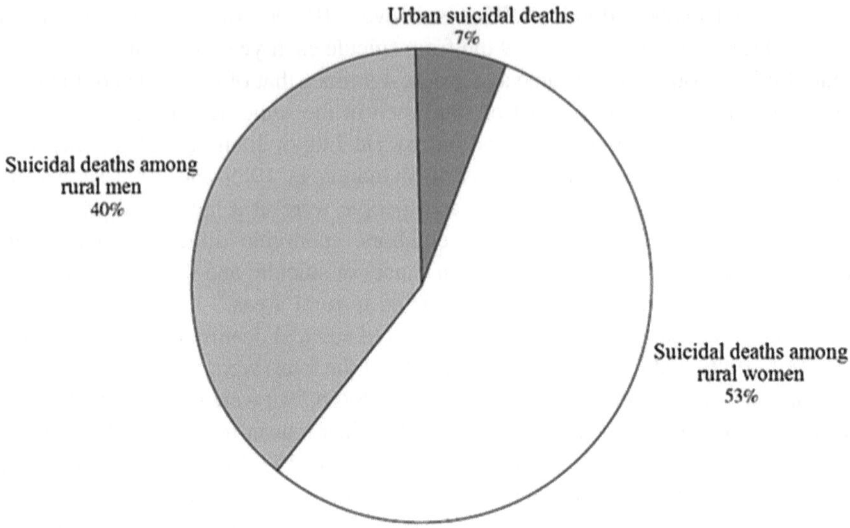


**Fig. 1** Annual suicidal deaths in China, 1990–1994

example, if a woman whose life expectancy is 75 years die at the age of 25, her PEYLL is 50. WYLL refers to the years of working life lost to illness, accident, suicide, etc., when compared to the years he/she is expected to work. For example, if a woman who can be expected to work between the ages of 16 and 55 dies at the age of 25, her WYLL is 30. Among all rural suicides by women, those by young wives or mothers are the most harmful to their families. Unfortunately, this group of women also comprises the majority of all rural women who commit suicide. With these women gone, their families usually suffer huge economic loss.

Society is made up of individuals and families. The destruction of these "cells of society" naturally endangers the entire social organization in rural China. The suicide of a relative is an important psychosocial factor that in turn causes suicide among youth. It is difficult to imagine how more than five hundred thousand people in rural areas in China are physically and mentally hurt because of the suicides of their mothers, wives, daughters, or sisters, and how rural residents living in the shadow of such loss face life. A considerable number of these individuals become new candidates for suicide. According to a study conducted by the Beijing Suicide Research and Prevention Center and Chinese Center for Disease Control and Prevention, 55% of those who committed suicide in China are related to at least one person (by blood or friendship) who had attempted/committed suicide before.[12] In China's villages, many families have become impoverished or fallen back below the poverty line because of the suicide of a family member.

[12]The Secret behind Suicides of the Chinese. *Lifeweek*, 2002(50).

The urban–rural difference in suicide mortality rate also shows the differences in social roles, economic status, and educational attainment among urban and rural women in China. The differences in a social environment, education, working conditions, living standards, nutritional status, and medical and health conditions between urban and rural areas are obvious. An important reason for the high mortality rate of rural suicides (apart from the accessibility of pesticides) is the lack of adequate healthcare services in rural areas.

## *1.2 "Impulse Suicides": A Hallmark of Suicides Among Rural Women*

A prominent feature of suicide among rural women in China is that there are more impulse suicides. In a study by the Beijing Suicide Research and Prevention Center titled "Suicide attempts: a study containing detailed psychiatric evaluations," it is shown that among those who have attempted suicide (and "failed"), 37% had thought about the act for five minutes or less, 46% had pondered for up to ten minutes, and 60% had thought about it for up to two hours. In other words, the time it took for one to make a grave decision like suicide is not as long as we might imagine. More than half of those surveyed had made their decisions quickly and had chosen to give up their lives without hesitation.

Another study on suicide among rural women over the age of 15 shows that the vast majority of rural women did not think about it carefully before committing suicide. Specifically, 58.8% of those surveyed had thought about it for no more than two hours before the act, 40%, less than ten minutes, and 11%, no more than one minute. Most suicide attempts had occurred with the consumption of pesticides (or rat poison) stored in victims' homes. Most of those surveyed had experienced serious negative life events one month before the suicide attempt (especially two days before suicide). Quarrels between husband and wife were especially common. Thus, we see that the proportion of impulse suicides in China's rural areas is very high, and that suicides often occur after severe family strife; the presence of poisons such as pesticides stored in the home makes suicide easy to attempt.[13]

Zheng Rongchang, et al. studied 260 rural women who died of suicide and found that 133 suicides (or 51.15% of the total) were committed during peaks of emotion; 66 (25.38%) were committed by clear-minded victims; and the emotional state of the victims in 61 cases (23.46%) was unknown (see Fig. 2).[14]

[13]Li et al. (2002).

[14]Xie (1999b, p. 5).

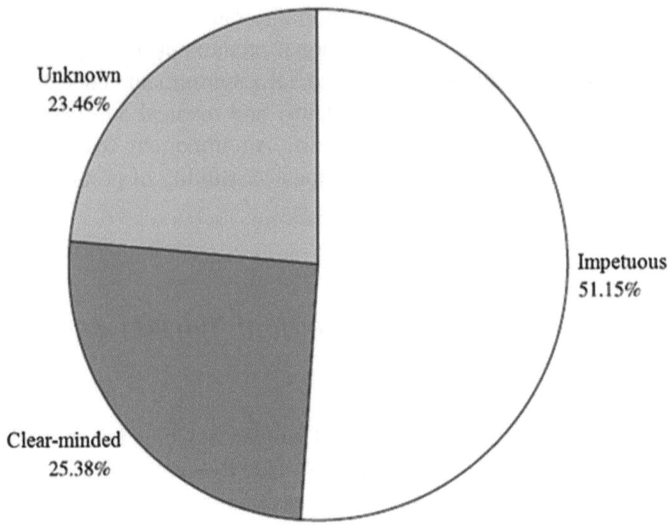


**Fig. 2** Emotional status of rural women when committing suicide

In China, rural women have basically adopted non-violent means of suicide, such as poisoning, hanging, hunger strike, and the refusal of medical treatment. They do so only for the purpose of threatening, self-liberation, or defense against slander.[15]

In rural China, both strong-willed women and women with mild temperaments often commit suicide in the heat of the moment or when they feel helpless. Some have even done so out of "spite" or as a "threat." "Cry, make a fuss, head for the rope" is a traditional "trump card" that rural women often use. However, this frequently comes at the price of the protagonist's life.

In rural China, pesticides are commonplace in the home. When a family strife arises, people take pesticide bottles in hand and the poison is drunk in the heat of the moment. Pesticides currently used in China are generally highly lethal. This, together with the fact that there are serious flaws in the rural public health system, means that suicide mortality rates are high. "Cry, make a fuss, take pesticides" has become the new "three-step program" for rural women seeking to resolve family strife. Comparatively speaking, "taking pesticides" is even more lethal than "heading for the rope."

Thus, we must work to effectively strengthen the management of pesticides, and put rules in place to promote the use of less toxic pesticides. These are important ways of reducing the suicide mortality rate in rural areas.

It is generally accepted that the slower pace of life and the closeness to nature in rural areas can effectively improve people's mental state. However, the high suicide

[15]Yan (2008).

rate in rural China reveals a grave reality. We can say that everyone who has lived in the countryside can recount suicides in their village. Sadly, a rural woman drinking pesticide is perhaps no longer anything surprising. It is also not uncommon for rural youth to commit suicide out of despair about the fact that there is a little hope for them to change their destiny they are born to have. Poverty, loneliness, and the boredom of life may also loom large and drive young people toward suicide.

It should be noted that poverty is not the top reason for the high suicide rate among rural women in China. The rural suicide rate kept rising from the 1980s to the 1990s: going up from the 15.40 per 100,000 individuals of 1980 to the 29.10 per 100,000 individuals of 1991. During this period, although not as much as in urban areas, the overall living standard in rural China still saw improvement that was widely acknowledged. Therefore, poverty cannot be considered as the main cause of the high suicide rate among rural women. In a study of rural Quanzhou County, Guilin, Guangxi, He Zhaoxiong found that most of the 194 women who had committed suicide in 1981 came not from poor families.[16]

Thus, heightened attention should be paid to the non-economic motivations of suicide.

## 2 "Contagiousness" of Suicide and Collective Suicides

### 2.1 *"Contagiousness" of Suicide, and the Werther Effect*

Whether "copycat" suicides contributed greatly to the suicide rate is a disputed subject but it is widely accepted that imitation does cause suicidal behavior and that suicidal behavior can be contagious. Adolescence is the period of life when people are most willing to imitate the behavior of others. Studies of numerous suicide cases revealed that the tendency to imitate clearly has a share in the ideation and the selection of method adolescent suicides. Many young people who committed suicides did because of the similar behavior of their relatives or classmates around them. Those who have not heard of such examples have often read about suicidal cases in books or magazines and tend to imagine doing the same.[17]

In Durkheim's opinion, suicide can be induced by a role model. Phillips D. P. calls this the "Werther effect"[18] after the protagonist of the Johann Wolfgang von Goethe novel *The Sorrows of Young Werther* who shoots himself after falling out of love. (This was a book that had triggered a chain of suicides among German youths after its publication.) Japanese sociologists call this the "Okada Yukiko syndrome."[19]

---

[16]He (1996).

[17]Liu and Li (1990).

[18]Fuse (1990).

[19]*Liberation Daily,* December 23, 1986, 3.

On April 9, 1986, 18-year-old Japanese singer Okada Yukiko committed suicide by jumping off a building. This triggered a wave of suicides among Japanese youths, pushing up the number of young women who committed suicide by jumping by more than threefold. On April 1, 2003, Hong Kong singer and movie star Leslie Cheung committed suicide by jumping off a building and six fans of his did the same in a time span of just nine hours. After the American singer Michael Jackson died on June 25, 2009, 12 of his fans followed him within three days.

In China, reports of copycat suicides are not rare either. For example, an eight-year-old girl in Tianjin loved fantasy dramas such as *White Snake Legend*, and in particular, the storyline of a character coming back to life after hanging. On June 12, 1995, this first-grade student and the only child suddenly asked her grandmother to leave her alone to play and her body was later found, slumped, hanging from an apron fixed upon a cupboard handle.[20]

## 2.2 The Serious Problem of Collective Suicides

Collective or mass suicides are generally premeditated acts of a simultaneous or continuous planned by someone and followed by others. The means used for collective suicides are generally violent and fatal. Such events have serious consequences and a profound impact on society. The contagiousness of suicidal behavior is a major cause of collective suicides.

Particularly noteworthy in the Chinese context is that in some youth gangs, suicide may be driven by beliefs in "brotherhood" and "loyalty." Once a member of the gang develops suicidal ideation, other members can be easily persuaded to do the same especially one it is the "boss" who suggests the ideation.

Collective suicides among females have also occasionally occurred in China. During the Ching Ming Festival of 1983, in a remote mountain village of only eleven households, eight girls led by one named Zhou Chaxiang tied themselves together and drowned themselves in a lake. The reason given for suicide is that "they do not want to go into the mountains to chop firewood every day." Four girls from Yuekou Town, Nancheng County, Jiangxi, drowned themselves on their way from chopping firewood.[21] Between 1983 and 1987, in Fuzhou of Jiangxi Province, there were ten cases of collective suicide of young women, causing 35 deaths. The oldest of the victims was 22 years old and the youngest, 13. All of these women had killed themselves as they no longer wanted to live in poverty and wanted to "reincarnate" into better lives.[22] In 1989, four young women under the age of 20 in Majia Village, Shenzhen Town, Yong'an, Fujian Province, collectively drowned themselves in a lake due to despair about marriage and the future. In 1992, again in

[20]Wen (1998).

[21]*China Women's News*, November 13, 1989.

[22]He (1997a, p. 460).

Yong'an, six girls jumped together into a river and killed themselves. The sextet had watched the movie *The Cowherd and The Girl Weaver*, thought about the many sufferings and their own misfortunes in the world, and decided to kill themselves thinking they might be able to enter heaven as fairies in this way.[23]

In recent years, online collective suicides have spread all over the world and drawn great attention.

In November 2009, an invitation to commit a collective suicide was suddenly extended in an online community in Hong Kong. Someone created a group called "I want to practice committing suicide" and only young people were invited to join it. More than 180 people were found to have joined the group and agreed to attempt suicide together in December before Christmas. One member, a high school girl, even proceeded ahead of schedule and attempted jumping off a school building in early December. The group was deleted by community administrators and the case was investigated.[24] In November 2010, in order to save a Hubei girl who had joined a suicide group on the instant messenger application QQ, a reporter joined the group in disguise. The group description read: "Living in this world only brings forth pain, and so it is better to leave early. The group only accepts members who wish to die … The group master has bought a map, please enter your address into the group 'business card folder' so that the group master can select a place for our collective suicide … Thank you for your cooperation!" Even more shockingly, the group master even swore in the group: "If I don't die, my entire family will!" 81 group members from all over the country were actively discussing when and where to commit their collective suicide.[25]

## 2.3 *Family Suicides Led by Adult Women*

It is common for multiple family members to commit suicide together in China after family strife because the Chinese ethics put more emphasis on family ties. This is particularly true for women, and the majority of such suicides are caused by conflicts between mother-in-law and daughter-in-law, between mother and daughter, between mother and son, and between sisters.

Suicidal behaviors are often closely related to one's family or more specifically, one's family history or family relations. In the social aspect of suicide, there are murder-suicide (suicide after killing family members) and joint suicide (completing the killing at the same time). In the psychological aspect, a suicide may be a copycat suicide or a forced choice. Familial transmission of suicidal behavior means people commit suicide by mimicking a family member or do so because of family strife. Suicide committed after killing other family members is often the result of

[23]Xie (1999c, p. 18).

[24]Wang (2009).

[25]Niu (2010).

intensified family strife, mental illness, poverty, despair, or sense of "pity." Joint suicide is mostly seen in the case of parent and child or husband and wife purposefully ending their lives at the same time (e.g., by drowning, with gas, by self-poisoning, self-immolation) or ending one's life after killing the other.[26]

In China, a common cause for joint suicide, murder-suicide, parent–child suicide, or extended suicide is family strife that occurs between husband and wife, mother-in-law and daughter-in-law, or sisters-in-law.

In most cases of parent–child suicide, the mother forces her children to commit suicide or kills her children (perhaps with poison) before committing suicide. These are in fact murder-cum-suicides by the mother. Such cruel cases do occur sometimes.

At about 6 pm on August 26th, 2016, Yang Gailan, a 28-year-old woman from the Agushan Village of Jinggu Town, Kangle County, Gansu Province, used an axe to slay her four children (including one 6 years old, two twins 5, and the youngest 3) on a winding narrow path behind her house. When finding her children still alive, she forced them to drink pesticides and then she herself committed suicide. On September 4th, 2016, Yang's husband also committed suicide by taking poison. A family of four generations with eight members has six of them gone forever.

According to a study by Liu Jicheng and Li Yuanzhi, family strife is a major cause of suicide in China. The types of family strife cited as causes of suicides are conflicts between mother-in-law and daughter-in-law (40.7%); between husband and wife (22.5%); between parents and children (12.1%); between the daughter and daughter-in-law (8.8%); between siblings (7.1%); between daughters-in-law (5.0%); between father-in-law and daughter-in-law; and "others (3.3%)."[27]

These numbers show that conflicts between mother-in-law and daughter-in-law is the top cause of suicidal deaths (mainly in rural areas). There is always strife between mother-in-law and daughter-in-law in traditional Chinese families. In a 1980s survey of 50 households in Shanghai, 18% of the respondents reported good relationships between mother-in-law and daughter-in-law, 52% reported tensions, and 30% reported severe tensions. Gao Zhixu, et al. surveyed 108 elderly women from six neighborhoods in Shanghai and found that 18% of these women suffered tension in their relationships with their daughters-in-law, 28% enjoyed good relationships, and 54% described their relationships with their daughters-in-law as "so-so."[28] With dramatic changes going on in Chinese society, we are in a time of fierce clashes between the old and the new, but the typical causes of strife between mother-in-law and daughter-in-law have not dissipated.

The most common causes of strife between mother-in-law and daughter-in-law are as follows: (1) Differences in habits and lifestyle. Coming from different families, mother-in-law and daughter-in-law may not be able to coordinate. For the mother-in-law, the daughter-in-law is not her daughter after all, so she has to be careful with any attempts to "discipline" the daughter-in-law. In the eyes of the

---

[26]He (1997b, p. 494).

[27]Liu and Li (1992a, p. 86).

[28]Gao et al. (1987).

daughter-in-law, her mother-in-law is not her own mother and is, by default, biased. Thus, if the two are unable to understand each other, respect each other, and adapt to each other's personality traits and living habits, negative feelings can develop easily. (2) More than a hundred million young and middle-aged laborers (mainly males) from rural China are working in cities. Young and middle-aged women are left behind to bear the heavy burden of childbearing, child-raising, labor, and family support. When the husband is not at home, the possibility of strife between in-laws increases. (3) Emotional barrier and distance between mother-in-law and daughter-in-law. The mother-in-law typically enjoys a close relationship with her son prior to the latter's marriage. However, once the son is married, he may shift his focus to his wife. This is unacceptable to some narrow-minded mothers-in-law. This is particularly true in the countryside. Many mothers-in-law experience ambivalence from the day their sons get married: on the one hand, they are happy that their sons have established families of their own, but on the other, they feel that they have been "robbed" of their sons by the wives and that they themselves are replaced by their daughters-in-law at the master of the family. Some mothers-in-law even become jealous of their daughters-in-law, making strife more likely. (4) The influence of traditional and feudal attitudes about the family. Mothers-in-law and daughters-in-law are born and raised in different eras and environments. Some mothers-in-law (especially in rural areas) still hold feudal beliefs about how women should behave and expect their daughters-in-law to act accordingly. When the mother and son do not agree on the son's marriage, the mother-in-law will probably be more demanding on the daughter-in-law.

Today, the attitude toward women are more open, and the majority of daughters-in-law are reluctant to follow old traditions and moral code. In addition, younger women are mostly economically independent and no longer dependent on the husband (or his family). They have a greater sense of self-reliance. Such quiet transformation of the role of contemporary women in the family has increased the possibility of strife between mother-in-law and daughter-in-law, and often the problem is taken to the other extreme: mistreatment of parents-in-law by the daughters-in-law occurs from time to time and has become a major reason for suicides by elderlies. On April 8, 2007, an elderly couple over the age of 60 in Zhuyuan Village, Zhima Town, Zunyi County, Guizhou Province committed suicide by taking poison after suffering beating and other forms of mistreatment by their son and daughter-in-law. The unfilial son and daughter-in-law were kept in detention by the public security authorities for a criminal offense.[29]

Another important cause of suicide by women caught in family disputes is strife between husband and wife. According to Zheng Rongchang, et al., among 260 cases of suicidal deaths of women, 121, or 46.5% of the total, were caused by

[29]Luo (2007).

spousal conflict.[30] Marital relationship is one of the most intimate relationships a person can have. However, as society develops, the family, which is the most basic unit of society, has become increasingly unstable and more prone to disintegration. It is an indisputable fact that marital tension is becoming more and more common and divorce rates have continued to claim in China. There are many reasons for this and one of them, domestic violence, is worth special attention because of its close link to elevated suicide risk for married women. That is A survey shows that 50% of spousal conflict-induced suicides by married women occur soon after violent behavior by the husband toward his wife.[31]

## 3 Suicides for Love

Dying for love is something people have been doing since the ancient times. In traditional China culture, martyrdom on account of love, lofty pursuits and chastity has been considered highly praiseworthy.

Since the early modern times, suicide for love among young Naxi boys and girls in Yunnan Province has shocked the world.

In China today, dying for love still accounts for a fair proportion of suicides committed especially among young people.

### *3.1 Suicide Triggered by Breakups of Romantic Relationships*

The breakup of a romantic relationship is a primary cause of suicides among youths. A survey by Hu Qingyun, et al. found that of the 78 young women who committed suicide between January and November 1986, 63 or 81% did so due to such breakups.[32]

There are many reasons why breakups of romantic relationships might lead to suicides. Acute agony is a big one. Also, some resort to suicide out of spite, in order to make the other one feel guilty for the rest of his/her life. A typical case is a female victim who poisoned herself to death on flight MU5368 from Shenzhen to Shanghai on July 20, 2000.

Suicide for lost love accounts for a significant proportion of suicides among college students. A study shows that 20% of college students who commit suicide do so after a breakup, and 73.3% of them are female.[33]

[30]Xie (1999d, p. 34).

[31]Zhang (1988).

[32]Liu and Li (1992b, p. 90).

[33]Jiang et al. (2002).

Another type of suicide for lost love occurs to girls who are jilted after having sexual intercourse. The victim, influenced by traditional ideas on chastity, commits suicide as she believes herself to have lost everything with the loss of her "chastity." A suicide would, in her opinion, restore her honor and make a statement. The victim is unable to face the world with the knowledge that she has given both her heart and body to the man who had jilted her. There are many reasons as to why a female would commit suicide after being jilted. Apart from sheer despair, committing suicide may also be a way to cry out the victims' spite, fight, and loyalty.

The broken-hearted can develop an extreme sense of despair, loneliness, and emptiness after having lost their loved ones with no one else to fill the gap. At this critical moment, the more extreme ones among the broken-hearted typically exhibit the following psychological and behavioral characteristics:

First, suicide. These individuals may experience a loss of self-esteem, or other negative feelings like pessimism, weariness with the world, emptiness, humiliation, remorse, etc., due to the loss of love and resort to suicide to relieve themselves of such mental burdens.

Second, revenge. This is a rather common way of venting. The desire for revenge can be triggered by the thwarting of an extreme sense of possession. Emotions such as the fear of punishment for one's mistake or crime, remorse, and pessimism after seeking revenge can lead to retaliation, self-blame, and then suicide. Such cases of suicide may take the form of murder-cum-suicide.

Third, depression. The major manifestations are anxiety, indifference, emotional pain, and a dispirited demeanor. In severe cases, the person can exhibit symptoms of schizophrenia. Depression is also a main mental factor behind suicide.

On May 15, 2011, we tried searching for "shilian zisha" (or suicides due to lost love) on Google and shockingly got a total of 2.19 million results, most of which were reports of such cases.

## 3.2 Suicide for Love

Suicides for love are, in some cases, the result of despair after failure to get the freedom of marriage or the despair caused by the death of the beloved. Very often, many men and women who commit suicide for this reason include in their suicide notes classic lines that celebrate eternal romance, with melancholic allusions.

Today, with the progress of the times and the liberation of people's minds, suicide for love by young people failing to obtain freedom to marry whoever they want is not as common as before, but such cases are still common enough, especially in remote rural areas economically underdeveloped and deeply mired in feudalistic thoughts. Such suicidal behavior is most commonly seen in scenarios where a young person seeks to fight against his/her parents' decisions for his/her marriage. Arranged marriages are still common in certain areas due to the prevalence of feudalistic attitudes. Some young people who do not want to accept such arrangements may have fierce confrontations with their parents and even the whole family on this issue. These young people would rather die as a form of resistance than to surrender to the arrangements. Another common scenario of suicides for love is when there is strong interference with one's freedom of love (or marriage) from, for instance, one's parents, relatives, friends, work superiors, or teachers, for various reasons. The individuals thwarted then commit suicide out of despair. Some couples commit suicide together, while some do it alone. In other cases, suicide occurs as the protagonist seeks to "follow" a lover or spouse who has already left this world for various reasons.

"Voluntary homicide" is common in cases of suicide for love where a couple seeks to die together. In such cases, the "victim" and the "perpetrator" are deeply in love with each other and seek to commit suicide together. However, one party (usually the female) dare not take her own life and instead turns to the other party for help. So, the "perpetrator" first kill his/her lover and then commits suicide. Alternatively, the two may kill each other at the same time (by pulling the gun trigger simultaneously). It is more common though for the male of the couple to kill the female before committing suicide (like in the aforementioned movie-theater suicide case). In cases of "voluntary homicide," suicide notes are generally left to prove the "voluntary" aspect of the crime.

As social transformation continues in China, young people are romancing at a younger age, and instances of adolescent suicide in the name of love occur occasionally. More attention should be paid to the dangerous period when children fall in love easily. Adults should give appropriate guidance on this subject. Inappropriate and reckless intervention is generally counterproductive and can add to the risk of suicide. Youngsters today are experiencing more frustrations in love at a younger age. It may be difficult for adults to understand or imagine what the younger generation has encountered. To a certain extent, this is related to the critical attitude toward adolescent romance on the part of parents and school authorities, and in society in general. When young men and women fall into fruitless love, they tend to lose their senses and act in unimaginable ways. For many parents, early age romance is naturally something they object to. However, it is necessary for parents to be careful with how they approach this issue so as to minimize the danger caused.

## *3.3 Suicides Caused by Broken Marriages and Extramarital Relationships*

A broken marriage is undoubtedly painful, especially for the "passive" party who has no choice but to acquiesce. The different roles of men and women in marriage determine that a divorce hurts the woman more than the man. Suicide caused by divorce occurs to both men and women, but it is more common among women, especially rural women. A sense of guilt toward one's children and parents often develops due to social and family prejudice against divorcees. Divorced women, in particular, feel more pressure economically and non-economically for supporting the elderly and raising the young. Some women are more likely to feel lost and unmoored after divorce and commit suicide in despair.

In the vast rural areas of China, social transformation has brought about changes in people's mindset and in family structures. A large number of young and middle-aged migrant workers have left home to work in the cities, and this has a significant impact on marital relationships, pushing up rural divorce rate. In rural areas (perhaps urban areas too), feudalistic ideas about how women should behave are still fairly influential, and many women regard faithfulness to one man as an important principle in life. Once their marriage breaks down, the combination of the resulted mental imbalance, discrimination from the outside world, and the pressures of life can make things hard to bear and the temptation to "self-liberate" by suicide becomes stronger. Some rural women have developed the mentality of serious overreliance. They believe that men's place in the world lies in toil, and women's, in childbearing. So, these women tend to take it for granted that they have the right to stay at home and enjoy the fruits of their husbands' labor. Once their marriage is over, they feel as if the sky has collapsed on them, and they are plunged into despair.

The survey by Zheng Rongchang et al. shows that 46.5% of suicidal deaths of rural women can be attributed to strife between husband and wife and 3.8% to broken marriage (abandonment or forced divorce).[34] Thus, we see that strife between husband and wife are a major cause of suicides by rural women.

Extramarital affairs, which generally refer to covert or overt sexual relationships where either or both persons involved are married to somebody else and which are either live-in relationships or relatively stable otherwise, are one of the main causes of family strife and a key trigger of marriage breakdowns. This kind of sexual relationship is contrary to China's traditional moral values and the morals of the day. Cohabitation is also not allowed under the current law of marriage. There are two types of suicides caused by such relationships. The first is where the relationship is uncovered, bringing tremendous pressure on the two people involved. The protagonists may then commit suicide either out of despair or for love. For instance, in August 1987, an unmarried live-in couple in Chongqing died from self-immolation after their romance was made public. On November 9, 2000, a married woman in Gengzhuang Town, Haicheng City in Liaoning and her 19-year-old unmarried lover committed suicide by drinking pesticide after their affair was brought to light.[35] The other type occurs due to the damage to family harmony brought about by the extramarital affair or extramarital sexual relationship. The spouse of the offending partner, hurt, resorts to suicide. In most of such cases, the partner committing suicide is the female one. These cases are quite common, so we shall not dwell on them here. "The other woman" has become

[34]Xie (1999e, pp. 34–38).

[35]Wang (2000).

common as Chinese society changes. We will not provide a moral-based critique here. The occurrence of extramarital relationships has its roots in a complex web of social, familial, and individual reasons. Currently in China, this is a one cause of suicide. Individuals who commit suicide in such scenarios are generally the spouse who has been cheated on. They choose to kill themselves as a form of protest, out of despair, shame, or resentment. "The other woman" (or man) is an individual who seeks his/her happiness while causing pain to his/her lover's spouse for reasons such as emotional needs, financial needs, social status, and revenge (of course, some extramarital affairs are born out of marriages that exist in name only, which make such affairs understandable, if not legal). In recent years, the phenomenon of keeping another women (or men) in extramarital relationships has been spreading among wealthy people. These relationships, not based entirely on affection, have a major impact on families and have drawn the attention of legislators. A significant number of spouses who have been cheated on emerge as "losers" in "struggles" against "the other woman/man." These spouses often commit suicide feeling wronged. In addition, "the other woman/man" may also commit suicide for being kicked out of the relationship or the inability to keep the relationship going, or guilt. "The other woman" runs the risk of reputational ruin. Once her lover changes his mind and goes back to his wife, or once she finds that she has been lied to and there is no hope of growing old with her lover, she is likely to commit suicide.[36] A survey by Zheng Rongchang et al. show that of the 260 rural women who had killed themselves three (or 1.15% of the total) did it because of extramarital relationships. All three had killed themselves after they were beaten up by their husbands when their affairs came to light.[37]

## 4 High Suicide Rate Among Women

It is generally believed that suicide is the result of multiple factors, including sociological, psychological, moral, biological, psychiatric, and genetic factors. Suicide is the product of the interactions between personal factors and stress against the backdrop of the relationship between personal factors and protective factors.

China was once the only country reporting a higher suicide rate among women than among men to the WHO. As mentioned earlier, there are many reasons for suicides. In studying the issue of suicide in China, we will have to consider historical and cultural factors as well as economic and psychiatric issues. These various factors may exist at the same time or interact and lead to suicidal behaviors. After examining suicide cases of various kinds, we can see that while in some cases social pressures are at play but not psychiatric issues, in some others only

[36]Liu and Li (1992c, p. 93).

[37]Xie (1999f, p. 46).

psychiatric issues were at play, not social pressures. In even more cases, both categories of factors were at play and eventually combine to lead to suicide.

Therefore, it is clearly not reasonable to attribute the high suicide rate among Chinese women today to social transformation. It will be more reasonable for us to conclude that suicide is caused by the interplay between psychological factors (endogenous factors) and social factors (exogenous factors). Mental illness among women (excluding hereditary mental illness) can be regarded as a kind of psychological state arising from social pressures (including those from social transformation). The growing prevalence of mental illness among women can also increase the social pressures experienced by other members of society (the media often adds to such pressures).

There have been many explanations for the high suicide rate among Chinese women but none seems to be sufficient and convincing enough.

Why has the suicide rate among rural Chinese women been high? We believe the following factors have contributed to it.

## 4.1 Double Roles and Double Discriminations

Over the years, China's rural women have found themselves in the midst of grave family strife and social crises. The dramatic changes of the Chinese society since early modern times have placed rural women in amid lasting tensions and intense conflicts. Of course, the emancipation of women is without doubt a major achievement of the democratic revolution against feudalism but emancipation without a sound ideological and economic foundation may exactly be the cause a split in the minds of rural women in China. Within mainstream Chinese politics, the idea that "women hold up half the sky" has been strongly advocated and as a result, Chinese women pursue independence with enthusiasm that is hardly seen elsewhere. However, traditional Chinese culture is a deep-rooted tree, lush and thriving as it has always been. The revolution was not able to uproot it though it overthrew both imperialism and feudalism. Therefore, in a sense, Chinese women still have to assume the role they have been playing in the past several thousand years.

Thus, an unexpected consequence of the emancipation of Chinese women may be that "a number of rural women find themselves in an 'in-between' zone that is neither 'male' nor 'female' in terms of their role in society. This way, women end up struggling between the 'modernity' of society and the 'feudal' aspects of the family, as well as between the 'modern' aspects of the family and the 'feudal' aspects of society. Disorder, arise therefrom and ends with suicide."[38] An adult woman bears the double burdens of being a housewife and an active member of society. Emancipation, quite unexpectedly, turns the personality of some women from "soft and tender" to "hard and rigid." Unfortunately, what is hard and rigid is

[38]Li and Zuo (2010).

often brittle, so these women are more likely to commit suicide in the case of some major negative events in life. They are no longer like the older generations of women who would probably endure and suffer in silence for the greater good.

Even more peculiar to the Chinese context is the fact that rural women are doubly discriminated against due to their dual roles as "rural residents" and "women." They may suffer gender discrimination as women and may also be discriminated against because of they are rural residents. These women are almost destined to be disadvantaged. If farmers and women are two topics that have long been drawing extensive attention, rural women are unfortunately caught in the dire situations that both groups find themselves in. For Chinese women, marriage, children, and family obligations make up an overwhelmingly large part of their lives, if not their entire lives. This is especially true for rural women.

The line "you will be extraordinarily unfortunate because you are a woman" seems to suit China's rural women the best. Their misfortune also lies in the fact they can neither escape nor change their circumstances. They usually have no access to good education, lack the means to support themselves, are accustomed to obeisance, and have not developed autonomy and independence. All these are insurmountable obstacles for rural women in China. To make things even worse, rural women in China usually live in shortage of both material and spiritual resources, and thus have hardly any chance to find and fight their way out of the mire.[39]

The de facto lack of and inequality in access to education for rural women in China has directly led to the general low educational attainment in this group and the lack of independence and clear values of their own. Statistics show that in 2000, there were a total of 61.81 million illiterate females in China, 70% of the total illiterate population in the country. Within the female population, 80% live in rural areas.[40] According to the second survey on the Social Status of Chinese Women conducted in 2000, 8.5% of rural women received senior high school or a higher level of education, which is 6.9% points lower than the share of men; 41.3% received junior high school or a higher level of education, which is 21.8% points lower than for their male counterparts; and 13.6% were illiterate, 9.6% points higher than that for men. In 2013, the female illiteracy rate fell to 10.43%.

A major material cause of the high suicide rate among China's rural women is the de facto lack of and inequality in property rights, primarily manifested by land contracts. If the de facto lack of and inequality in access to education make rural women mentally prone to committing suicide, the de facto lack of and inequality in property rights (primarily right to land contracts) lay the material foundation for the high suicide rate in this group.[41]

---

[39]Xu (1999).

[40]National Bureau of Statistics of the People's Republic of China. *The Development of the Education Sector*. http://www.stats.gov.cn/tjfx/ztfx/jwxlfxbg/t20020530_20836.htm. Accessed: 10 January 2012.

[41]Liu (2004).

Chinese women, whether they live in urban or rural areas, have to labor both inside and outside of the home. Thus, women experience more social tension relating to their career and labor than men. They take on more roles in society, and switching between these roles imposes greater pressure and makes women more vulnerable to mental imbalance than men. In addition, the low social status of women is another key cause of the high suicide rate. Although in recent years, the status of women in society and in homes has improved greatly, women are still in a position of passivity and subordination compared to men. This is also a reason for the higher suicide rate among women than among men.[42]

The high suicide rate among rural women in China is in a way a reflection of the differences between urban and rural women in China in terms of social roles, social organization, economic status, and educational attainment. The problems of agriculture, farmers, and rural areas have long existed in China, and the differences between urban and rural areas in terms of the social environment, education, working conditions, living standard, nutrition, healthcare, etc., are clear.

## 4.2 *Flaws in Traditional Attitudes*

An ideal person in traditional Chinese culture eschews individual expression, and an ideal Chinese woman is characterized by dependence and submission. This still has its influence today (especially on rural women) through the collective unconscious that has survived all the years. Traditional Chinese culture demands that women take on introverted personalities and undergo self-abnegation. As a result, women are more likely to turn their aggressivity toward themselves amid self-sacrifice and quiet suffering, and then react in the most extreme way, i.e., suicide.

In traditional Chinese culture, the "three obediences and four virtues" are the golden rule for women's behavior. The "three obediences" refer to obedience to one's father for an unmarried woman, to the husband for a married woman, and to the son for a widow. The "four virtues" are wifely virtue, wifely speech, wifely manner, and wifely work. Specifically, women are required to behave morally and be able to serve as moral examples; they must have a dignified and proper appearance and must not appear frivolous; they must be able to understand what their counterparts are saying in conversation and know what they can say and what they ought not say; they must be able to keep the home in good order, including by tending properly to her husband and children, caring for the elderly and young, and

[42]An and Jia (2007).

living frugally. It is also said that "the husband's words are the wife's law." This saying emphasizes the dominant position of the man *vis-à-vis* the woman.

In ancient times, the lives and deaths of most women, the sex of lower social status, were consigned to oblivion. Only a handful were the exception to the norm. "Female martyrs" (*lienü)* women who killed themselves in order to preserve their chastity have throughout history been regarded as paragons of virtue. According to historical records, there were no more than one hundred of those prior to the Song Dynasty, a few hundreds after that, and more than 10,000 in the Ming and Qing dynasties. In Shexian County, Anhui Province, there are more than 6000 halls dedicated to the commendation of chaste women and numerous more archways erected for the same purpose.[43]

Traditionally, Chinese women generally subscribed to beliefs about the duty of fidelity in marriage or other domestic relationships. The combination of such beliefs and inherent weaknesses of femininity left those women whose romantic pursuits were thwarted few choices besides suicide. Even today, this accounts for a significant proportion of female suicides in rural China. Growth in the number of women who are abandoned due to extramarital affairs and pregnancies out of wedlock has also contributed to higher numbers of female suicide. In the West, it is traditionally believed that pregnant women usually do not commit suicide, but in China, both attempted suicide and suicidal deaths are not uncommon among would-be mothers, especially those who are pregnant out of wedlock or who have married against their family's wishes.

Traditional Chinese women (especially rural women) are not only accustomed to being dependent on men but are even more accustomed to being dependent on their families and clans. As such, in families with complex and overly dense interpersonal relationships, the eruption of family strife and disputes are bound to become a possible cause of the high suicide rate among Chinese women.

Since early modern times, Chinese women have experienced dramatic social and cultural changes in terms of what personalities are valued as society shifted from feudalism to new democracy, planned economy competes with a market economy, and a mindset of the agricultural era co-exists with an industrial society. These together put Chinese women in multiple splits.

## 4.3 Proliferation of Agrochemicals and an Inadequate Public Health System

Following the implementation of the household contract responsibility system in rural areas, agrochemicals started to be distributed to households for use. For

[43]Ye (2006).

women living in China's rural areas, these highly lethal and quick-acting agrochemicals are available at their fingertips. This is an important reason why agrochemicals are a primary means of suicide for Chinese women in rural areas. At present, there are three broad types of poisons that pose a serious threat to the lives of rural residents in China: organophosphorus pesticides, carbamate pesticides, and barbiturates. It is necessary for the supervision of highly toxic pesticides to be strengthened in rural areas as well as for the development and promotion of low-toxic pesticides as soon as possible. Good news is in 2003 the Chinese government banned the production and sales of certain highly toxic rat poisons and put in place criminal liabilities for those caught in the production and sales of such poisons.

One reason for the high mortality rate of rural suicides is the inadequacy and backwardness of rural medical care. These conditions have led to deaths in cases where emergency medical care could otherwise have saved lives.

The majority of the existing rural cooperative medical organizations in China are rural clinics that were established prior to the implementation of the household contract responsibility system in rural areas. These clinics played an irreplaceable role in the time of people's communes. In 1965, Mao Zedong called for shifting the focus of medical and health work to the countryside, and as a result, a large number of rural health workers ("barefoot doctors") were trained within a short period of time. They do both agricultural work and medical work. These "barefoot doctors" played a key role in primary health care in rural areas at the time. Meanwhile, there was also significant development with medical cooperatives. Health stations, "barefoot doctors" and cooperative medical care became the "three magic weapons" of rural health work at that time. Although the skills of these "barefoot doctors" was once widely questioned, they are indeed more helpful than none. Currently, we are seeing the disappearance of large numbers of rural medical cooperatives.

The average amount of health resources available to the rural population in China is much lower than the national average: the rural population, which accounts for 80% of the total, had accessed to only 20% of all medical resources and facilities. Many of the medical facilities and personnel lay idle or are underused in cities while rural clinics have poor basic medical facilities and lack high-caliber medical personnel, and thus failing to meet the healthcare needs of the vast rural population. This results in an imbalance in the allocation of health resources between urban and rural areas.

On January 10, 2005, at the National Health Work Conference, Gao Qiang, then vice minister of health, noted that while China is home to 22% of the world population, it had only 2% of the world's medical and health resources, which are unevenly distributed throughout the country, with 80% in urban areas and 20% in rural areas, and 44.8% of China's urban population and 79.1% of its rural population did not have any medical insurance coverage.[44] Further, according to statistics, the per capita health expenditure is RMB38.3 in urban areas and only

[44]Gao (2005).

RMB9.9 in rural areas. Investment in rural healthcare only accounts for 16% of total healthcare investment. In June 2000, the WHO ranked China 188th among 191 member states in terms of the equity of its health funding. Lacking good governance, the healthcare industry is plagued by widespread corruption. Complaints of poor accessibility to, and the high costs of, healthcare, became rife. Nearly 40% of patients have reported choosing not to seek medical attention due to the high cost of medical care and financial difficulties. More than half of rural residents cannot afford to seek medical care.

With the weakening of the rural collective economy, the cooperative healthcare system based on collective public welfare funds is severely undermined and the rural healthcare systems have essentially been paralyzed or even collapsed. According to the third National Health Services Survey, in 2003, 79% of rural residents did not have any medical insurance, 38.6% did not see a doctor when sick because of financial difficulties, and 75.4% ought to have been hospitalized but were not.[45] Healthcare cost grows faster than farmers' income, and farmers lack the minimum insurance coverage for healthcare. Many rural residents dare not seek any medical service due to the dramatic increases in medical cost and the high prices of drugs. Many rural clinics support themselves with the earnings from drug sales, and it is not uncommon for rural residents to fall or lapse back below the poverty line due to illness.

It is gratifying that through Chinese government's unremitting efforts, the public health and medical care systems in rural China have been improved significantly in recent ten years. "Healthy China" has become a national strategy.

## *4.4 Family and Marital Problems: The Top Cause*

The top cause of female suicide in rural China is family strife, and the majority of cases involve strife between husband and wife. The friction between mother-in-law and daughter-in-law which is to China, especially the Chinese countryside, is another important cause. A major reason for the high suicide rate among rural women in the 15–39 age group in China is that women in this age group have to surmount five major hurdles in life.[46] The first is choosing a spouse. Matchmaking is still a major means to marriage for the majority of rural women. In addition, despite being banned, child brides, "marriage exchanges" (marriage arrangements where the daughter of one family marries the son of another family in exchange for the daughter of this other family who shall marry the son of the first family), wife-buying, and the kidnaping of women for marriage remain common. We can imagine the life of women forced into these sorts of marriages. As Karl Marx once said, "a marriage that is not built upon the foundation of love is an immoral one."

[45]Zhang (2004).

[46]Da (2001).

Many women who could not endure these arrangements have taken to suicide in desperation. The second "hurdle" is dowry. Dowry is an important signifier of a rural woman's status. At the same time, it can be a source of tension between mother-in-law and daughter-in-law. Women who marry into a family with little dowry can expect to be treated less well in the future. Suicides due to disagreements over dowry are not uncommon. The third "hurdle" is the relationship between the mother-in-law and the daughter-in-law. Traditionally in China, this has always been a relationship full of tension. This is a social problem that is known around the world. An old saying among Chinese women goes: "30 years of being a daughter-in-law, then 30 years of being a mother-in-law." In the position of a mother-in-law, it is the turn of a woman to impose high standards for her daughter-in-law, perhaps even more stringent than what she herself experienced when she was young. Such a vicious cycle has oddly become a part of the interpersonal relations within traditional Chinese families. For many young rural women, interactions with their in-laws can be a major headache. The fourth "hurdle" is reproduction. Rural women are unable to fully enjoy the rights of free matrimony as provided under the law. While this may not be a serious problem, the issue of fertility can be a clearer reflection of the hardships rural women in China face. That one should give birth to boys rather than girls is an expectation that comes not just from the husband's family but also society in general. Depression is more common among childless women, who also have high rates of suicide ideation.[47] Those unfortunate enough to be infertile are likely to take the tragic route of suicide. In addition, regardless of whether one gives birth to a boy or a girl, the basic national policy of family planning is the first consideration. Rural women must thus bear two kinds of conflicting social responsibilities and the psychological and physiological pressures of not fulfilling their responsibilities. The fifth "hurdle" is family burdens. Young and middle-aged women who support their families in rural areas bear the heavy responsibilities of childbearing, child-raising, production, and caring for the elderly. It is very likely that they suffer setbacks in these various areas.

At the same time, domestic violence is also a widespread problem that cannot be ignored. In modern families, family members demand equality. There should be equality between men and women. Husband and wife must respect each other and this respect should be won through actions. Husband and wife should be able to enjoy the rights that they are entitled to and at the same time, fulfill their family obligations as much as possible. Only with mutual care, understanding, help, respect, and love can a husband and wife build close and harmonious family relationships. Today, around the world, social issues caused by family crises are becoming increasingly severe. Family crises intensify and the problem of domestic violence is serious. Domestic violence has also been growing in China. A survey by relevant authorities shows that domestic violence in China increased by 25.4% in the 1990s over the 1980s. In 1995, the All-China Women's Federation's (ACWF's)

---

[47]Song (1998).

Letters and Calls Office received a total of 128,900 letters requesting the protection of women's rights and interests, as well as 1600 visits for the same purpose. Among these, 30% were related to domestic violence, a figure that is 30 times higher than that of 1994. In addition, the ACWF also found that 50% of the letters and visits it received in 2000 were related to marriage and family issues. In particular, 15.5% were related to domestic violence.[48]

These are the characteristics of domestic violence in China at present: First, the regional division in the prevalence of domestic violence is disappearing. Domestic violence was previously seen mainly in rural areas, but it is now growing in frequency in urban areas. Second, the distribution of domestic violence across population groups with different educational attainments has changed. A survey shows that domestic violence is becoming increasingly common among individuals with higher educational attainments. Third, domestic violence has taken on more diverse forms. In modern society, women often encounter mental abuse, sexual abuse, and financial abuse on top of physical abuse, and these new forms of violence can be even more harmful. Fourth, domestic violence has caused extreme reactions among women as retaliation, including suicide. On August 19, 2009, a 28-year-old woman in Qingdao who had been married for only a year killed herself because of abuse from her husband. She was four-months pregnant then.[49]

Fundamentally, domestic violence in China is directly related to traditional Chinese culture (especially in rural areas). In ancient China, the rights of the male were absolute, alongside the patriarch's rights and the rights of the husband. Domestic violence was legitimized by the morals of the times. In modern society, marital violence[50] is a natural extension of this historical legacy. The strict hierarchy and gender discrimination in traditional culture, pillared by the concepts of the rights of the patriarch and of the husband, are the ideological fount that continues to nourish marital violence in modern times.

---

[48]Wang (2004).

[49]28-year-old Pregnant Woman Dies after Beaten by Husband. *Sina.com*. August 28, 2009.

[50]In the academic world, there is no universally accepted definition of "marital violence". The term generally refers to one party in a marriage being harmed by his or her spouse through verbal, physical and sexual violence. It is also known as "spousal violence". "Violence" refers to behaviors that cause fear, the sense of being unsafe, or conflicts, etc. Cases of marital violence can be classified into three categories. (1): Physical violence: includes all attacks on the body of the target, such as beatings, shoving, slaps on the face, kicking, and the use of tools for attacks. (2) Mental violence: the harming of another person's psychology and emotions through inhumane and inappropriate ways, by means of threats, malicious libel, insults, and language that damages the target's self-esteem. (3) Sexual violence: deliberate attacks on sex organs and coerced sexual intercourse or contact, etc. For more details, refer to Zhang and Liu (2004).

## 4.5 Migrant Workers and the Risks of Their Families

A family is a discrete unit of society that comprises members each of whom plays different functions and who depend on each other based on mutual trust. The family is the basic element of society and at the same time it is directly influenced by society, dependent on society, and must align itself with developments of society. With the changes in China's social structure since the launch of the reform and opening-up policy, the influence of society on families has given rise to diverse family structures and the changes in family relations have brought on a number of problems and conflicts.

On the one hand, following the implementation of the household contract responsibility system in rural China, families became smaller in size and more isolated from one another, and individuals became more indifferent to one another, making it easy for rural women to fall into helplessness. Further, the pace of rural life is accelerating, with a large number of rural laborers flooding into cities. More than a hundred million migrant workers left home and this tide and its associated risks are growing. The difficulties thus caused have continued into the new century.[51]

On the other hand, discrimination against migrant workers in cities due to their identity (manifested by temporary residence permissions and the custody and repatriation system) and discriminative treatment are widespread. The low level or even lack of social security for these workers pushes up the cost of the migration of rural surplus labor. In 1988, the *Workers' Daily* reported that the treatment of lower-tier female workers in certain foreign-owned enterprises was strikingly similar to the treatment of indentured workers as described by Xia Yan more than half a century before.

As migrant workers rushed into cities, a large number of rural girls at schooling age come into the city and are constantly on the move with their parents. They do not stay long in any one place and have little access to education. Even worse than that, they usually experience discrimination and suffer from mental imbalance. In recent years, the second-generation migrant workers have emerged in society as a group. They do not belong to cities and neither can they go back to their rural homes and fit in. It is therefore of great concern how this group is going to live their lives. In other cases, girls do not follow their parents into cities and are instead left behind at home. These girls tend to be more fragile in the face of failure and frustration given that they lack the love and care from their parents.

Compared with urban families, rural families in China used to be super stable with three or four generations living together. Since the 1990s, such traditional large, extended families that have existed in rural China for millennia, serving as the cornerstone of social stability, have started to hollow out as large numbers of migrant worker left the countryside that had been their home for generations. The social structure in rural China is thus changing rapidly, and China is currently in an

[51]Song (1996).

urbanization process which has brought about the largest ever migration of people. Rural families are also undergoing unprecedented transformations, and new family structures are gradually replacing the old one as the "new normal" in rural areas. Problems thus arise. As the social structure changes, more than a quarter of families are not "intact" as family members work and live separately from one another (e.g., separation of parents and their children, or of husband and wife). The hold of the two elements that tie Chinese people together, blood relations and the hometown, has been loosened.

According to *Analysis and Forecast on China's Social Development (2007),*[52] the average household size in China declined rapidly for a number of reasons: the sustained implementation of the family planning policy, the growing migrant worker population, postponed marriage, postpone childbearing, the increase of the nuclear families, and the growth of empty-nest households. Now the typical structures of rural families are the empty-nest structure and the migrated marriage structure. The first covers three groups of the population that require attention: empty-nest elderlies, left-behind wives, and left-behind children. The latter covers two types of migrated families: the passive type and the active type.

As a large number of young and middle-aged laborers move into cities, women are left behind and have to engage in agricultural production which is undoubtedly an extra burden on their shoulders. According to a study conducted in the late 1990s, among 1022 men and women of eight villages, only 389 were fully or mostly engaged in agricultural production and two hundred and forty of them were women. In other words, only 38% of the 1022 people surveyed engaged mainly in agricultural production and 62% of them were female.[53] These women also had to perform household labor such as feeding animals, looking after children, caring for the elderly, cooking, laundering, so on and so forth.

On top of the roles of wife and mother, these women also had to bear the burdens that should have been shared between husband and wife, such as productive labor, raising the children, and looking after the elderly. As their husbands are away from home for long periods of time, the traditional tension between these women and their mothers-in-law may intensify at any time, meaning that these women are more likely to feel frustrated. The heavier burden only makes things worse for them and they thus become more likely to commit suicide.

It is very common in rural areas today that the husband is absent from home and work in cities and the wife, left behind and alone, do all the agricultural labor, raise children, care for the elderly, and even do construction work such us road building or bridge building as assigned by the collective. The husband may return home once a year or even once every couple of years. These women are subject to physical pressures as well as tremendous emotional and mental pressures. These left-behind women no longer have the stable family life of yore and are repressed in both physiological and psychological terms over long periods of time.

---

[52]Ru et al. (2006).

[53]Huang et al. (1997).

Communication and affection enhance the bond between husband and wife and alleviate the pressure of the fast-paced modern life for both husband and wife. It is an important factor that keeps marriage stable. Conversely, the lack of communication between husband and wife can lead to the breakdown of the marriage. The long-term separation of left-behind women from their husbands over great distances can hamper communication and even lead to distrust, thereby leading to crises in the relationship. The divorce rate in rural areas has been going up in recent years and many cases involve migrant workers.

A survey of four cities and nine counties in Anhui Province reveals that the long-term separation of couples and the expansion of one party's social circle can increase the occurrence of extramarital affairs. Among the cases seen during a spot check of cases handled by the county-level people's courts in Bozhou and Anqing, rural divorce cases accounted for 80% of the case load and all such cases have one party who is a migrant worker away from home for long.[54]

The massive migration of rural laborers has a tremendous impact on the marital relationships of rural families in China. It makes the stay-home women in rural areas who have to support the entire family along more likely to suffer setbacks on various fronts. Under the influence of traditional attitudes, rural women tend to be more vulnerable in the face of a breakdown of their marriage, and change of heart on the part of the husband who has gone to cities to work can be a great blow to these women. According to a survey, 71.04% of women "object to" "the other woman," 6.27% reported feeling "dejected," and 8.36% said that they were living in "agony"; nearly half of all rural women surveyed stated that they would not divorce their spouses: 42.08% said that they would "object" to a divorce, 28.05% said that they would "approve," 14.63% were "skeptical," and 19.07% would be "dejected"; as for marriages arranged by parents, 85.37% expressed objection, 4.18% said they would fight against such marriages "with death," and 18.80% expressed empathy with those who had committed suicide due to marriage issues. "The other woman," arranged marriages and divorce are all risk factors for suicide by rural women.[55]

## 4.6 *Widening Wealth Gap, Flaws in the Social Security System, and "Farmer Exploitation"*

Poverty is another cause of suicide among rural women. At the end of 1995, 65 million people lived below the poverty line in China's impoverished rural areas and the figure for 1998 was 42 million. On April 22, 2009, at the eighth meeting of the Standing Committee of the Eleventh National People's Congress, Li Xueju, then Minister of Civil Affairs, delivered a report on behalf of the State Council, pointing out that there was still a large agricultural population and more than 40 million rural

[54]Wang and Wu (2007).

[55]He (1997c, p. 543).

residents living below the poverty line in China.[56] The Chinese government is fully committed to poverty alleviation which has become a national strategy. Since 2017, the number of rural poor has fallen to 30.46 million, with the incidence of poverty dropping to 3.1% (National Bureau of Statistics, 2018-2-1). By 2020, China will lift the entire impoverished population in rural areas out of poverty and complete the building of a moderately prosperous society in all respects.

The gap between the highest and lowest income levels in China was expanded. Human factors and urban changes combined to widen the gap between the rich and the poor at a growing pace in China.[57] It is for sure that in the near future, 80% of China's wealth will be in the hands of the richest 20% of the population. According to economist Jin Yanshi, "in developing countries, the widening of the gap between the rich and the poor can be attributed mainly to circulation and trading markets. One involves the common urban–rural gap that widens over the course of urbanization, and the other has to do with the premiums and depreciation that arise in the course of asset trading. The former is normally understood as 'the urban exploitation of rural areas' while the latter is generally outside the scope of theoretical analysis. The shift toward a market orientation over the course of urbanization will invariably cause the wealth gap to grow wider disproportionately."[58]

When the very basic needs such as food and clothing are not yet ensured, survival itself can be a cause of suicide.

In rural China, the sales of falsely labeled seeds have led to incidents of non-harvest from acres and acres of farmland. On March 30, 2010, a farmer hanged himself in the courtyard of a seed station in Queshan County, Henan. He had purchased falsely labeled rice seeds from the station and suffered a very poor harvest on the nearly 300 *mu* of farmland as a result. He hanged himself after failing to obtain compensation after half a year of strenuous efforts to seek it.[59]

Fake fertilizers, fake pesticides, and the unscrupulous trafficking of women and children also spell disasters for many rural women.

The 2010 case of illegal fundraising by Nanshan Company of Suihua, Heilongjiang Province affected individuals in all three northeastern provinces of the country. More than 10,000 investors were harmed. In Harbin alone, the case involved RMB 850 million "invested" by 8400 persons. Many of these people and their families went bankrupt, dozens of them committed suicide out of despair or died under the sudden heavy blow, and numerous families were torn apart or turned into groups of beggars in the streets.[60]

The social security system in rural China is currently incomplete, with mainly the following problems: First, there is a development imbalance. The rural minimum living allowance system, the new rural cooperative medical insurance system,

[56] Li (2009a).
[57] Tong (2011).
[58] Jin (2010).
[59] Wu (2010).
[60] Liang (2010).

medical assistance, and other systems are all in the initial stage of development. The system of social security for farmers whose land has been expropriated and the system of social insurance for migrant workers are gradually being introduced. The new rural social pension insurance system is still in the pilot stage. There is a lack of cross-regional coordination and rural social security coverage levels differ quite significantly between eastern, central, and western China. Uneven development between urban and rural areas makes rural areas lag significantly behind cities in terms of social security. Moreover, rural areas are also seriously in lack of social welfare services. Second, system building lags behind in rural areas. Overall, social security is underdeveloped in China's rural areas due to factors such as the level of economic and social development achieved, the bifurcation between urban and rural areas, and the relatively late start of efforts at system building, thus the system now features relatively narrow coverage, low levels of protection, and limited funding. In some areas, there are even problems with the proper implementation of relevant policies. In particular, the flaws of the rural social insurance financing mechanism prevent many rural residents to join the schemes. Third, there is a lack of a strong legal framework. At present, China's rural social security system is only governed by the *Regulations on the Rural Five Guarantees Work* and issues not covered follow only relevant policies, with no legal document of any kind to refer to. Without the necessary legal foundation, rural social security work remains poorly regularized and more efforts need to be made for improvement. Fourth, policy support and information sharing are insufficient. With regard to rural social security, system coordination and policy support are insufficient and communication and information sharing also need to be enhanced. In addition, more needs to be done to improve collaboration and form stronger synergy. Fifth, weak management at the basic level. At the village level, social security authorities are not well-established and are manned mostly by less capable staff. These authorities have access to only the minimal level of facilities. On average, each official in charge of the new rural cooperative medical insurance scheme at the county level is responsible for thirty thousand residents. Many townships and towns do not have a dedicated social security agency, and only one person has to take charge of a number of social security-related matters and this person may even work only part-time sometimes. Low management standards and flaws in the rural social security system have led to poor compliance with relevant standards and arbitrariness in eligibility review and fund granting. Sixth, the division of powers and financial expenditure responsibilities is not clear. The lack of a reasonable definition of the responsibility of expenditure at various levels of government has hampered the development of rural social security undertakings at various levels and lower-level governments usually depend heavily on higher-level governments for action, with very low initiative in completing their duties.[61]

Rural women in China seriously lack the ability to support themselves in financial terms. They are usually incapable of withstanding economic risks once a

[61]Li (2009b).

major change like a divorce or widowhood occurs to them. This, coupled with inadequate social security coverage, easily leave rural women in despair in the event of an unforeseen occurrence.

In recent years, as urbanization and industrialization speed up in China, land acquisition increases and demolitions and relocation for large-scale transportation and other infrastructure projects occur on a large-scale, bringing with them issues of compensation and livelihood on the part of farmers who lose their land. Reports of suicides caused by forced demolition and relocation are commonplace.

Encouragingly, the Chinese government resolutely announced on December 29, 2005, that the *Agricultural Tax Regulations* would be abolished from January 1, 2006. This means for the first time in more than 2600 years, Chinese farmers would not have to pay any agricultural taxes. The corresponding pieces of legislation on land acquisition and demolition are also being improved. In May 2011, the State Council issued an urgent circular, calling on all regions and authorities to conscientiously implement the regulations on the expropriation of and compensation for acquisition of houses on state-owned land and the urgent circular of the General Office of the State Council on further strengthening the management of land acquisition and demolition to effectively protect the legal rights and interests of the masses in a bid to prevent any forced evictions and the use of violence in such evictions.

## 4.7 Flaws in Rural Social Organizations and a Less Integrated Society

A major change in the social structure of rural China in transition is that the basic unit of resource allocation has changed from a production team to a family or household. As a result, an array of social organizations is damaged and even paralyzed. In the time of people's communes, a people's commune, organized on the basis of a production team, performed administrative functions on behalf of the government and served as the basic unit of resource allocation. The commune was responsible for organizing agricultural production and distributing resources at the village level, and it kept track of matters relating to life and death in the village, including disputes in neighborhoods, and family strife. It was what rural residents believed they could rely on.

Following the dissolution of the people's communes, farmland was assigned to households and Chinese villages gradually "depoliticized." However, the powerful political forces and mainstream ideology over the decades before the reform and opening up had already uprooted the weak endogenous values of rural traditions, rural self-organization, and local and customary norms. After the 1980s, the gradual withdrawal of the state-centered political ideology caused more severe disorder and even a vacuum of values in the rural society. As such, individualism and the rational calculations brought on by the market economy, meeting no resistance, soon became the mainstay of the rural mindset as well as the basic logic of action for individual farmers.

With the implementation of the household contract responsibility system, the household has become the basic unit of production and accounting. The production team morphed into a village committee or a villagers' group, and its function of organizing production and distribution disappeared. Its function of mediating various interpersonal relationships in rural areas, including family strife, was also diluted. There is no longer any other organizational connection between families except for blood relations, while various risks intersect and stack. Production risks and the risks of everyday life are borne by families or individuals. The wealth gap across families and between individuals appeared and widened, and the Matthew effect became commonplace in rural areas. The lack of rural social organizations exacerbated various conflicts and problems. In some counties and townships, officials raised funds and assigned financial and labor obligations arbitrarily and then forced rural residents to complete relevant assignments.

In addition, the role of traditional organizations such as women's federations, rural cooperative medical organizations, and "five guarantees" committees in rural areas have generally been weakened, and rural residents lack the support and help from social networks.

At present, there are about two million social organizations of all kinds in rural China, including economic cooperation organizations, public interest organizations and mutual aid organizations. For example, there are associations of various economic specialities, senior citizens' associations, temple fair committees, lantern festival committees, water use associations, and environmental protection associations. They are an important force in rural society. Currently, in academic circles, these organizations are generally known as "rural civil society organizations" or "rural NGOs." There has yet to be an academic consensus as for what rural social organizations are and what are the key types of such organizations. Some scholars are already paying attention to the negative effects that such rural social organizations may bring: They may weaken the formal organizations within rural society or create high levels of political pressure on rural residents when the demands of certain organizations exceed the allowance under the existing system, and certain social organizations may turn into "local warlords" that seek to protect the illegal interests of their members and resist the implementation of national laws and regulations, exploit vulnerable groups by on behalf of rural elites, and even become gangs.[62]

In addition, education is also underdeveloped in rural areas as much needs to be done before the "Two Basics"[63] can be fulfilled. A fairly large proportion of the population is still illiterate or semi-literate, and the general quality of the rural

[62]Liu (2009).

[63]The "Two Basics" policy is the drive to "basically eradicate" illiteracy among the young and middle-aged and to "basically universalize" the nine-year course of compulsory education. The policy was laid out by the Ministry of Education as part of efforts to implement the Decision of the State Council on the Further Strengthening of Education Work in Rural Areas.

population is low. Feudal thoughts and superstition, and even cult beliefs, spread easily in certain areas. These are also indirect causes of suicide among rural residents.

A basic view in sociology is that human beings are social animals who cannot live in isolation or merely in families; they must belong to a wide variety of social organizations. However, in the vast rural areas of China, apart from families, there are few other social organizations due to the lack of the tradition and ability of Chinese farmers to form such organizations on their own. And it takes time for villagers' committees, the substitute of production teams of the people's commune era, to become an organization that rural residents feel reassured to rely on.[64]

## References

An, L., & Jia, H. (2007). An analysis of suicidal deaths among Chinese women in various areas. *Chinese Journal of Health Statistics, 1*, 31.

China Population Information Research Center. (2002). WHO official speaks about China's suicide rate. *Population Information Newsletter, 2*.

Da, D. (2001). An examination of the factors that have an impact on suicide among Chinese women. In *The Fifth National Conference on Crisis Intervention and Suicide Prevention*, Changsha.

Fuse, T. (1990). *Introduction to suicide studies* (pp. 136–137). Seishin Shobo.

Gao, Q. (2005). *Work report at the 2005 national health work conference*. http://www.moh.gov.cn/publicfiles/business/htmlfiles/mohbgt/pzxdt/200806/36636.htm. Accessed May 11, 2008.

Gao, Z., et al. (1987). An epidemiological study of suicidal deaths among the elderly. *Chinese Journal of Gerontology, 7*(1), 8.

He, Z. (1996). *Suicide and life* (pp. 200–201). Guangzhou: Guangzhou Publishing House.

He, Z. (1997a). *The pathology of suicide* (p. 460). Beijing: China Traditional Chinese Medicine Press.

He, Z. (1997b). *Pathology of suicide* (p. 494). Beijing: China Press of Traditional Chinese Medicine.

He, Z. (1997c). *The pathology of suicide* (p. 543). Beijing: China Traditional Chinese Medicine Press.

He, J., Yonghua, J., Bilei, X., et al. (2002). Study on the impact of comprehensive intervention on rural suicides. *Chinese Mental Health Journal, 2*, 30–31.

Huang, P., et al. (1997). *In pursuit of survival: A study of contemporary rural migrant population in China*. Kunming: Yunnan People's Press.

Jia, L. (2003). An analysis of the statement of Chinese government investment in public health. *Health Economics Research, 12*.

Jiang, C., et al. (2002). Psychology of suicides among college students and crisis intervention. *Chinese Journal of School Doctor* [*sic.*], *16*(1), 77.

Jin, Y. (2010). Process of urbanization bound to amplify polarization to an unreasonable extent. *Shanghai Securities News*, July 6.

Jing, J., Wu, X., & Zhang, J. (2010). Migration of women in rural areas and the decline ofsuicide rate in China [J]. *China Agricultural University Journal of Social Science Edition, 27*(4), 20–31.

[64]Xie (1999g, p. 58).

Kang, Q. (2002). An analysis of suicide among women in rural areas in China. *Journal of Jishou University (Social Sciences Edition), 1.*
Li, X. (2009a). *Report of the State Council on the development of the rural social security system.* http://www.gov.cn/gzdt/2009-04/23/content_1294027.htm. Accessed February 13, 2010.
Li, X. (2009b). *Report of the state council on the development of the rural social security system.* http://www.gov.cn/gzdt/2009-04/23/content_1294027.htm. Accessed April 11, 2010.
Li, X., Yongchen, Xu, et al. (2002). Characteristics of patients who have attempted suicide treated by general hospitals in rural areas. *Chinese Mental Health Journal, 16*(10), 684.
Li, B., & Zuo, G. (2010). The disorder model: An examination of the reasons for suicide among China's rural women. *Journal of Shijiazhuang University, 1,* 80.
Liang, S. (2010). *Forty arrested for illegal fundraising by Nanshan company in Heilongjiang.* Xinhuanet.com.
Liu, H. (1995). A comparative study on suicidal deaths among urban and rural women in China. *Chinese Journal of Behavioral Medical Science, 4*(2), 78.
Liu, B. (2004). An analysis on the reasons behind the high suicide rate among rural women. *Journal of China Agricultural University (Social Sciences Edition), 4*, 65.
Liu, Y. (2009). Building rural social organization mechanisms toward social self-governance. *Southeast Academic Research*, *1.*
Liu, J., & Li, Y. (1990). *Unveiling the mystery behind suicide* (p. 120). Chengdu: Sichuan Science and Technology Press.
Liu, J., & Li, Yuanzhi. (1992a). *Unveiling the mystery behind suicidal behavior* (p. 86). Chengdu: Sichuan Science and Technology Press.
Liu, J., & Li, Y. (1992b). *Unveiling the mystery behind suicidal behavior* (p. 90). Chengdu: Sichuan Science and Technology Press.
Liu, J., & Li, Y. (1992c). *Unveiling the mystery behind suicidal behavior* (p. 93). Chengdu: Sichuan Science and Technology Press.
Lu, Q. (2011). Investigation into suicide of Shandong vegetable farmer. *Lifeweek*, April 29.
Luo, P. (2007). Parents kill themselves by poisoning due to mistreatment by children. *Guizhou City News*, April 14.
Niu, T. (2010). Young woman from Hubei joins online suicide group for collective suicide. *Chutian Metropolis Daily*, November 18.
Ru, X., Lu, X., & Li, P. (Eds.). (2006). *Analysis and forecast on china's social development (2007).* Beijing: Social Sciences Academic Press.
Song, L. (1996). Migration of China's rural labor force and countermeasures. *Sociological Studies, 2.*
Song, A. (1998). Study on the correlation between characteristics of and social support for infertile women. *Medicine and Society, 11*(3), 25.
Tong, D. (2011). *Migration of the century: Shift toward mega-cities that will determine China's fate* (p. 176). Beijing: China Development Press.
Wang, S. (2000). 19-year-old boy and woman in her forties criticized for romance, kill themselves with poison. *Liaoshen Evening News,* November 13.
Wang, S. (2004). Reflections on the management of domestic violence in China. *Journal of Women's Academy at Shandong, 1.*
Wang, J. (Ed.). (2006). *Report on women development in China (No. 1).* Beijing: Social Sciences Academic Press.
Wang, W. (2009). *Two hundred Hong Kong youths seek collective suicide*. Xinhuanet.
Wang, K., & Wu, D. (2007). *Four generations under one roof" shattered by the migrant worker wave: A study of family relationships in rural areas at a time of social transformation.* http://www.sociology.cass.cn/shxw/xstl/xstl39/t20071128_14499.htm. Accessed February 10, 2010.
Wen, Z. (1998). *Transcending death: Prevention and control of suicidal behavior* (p. 37). Shanghai: Shanghai Medical University Press.
WHO. (1989). *World health statistics annual* (pp. 364–375).
WHO. (1990). *World health statistics annual* (pp. 346–369).
WHO. (1990). *World health statistics annual* (p. 117).

Wu, Y. (2010). *Farmer commits suicide in seed station after failing to obtain compensation for falsely labeled seeds*. http://news.sina.com.cn/s/2010-04-01/042917305612s.shtml. Accessed October 5, 2011.

Xie, L. (Ed.). (1999a). *Report on suicides among rural women in China* (pp. 6–8). Guiyang: Guizhou People's Press.

Xie, L. (Ed.). (1999b). *Report on suicides among rural women in China* (p. 5). Guiyang: Guizhou People's Press.

Xie, L. (Ed.). (1999c). *Report on suicides among rural women in China* (p. 18). Guiyang: Guizhou People's Press.

Xie, L. (Ed.). (1999d). *Report on suicides among rural women in China* (p. 34). Guiyang: Guizhou People's Press.

Xie, L. (Ed.). (1999e). *Report on suicides among rural women in China* (pp. 34–38). Guiyang: Guizhou People's Press.

Xie, L. (Ed.). (1999f). *Report on suicides among rural women in China* (p. 46). Guiyang: Guizhou People's Press.

Xie, L. (Ed.). (1999g). *Report on suicides among rural women in China* (p. 58). Guiyang: Guizhou People's Press.

Xu, M. (1999). Rural women: A disadvantaged group worth paying attention to. In L. Xie (Ed.), *Report on suicides among rural women in China*. Guiyang: Guizhou People's Press.

Yan, M. (2008). A preliminary analysis on the social causes of the high suicide rate among rural women in China. *Journal of Tianzhong, 23*(6), 49.

Yang, G., Lingni, Z., Zhengjing, H., & Aiping, C. (2004). Trends and geographic distribution of suicide in the Chinese population. *Chinese Journal of Epidemiology, 25*(4), 280–284.

Ye, Y. (2006). A few interpretations relating to traditional attitudes about women. *Journal of the Fuqing Branch of Fujian Normal University, 6,* 59.

Yu, D. (1997). *The door between life and death* (p. 187). Beijing: New World Press.

Yuan, Z., & Yu, G. (2008). *Seven cases of suicide by hubei farmers burdened with heavy loads*. http://news.sohu.com/90/82/news147748290.shtml. Accessed December 5, 2008.

Zhang, Y. (1988). Suicide: A social problem and taboo. *Marriage and Family, 11,* 34–35.

Zhang, Y. (2004). Supply of and funding for public health services in rural areas. *China Rural Survey, 10,* 5.

Zhang, L., & Liu, M. (Eds.). (2004). *A study of domestic violence in China* (p. 8). China Social Science Press: Beijing.

Zheng, R. (1998). Report on suicide among women in rural areas. *Southern Weekly,* May 15.

Zhu, Y., & Zhou, T. (2004). Half of Chinese rural residents unable to seek medical care due to financial reasons. *Zhejiang Daily*, November 6.

# Chapter 3
# Youth Suicide in China

Although youth suicide may not currently constitute an independent topic of study (rather, it is generally considered part of the general topic of suicide categorized by age group), we believe that adolescent suicide in China has specific characteristics while sharing common features with suicide by people of other age groups. The prevention and control of youth suicide in China should also be done in ways that suit this age group specifically. At a time of unfolding social transformation in China, we should study the high youth suicide rate, as well as the current status, nature, and development of suicidal behaviors among young people; explore the physical, psychological, and social foundations; tackle head-on the huge shock wave of youth suicide on social mentality; and put forward practical and feasible countermeasures.

Youth suicide rate, the characteristics of young people who commit suicide, and the main means of and reasons for their suicides that vary from society to society all give us clues to better understand the underlying social issues and ultimately to know the unique social structure that lies at the bottom of it. As a type of social behavior, youth suicide is inevitably closely related to the social and cultural customs of the nation, and to the national character.

Youth suicide is on the rise in China and around the world, and the harms it causes need no explanation. So, youth suicide is a major topic in the study of suicide.

## 1 Suicide Among Chinese Youths: A Fairly Grave Issue

According to the World Health Organization (WHO), suicide is the top cause of accidental deaths. In most countries with data available, suicide is one of the top ten causes of death and one of the top three for death at an early age.[1]

---

[1]Liu and Li (1996).



J. Li, *A Study on Suicide*,
https://doi.org/10.1007/978-981-13-9499-7_3

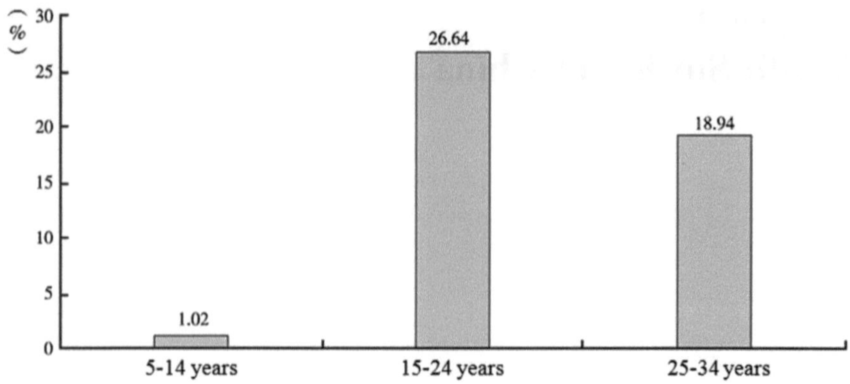


**Fig. 1** Share of youth suicide in total suicides in China, 1987–1989. *Source* WHO (1989)

## *1.1 Relatively High Youth Suicide Rate*

According to the WHO, the youth suicide rate in China is relatively high. Between 1987 and 1989, suicides among people aged 15–24 accounted for 26.64% of the total number of suicides and suicides in the 25–34 age group accounted for 18.94% of the total (see Fig. 1). What is striking[2] is that 1.02% of the total number of suicides were committed by children 5–14 years old.

According to *China Health Statistics Yearbook* published by the National Health Commission, in 2017, suicide was the fifth major cause of death among the 15–24 age group in China, the fourth among the 25–34 age group, and the fourth among the 35–44 age group.

The large proportion of suicidal deaths of young people has a significant impact on the years of life lost in China. According to data submitted by the Ministry of Health of China to the WHO, in 1998, suicide was the leading cause of death in China's 15–34 age group. The rate of suicidal death among people aged 15–24 was 10.63 per 100,000 individuals, that among 25–34-year-olds was 22.41 per 100,000 individuals, and that for the 35–44 age group was 18.19 per 100,000 individuals (see Fig. 2). For this last age group, suicide was the fourth cause of death.[3]

Moreover, suicide tends to occur to younger people in China today. The suicide rate among children and youths aged under 19 is higher in China than in many other countries.

According to the WHO, in 1988, the suicide rate of Chinese children aged 5–14 was 1.0 per 100,000 individuals for both boys and girls. The number of suicidal deaths in this age group accounted for 1.02% of the total, which translates to 2142 deaths based on a total of 210,000 in the year. In the next year, the suicide rates for

[2]World Health Organization (1989).

[3]http://www.hotlife.com.cn/learning/yx-ml/information/WHO/1.htm. Accessed: 10 June 2011.

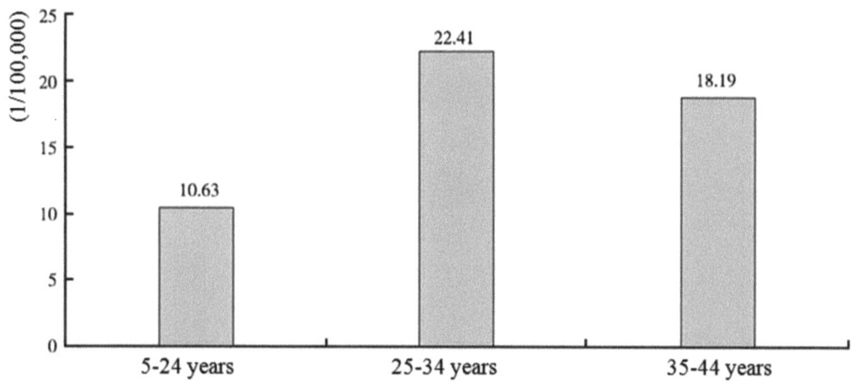


**Fig. 2** Suicide rates among Chinese youths, 1998. *Source* http://www.hotlife.com.cn/learning/yx-ml/information/WHO/1.htm. Date retrieved: June 10, 2011

children of this age group decreased to 0.50 per 100,000 individuals for boys and 0.80 per 100,000 individuals for girls.[4] But in 1999, the rates picked up again with an overall rate of 0.80 per 100,000 individuals, 0.90 per 100,000 individuals for boys, and 0.80 per 100,000 individuals for girls. Suicidal deaths in this age group accounted for approximately 0.9% of the total of that year.[5]

According to the Center for Statistics and Information of the Ministry of Health, the suicide mortality rates of Chinese residents aged 5–19 in the period 2003–2009[6] are as follows.

For the year 2003, the urban suicide mortality rate for the 5–9 age group is 0.21 per 100,000 individuals (0.18 per 100,000 individuals for boys and 0.21 per 100,000 individuals for girls), that for the 10–14 age group is 1.10 per 100,000 individuals (1.25 per 100,000 individuals for boys and 0.92 per 100,000 individuals for girls), and that for the 15–19 age group is 1.93 per 100,000 individuals (1.75 per 100,000 individuals for boys and 2.11 per 100,000 individuals for girls); the rural rate for the 5–9 age group is 0.13 per 100,000 individuals (0.28 per 100,000 individuals for boys and 0.44 per 100,000 individuals for girls), that for the 10–14 age group is 1.05 per 100,000 individuals (3.30 per 100,000 individuals for the boys and 1.05 per 100,000 individuals for girls), and that for the 15–19 age group is 1.86 per 100,000 individuals (3.19 per 100,000 individuals for boys and 3.19 per 100,000 individuals for girls).[7] See Fig. 3.

For the year 2005, the urban suicide mortality rate for the 5–9 age group is 0.13 per 100,000 individuals (0.00 per 100,000 individuals for boys and 0.27 per 100,000 individuals for girls), that for the 10–14 age group is 0.90 per 100,000

[4]WHO (1989).

[5]http://www.who.int/mental-health/prevention/suicide/Charts/en/. Accessed: 13 March 2008.

[6]Data for 2004 could not be obtained despite attempts to seek out such data from multiple sources.

[7]Ministry of Health Statistics and Information Center (2004).

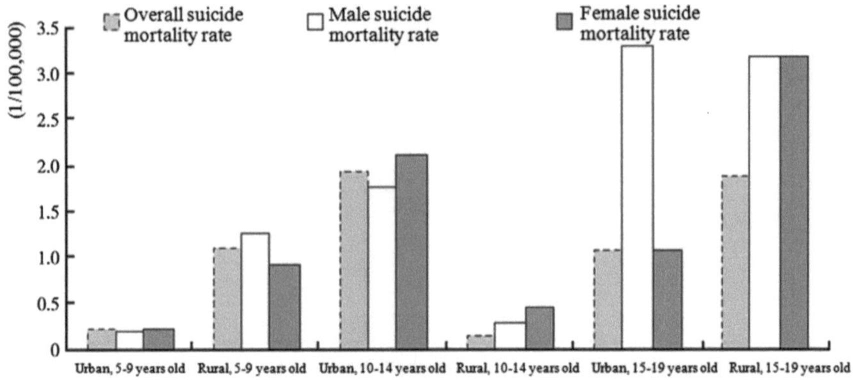


**Fig. 3** Suicide mortality rates among Chinese youths 5–19 years old, 2003

individuals (1.48 per 100,000 individuals for boys and 0.27 per 100,000 individuals for girls), and that for the 15–19 age group is 2.61 per 100,000 individuals (2.60 per 100,000 individuals for boys and 2.62 per 100,000 individuals for girls); the rural suicide mortality rate for the 5–9 age group is 0.72 per 100,000 individuals (1.03 per 100,000 individuals for boys and 0.00 per 100,000 individuals for girls), that for the 10–14 age group is 1.52 per 100,000 individuals (1.99 per 100,000 individuals for boys and 0.96 per 100,000 individuals for girls), and that for the 15–19 age group is 2.29 per 100,000 individuals (1.87 per 100,000 individuals for boys and 2.80 per 100,000 individuals for girls).[8] See Fig. 4.

For the year 2006, the urban suicide mortality rate for the 5–9 age group is 0.00 per 100,000 individuals (0.00 per 100,000 individuals for boys and 0.00 per 100,000 individuals for girls), that for the 10–14 age group is 0.24 per 100,000 individuals (0.31 per 100,000 individuals for boys and 0.17 per 100,000 individuals for girls), and that for the 15–19 age group is 1.80 per 100,000 individuals (1.88 per 100,000 individuals for boys and 1.71 per 100,000 individuals for girls); the rural suicide mortality rate for the 5–9 age group is 0.09 per 100,000 individuals (0.08 per 100,000 individuals for boys and 0.09 per 100,000 individuals for girls), that for the 10–14 age group is 0.97 per 100,000 individuals (1.47 per 100,000 individuals for boys and 0.42 per 100,000 individuals for girls), and that for the 15–19 age group is 3.47 per 100,000 individuals (2.63 per 100,000 individuals for boys and 4.38 per 100,000 individuals for girls).[9] See Fig. 5.

For the year 2007, the urban suicide mortality rate for the 5–9 age group is 0.06 per 100,000 individuals (0.18 per 100,000 individuals for boys and 0.00 per 100,000 individuals for girls), that for the 10–14 age group is 0.46 per 100,000 individuals (0.54 per 100,000 individuals for boys and 0.38 per 100,000 individuals for girls), and that for the 15–19 age group is 1.29 per 100,000 individuals (1.46 per

[8]Ministry of Health Statistics Information Center (2006).

[9]Ministry of Health Statistics Information Center (2007).

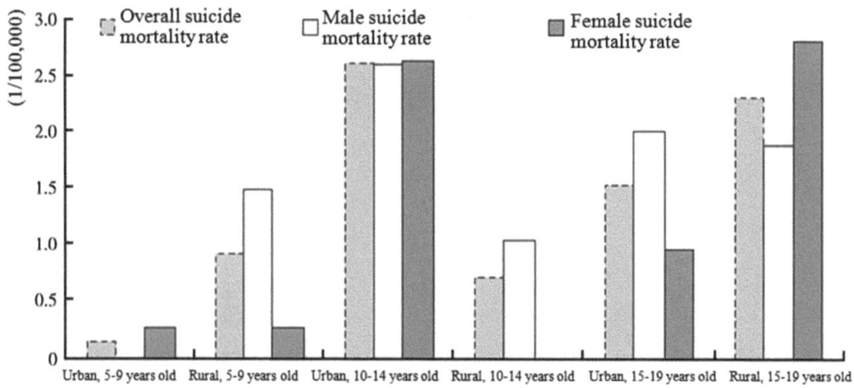


**Fig. 4** Suicide mortality rates among Chinese youths 5–19 years old, 2005

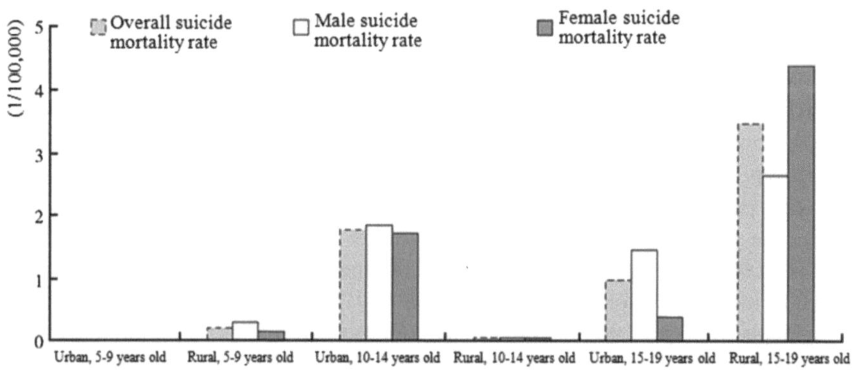


**Fig. 5** Suicide mortality rates among Chinese youths 5–19 years old, 2006

100,000 individuals for boys and 1.12 per 100,000 individuals for girls); the rural suicide mortality rate for the 5–9 age group is 0.08 per 100,000 individuals (0.16 per 100,000 individuals for boys and 0.00 per 100,000 individuals for girls), that for the 10–14 age group is 0.77 per 100,000 individuals (1.03 per 100,000 individuals for boys and 0.50 per 100,000 individuals for girls), and that for the 15–19 age group is 2.73 per 100,000 individuals (3.03 per 100,000 individuals for boys and 2.42 per 100,000 individuals for girls).[10] See Fig. 6.

For the year 2008, the urban suicide mortality rate for the 5–9 age group is 0.11 per 100,000 individuals (0.20 per 100,000 individuals for boys and 0.00 per 100,000 individuals for girls), that for the 10–14 age group is 0.80 per 100,000 individuals (0.46 per 100,000 individuals for boys and 0.16 per 100,000 individuals for girls), and that for the 15–19 age group is 1.57 per 100,000 individuals (1.57 per

[10]Ministry of Health Statistics Information Center (2008).

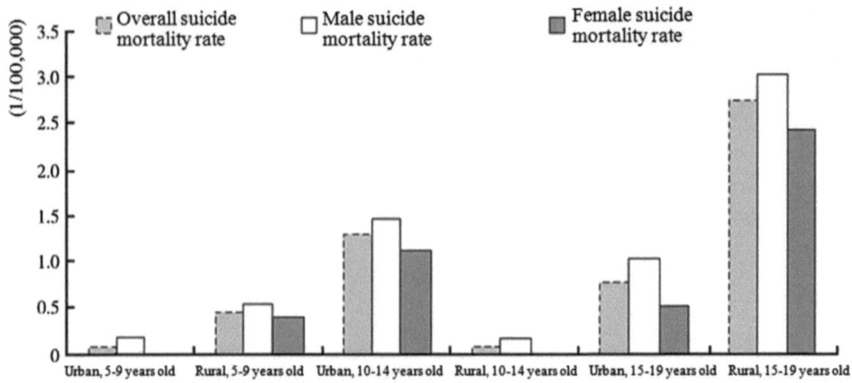


**Fig. 6** Suicide mortality rates among Chinese youths 5-19 years old, 2007

100,000 individuals for boys and 1.03 per 100,000 individuals for girls); the rural suicide mortality rate for the 5–9 age group is 0.00 per 100,000 individuals (0.00 per 100,000 individuals for boys and 0.00 per 100,000 individuals for girls), that for the 10–14 age group is 0.31 per 100,000 individuals (0.30 per 100,000 individuals for the boys and 0.32 per 100,000 individuals for the girls), and that for the 15–19 age group is 2.88 per 100,000 individuals (3.18 per 100,000 individuals for boys and 2.57 per 100,000 individuals for girls).[11] See Fig. 7.

For the year 2009, the urban suicide mortality rate for the 5–9 age group is 0.06 per 100,000 individuals (0.13 per 100,000 individuals for boys and 0.00 per 100,000 individuals for girls), that for the 10–14 age group is 0.37 per 100,000 individuals (0.26 per 100,000 individuals for boys and 0.50 per 100,000 individuals for girls), and that for the 15–19 age group is 1.41 per 100,000 individuals (1.27 per 100,000 individuals for boys and 1.55 per 100,000 individuals for girls); the rural suicide mortality rate for the 5–9 age group is 0.00 per 100,000 individuals (0.00 per 100,000 individuals for boys and 0.00 per 100,000 individuals for girls), that for the 10–14 age group is 0.40 per 100,000 individuals (0.39 per 100,000 individuals for boys and 0.41 per 100,000 individuals for girls), and that for the 15–19 age group is 2.38 per 100,000 individuals (2.67 per 100,000 individuals for boys and 2.07 per 100,000 individuals for girls).[12] See Fig. 8.

According to China Health Statistics Yearbook published by the National Health Commission[13], the suicide mortality rates of Chinese residents aged 5–19 in the period of 2010–2017 are as follows.

[11]Ministry of Health Statistics Information Center (2009).

[12]Ministry of Health Statistics Information Center (2010).

[13]National Health Commission of the P.R.C., China Health Statistics Yearbook. Date of inquiry: June 12th, 2019.

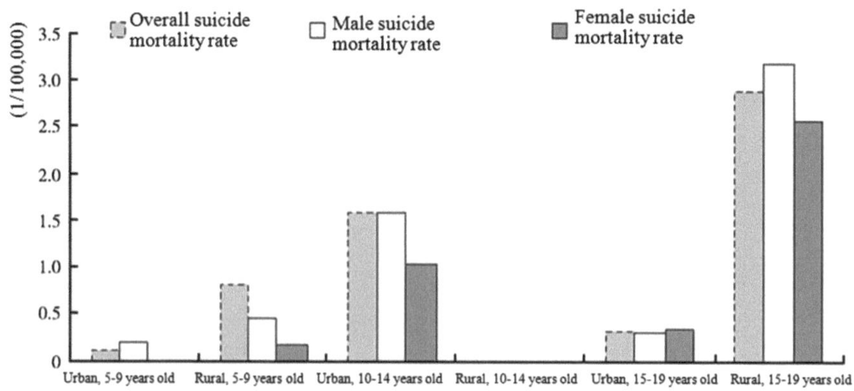


**Fig. 7** Suicide mortality rates among Chinese youths 5–19 years old, 2008

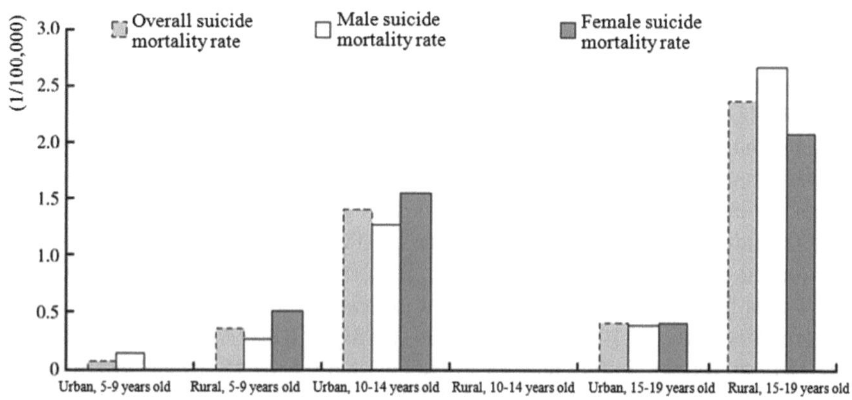


**Fig. 8** Suicide mortality rates among Chinese youths 5–19 years old, 2009

For the year 2010, the urban suicide mortality rate for the 5–9 age group is 0.00 per 100,000 individuals (0.00 per 100,000 individuals for boys and 0.00 per 100,000 individuals for girls), that for the 10–14 age group is 0.45 per 100,000 individuals (0.43 per 100,000 individuals for boys and 0.47 per 100,000 individuals for girls); and that for 15–19 age group is 2.03 per 100,000 individuals (1.97 per 100,000 individuals for boys and 2.09 per 100,000 individuals for girls); the rural rate for the 5–9 age group is 0.00 per 100,000 individuals (0.00 per 100,000 individuals for boys and 0.00 per 100,000 individuals for girls), that for the 10–14 age group is 0.26 per 100,000 individuals (0.33 per 100,000 individuals for boys and 0.19 per 100,000 individuals for girls), and that for the 15–19 age group is 2.32 per 100,000 individuals (2.10 per 100,000 individuals for boys and 2.58 per 100,000 individuals for girls).

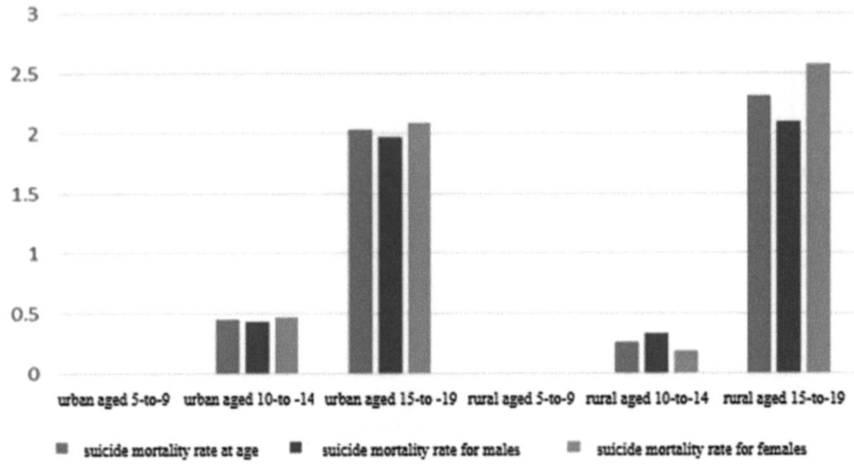


For the year 2011, the urban suicide mortality rate for the 5–9 age group is 0.08 per 100,000 individuals (0.00 per 100,000 individuals for boys and 0.16 per 100,000 individuals for girls), that for the 10–14 age group is 0.63 per 100,000 individuals (0.94 per 100,000 individuals for boys and 0.29 per 100,000 individuals for girls); and that for 15–19 age group is 1.45 per 100,000 individuals (1.91 per 100,000 individuals for boys and 0.98 per 100,000 individuals for girls); the rural rate for the 5–9 age group is 0.19 per 100,000 individuals (0.21 per 100,000 individuals for boys and 0.16 per 100,000 individuals for girls), that for the 10–14 age group is 0.85 per 100,000 individuals (0.88 per 100,000 individuals for boys and 0.81 per 100,000 individuals for girls), and that for the 15–19 age group is 2.44 per 100,000 individuals (2.90 per 100,000 individuals for boys and 1.92 per 100,000 individuals for girls).

For the year 2012, the urban suicide mortality rate for the 5–9 age group is 0.24 per 100,000 individuals (0.23 per 100,000 individuals for boys and 0.25 per 100,000 individuals for girls), that for the 10–14 age group is 0.72 per 100,000 individuals (0.61 per 100,000 individuals for boys and 0.84 per 100,000 individuals for girls); and that for 15–19 age group is 1.41 per 100,000 individuals (1.61 per 100,000 individuals for boys and 1.20 per 100,000 individuals for girls); the rural rate for the 5–9 age group is 0.14 per 100,000 individuals (0.13 per 100,000 individuals for boys and 0.15 per 100,000 individuals for girls), that for the 10–14 age group is 0.67 per 100,000 individuals (0.83 per 100,000 individuals for boys and 0.49 per 100,000 individuals for girls), and that for the 15–19 age group is 2.50 per 100,000 individuals (2.64 per 100,000 individuals for boys and 2.35 per 100,000 individuals for girls).

For the year 2013, the urban suicide mortality rate for the 5–9 age group is 0.09 per 100,000 individuals (0.06 per 100,000 individuals for boys and 0.13 per 100,000 individuals for girls), that for the 10–14 age group is 0.46 per 100,000

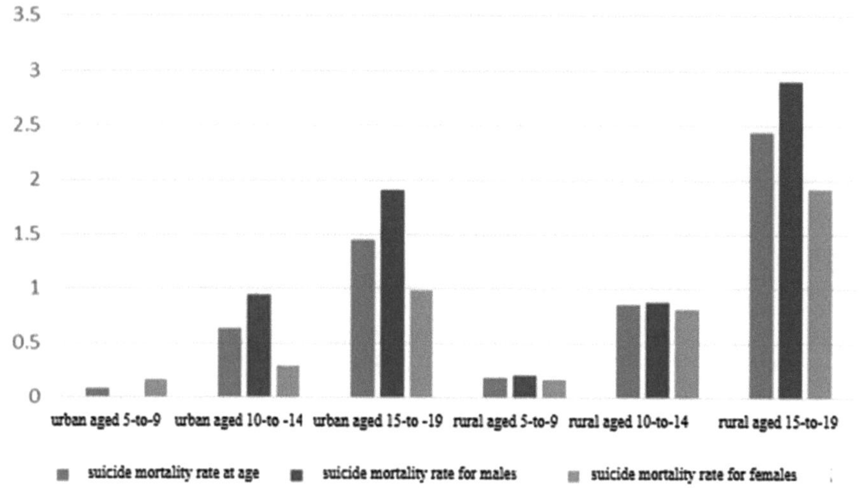


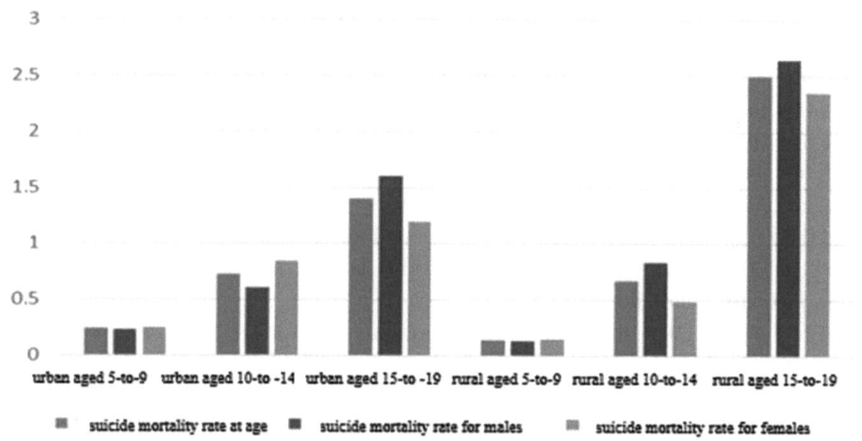


individuals (0.52 per 100,000 individuals for boys and 0.38 per 100,000 individuals for girls); and that for 15–19 age group is 1.83 per 100,000 individuals (1.79 per 100,000 individuals for boys and 1.87 per 100,000 individuals for girls); the rural rate for the 5–9 age group is 0.13 per 100,000 individuals (0.13 per 100,000 individuals for boys and 0.13 per 100,000 individuals for girls), that for the 10–14 age group is 1.09 per 100,000 individuals (1.09 per 100,000 individuals for boys and 1.08 per 100,000 individuals for girls), and that for the 15–19 age group is 3.03 per 100,000 individuals (3.34 per 100,000 individuals for boys and 2.68 per 100,000 individuals for girls).

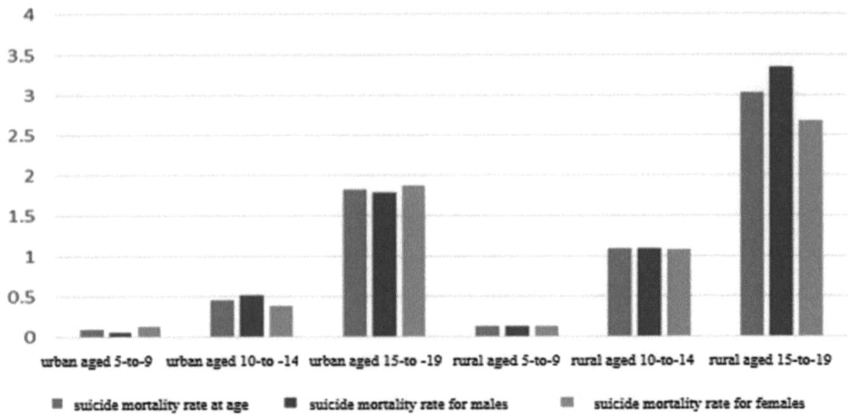


For the year 2014, the urban suicide mortality rate for the 5–9 age group is 0.05 per 100,000 individuals (0.05 per 100,000 individuals for boys and 0.05 per 100,000 individuals for girls), that for the 10–14 age group is 0.96 per 100,000 individuals (1.06 per 100,000 individuals for boys and 0.84 per 100,000 individuals for girls); and that for 15–19 age group is 1.92 per 100,000 individuals (2.21 per 100,000 individuals for boys and 1.60 per 100,000 individuals for girls); the rural rate for the 5–9 age group is 0.04 per 100,000 individuals (0.03 per 100,000 individuals for boys and 0.04 per 100,000 individuals for girls), that for the 10–14 age group is 0.90 per 100,000 individuals (0.93 per 100,000 individuals for boys and 0.85 per 100,000 individuals for girls), and that for the 15–19 age group is 2.60 per 100,000 individuals (2.89 per 100,000 individuals for boys and 2.26 per 100,000 individuals for girls).

For the year 2015, the urban suicide mortality rate for the 5–9 age group is 0.08 per 100,000 individuals (0.05 per 100,000 individuals for boys and 0.11 per 100,000 individuals for girls), that for the 10–14 age group is 1.08 per 100,000 individuals (1.14 per 100,000 individuals for boys and 1.00 per 100,000 individuals for girls); and that for 15–19 age group is 1.30 per 100,000 individuals (1.62 per 100,000 individuals for boys and 0.97 per 100,000 individuals for girls); the rural rate for the 5–9 age group is 0.03 per 100,000 individuals (0.03 per 100,000 individuals for boys and 0.02 per 100,000 individuals for girls), that for the 10–14 age group is 0.88 per 100,000 individuals (1.10 per 100,000 individuals for boys and 0.63 per 100,000 individuals for girls), and that for the 15–19 age group is 2.81 per 100,000 individuals (3.44 per 100,000 individuals for boys and 2.10 per 100,000 individuals for girls).

For the year 2016, the urban suicide mortality rate for the 5–9 age group is 0.02 per 100,000 individuals (0.05 per 100,000 individuals for boys and 0.00 per 100,000 individuals for girls), that for the 10–14 age group is 0.98 per 100,000 individuals (1.25 per 100,000 individuals for boys and 0.66 per 100,000 individuals

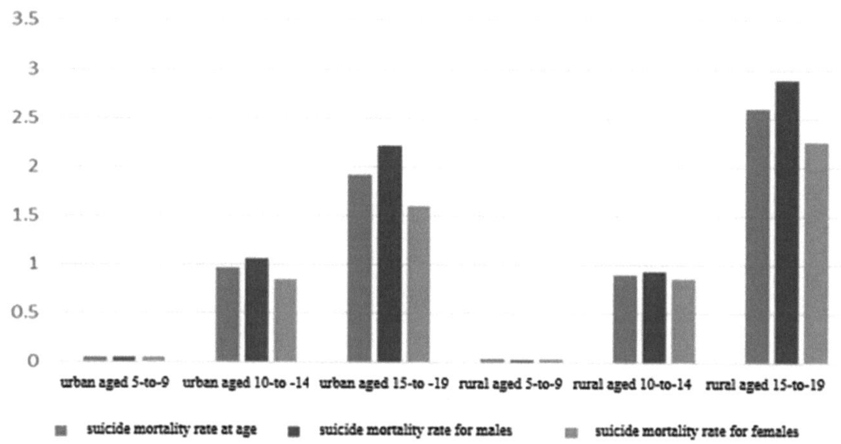


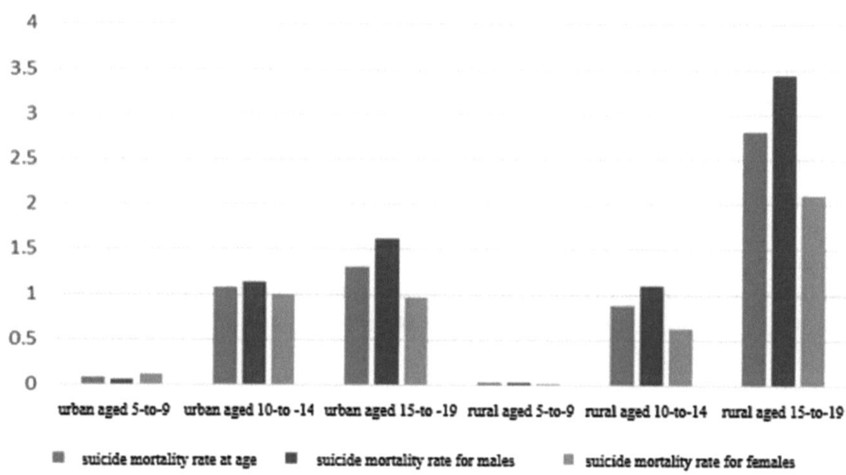


for girls); and that for 15–19 age group is 1.56 per 100,000 individuals (1.58 per 100,000 individuals for boys and 1.54 per 100,000 individuals for girls); the rural rate for the 5–9 age group is 0.03 per 100,000 individuals (0.00 per 100,000 individuals for boys and 0.06 per 100,000 individuals for girls), that for the 10–14 age group is 0.85 per 100,000 individuals (1.13 per 100,000 individuals for boys and 0.56 per 100,000 individuals for girls), and that for the 15–19 age group is 2.52 per 100,000 individuals (2.73 per 100,000 individuals for boys and 2.31 per 100,000 individuals for girls).

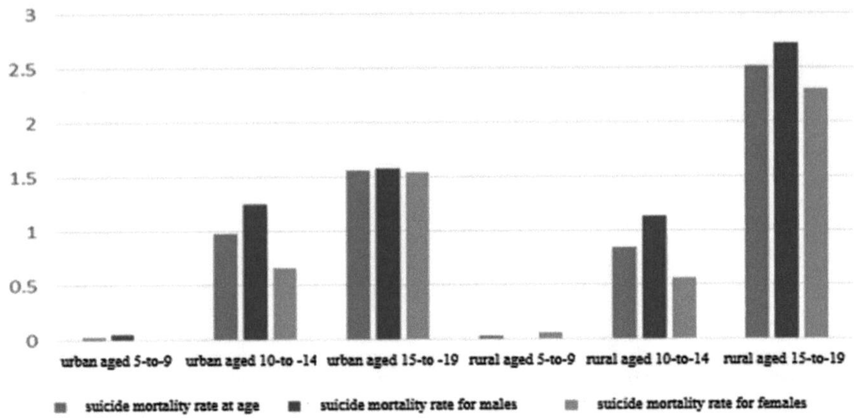


For the year 2017, the urban suicide mortality rate for the 5–9 age group is 0.09 per 100,000 individuals (0.17 per 100,000 individuals for boys and 0.00 per 100,000 individuals for girls), that for the 10–14 age group is 0.96 per 100,000 individuals (1.39 per 100,000 individuals for boys and 0.46 per 100,000 individuals for girls); and that for 15–19 age group is 1.40 per 100,000 individuals (1.81 per 100,000 individuals for boys and 0.96 per 100,000 individuals for girls); the rural rate for the 5–9 age group is 0.02 per 100,000 individuals (0.03 per 100,000 individuals for boys and 0.00 per 100,000 individuals for girls), that for the 10–14 age group is 0.94 per 100,000 individuals (0.96 per 100,000 individuals for boys and 0.92 per 100,000 individuals for girls), and that for the 15–19 age group is 2.49 per 100,000 individuals (2.73 per 100,000 individuals for boys and 2.21 per 100,000 individuals for girls) (Table 1).

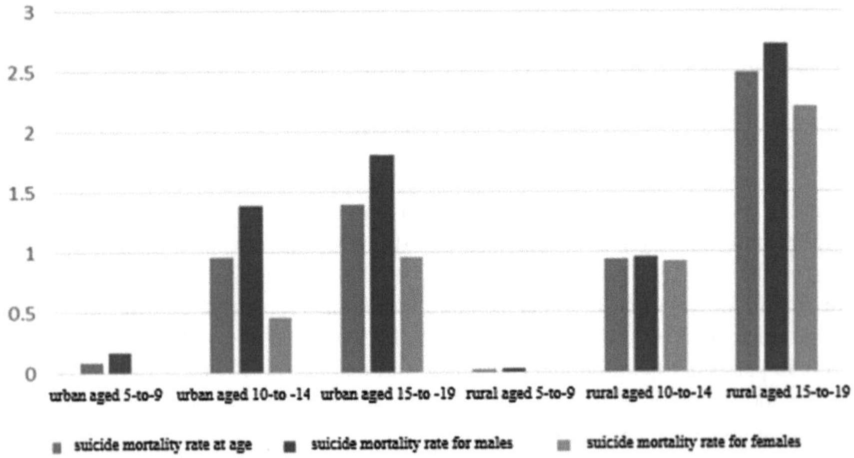

**Table 1** Gender ratio of Chinese youth suicide population from 2015 to 2017 (female = 100)

| Age<br>Year | 5–14 | 15–24 | 25–34 | 35–44 |
|---|---|---|---|---|
| 2015(male) | 131.82 | 169.50 | 144.56 | 146.99 |
| 2016(male) | 189.84 | 138.78 | 164.35 | 155.59 |
| 2017(male) | 184.78 | 160.73 | 184.98 | 162.55 |
| Average (male) | 168.81 | 156.34 | 164.63 | 155.04 |

In comparison with the above, no child suicide was reported in China prior to the 1970s.[14]

The frequent occurrence of campus suicides had a major impact. According to a survey by Social Survey Institute of China (SSIC), 26% of the college students surveyed had had thoughts of suicide.[15] In 2008, there were 63 suicides by students in universities under the direct supervision of the Ministry of Education, including 23 in Beijing and 23 in Shanghai. Fourteen college students in Beijing committed suicide in the first half of 2009, while in Guangdong three students from one university jumped from a height in February that year. In March and April, five consecutive cases of student suicide occurred in Hubei Province to doctoral candidates, postgraduate students and undergraduate students. According to the Education Bureau of Dongguan, Guangdong, in the second half of 2009 alone more than ten primary and high school students committed suicide. One of these cases caused quite a stir: An 11-year-old primary school student from Hunan Province hang herself with a red scarf in a rented house in Dongguan. A week later, a 12-year-old boy from a boarding school in Jinning County, Yunnan Province, also ended his life with a red scarf strung off a bed frame. This "red scarf knot of death" is an indictment of the missteps and inadequacies of parents, schools, and even society's psychological intervention as a whole.[16]

At the Third National Conference on Mental Health Work held in October 2001, then-Deputy Health Minister Yin Dakui stated, "Each year, around 250,000 people take their own lives around the country and the estimated number of attempted suicides exceed two million. Out of the 370 million children and adolescents aged below 17 in China, around 30 million are bothered by emotional and mental problems … By the year 2020, China's mental health burden will increase to a quarter of the overall national health burden."[17]

In December 2002, Beijing Huilongguan Hospital officially announced the results of a seven-year survey it conducted at the inaugural International Suicide Prevention Symposium held by the Beijing Psychological Crisis Research and

---

[14]Zhai (1997, p. 184).

[15]Fang (2010).

[16]Fang (2010).

[17]Yin (2002).

Intervention Center: Suicide was the fifth leading cause of death in China and the top cause of death in the 15–34 age group.[18]

### 1.2 Gender Ratio of Youth Suicide

In the Chinese mainland, more girls than boys commit suicide.

Generally, the suicide rate among boys is higher than among girls. Émile Durkheim, father of modern sociology and suicide studies, posits in *Suicide* that "more males commit suicide than females" and that "suicide is primarily a male phenomenon."[19] These statements have been taken as axioms in suicide studies.

In 1988, the male-to-female ratio for suicides in the 15–24 age group in the USA was 291.9:100, while that in the 25–34 age group was 438:100, roughly four men to one woman.[20] The opposite is true in the Chinese mainland, where women are overrepresented among those who commit suicide, especially in rural areas. More specifically, in the 15–24 age group, the female suicide rate is nearly twice as high as the male rate. According to the WHO, between 1987 and 1989, the male-to-female ratio worldwide for suicides in the 15–24 age group was 52.9:100, while that in the 25–34 age group was 75.6:100 (see Table 2 and Fig. 9).

The high suicide rate of young women, especially rural women, which is unique to China, is a prominent social problem.

In Hong Kong and Taiwan, the suicide rate is higher and is aligned with the international norm. According to Lester, the male-to-female ratio in Hong Kong is 121:100, and in Taiwan, 124:100.[21] The male-to-female ratio for suicides in Hong Kong in 1996 was 150:100.[22] The male-to-female ratio for suicides in Hong Kong among those aged under 19 was 113:100 (53.1–46.9%).[23]

## 2 Suicide Tends to Occur at a Lower Age

In China, suicides among children and adolescents are mostly attributable to school stress, family problems, and psychological issues. This calls for heightened attention and effective prevention. In the opinion of Hiroshi Uchimura, a high suicide rate among 15- to 24-year-olds may be a sign of social unrest.[24]

---

[18]Lin (2002).

[19]Durkheim (1998).

[20]WHO (1990, p. 117).

[21]Lester (1994).

[22]Suen (1996).

[23]http://www.sps.org.hk/sps-stat.htm. Accessed: 10 January 2012.

[24]Uchimura (1978).

**Table 2** Gender ratio of suicides among Chinese youths, 1987–1989 (female = 100)

| Year | Age | | | |
|---|---|---|---|---|
| | 5–14 | 15–24 | 25–34 | 35–44 |
| 1987 (male) | 110.2 | 51.9 | 76.8 | 93.9 |
| 1988 (male) | 114.0 | 55.6 | 82.3 | 89.8 |
| 1989 (male) | 65.2 | 51.6 | 69.8 | 85.9 |
| Average (male) | 97.9 | 52.9 | 75.6 | 89.4 |

*Source* WHO (1989, 1990, pp. 346–369)

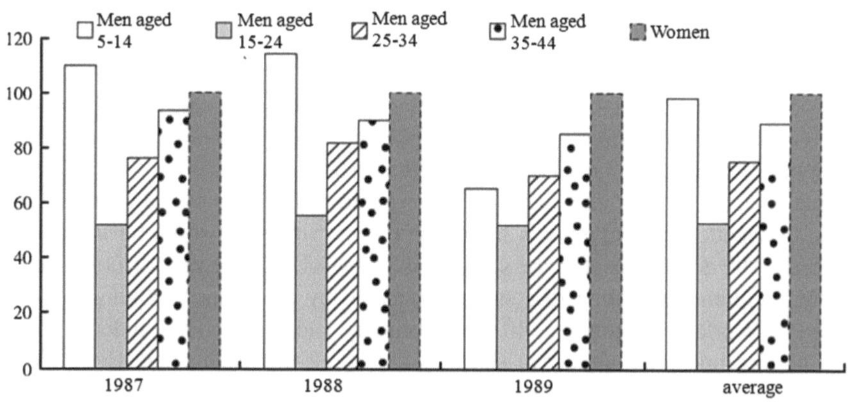


**Fig. 9** Gender ratio of suicides among Chinese youths, 1987–1989 (female = 100)

## 2.1 *Test-Oriented Education and Study-Related Stress*

In remarks made on November 27, 2010, at the 2010 National Primary and Secondary School Mental Health and Education Work Experience Exchange Meeting held in Sichuan Province, Wang Dinghua, Deputy Director of the Department of Basic Education of the Ministry of Education, said, "I am saddened by the number of suicides among primary and high school students across the country between January 1 and November 27. We have a total of 73 cases. The largest number of these occurred in Fujian province (19), followed by Sichuan province, with nine cases. Reports of such cases also came from Anhui, Shanghai, Guangxi, Shaanxi, and other places." Wang also said, "Today, schools and parents want children not only to enter university but it also needs to be a good university. More erroneously, they propound that 'a child must not lose at the starting line'." In Wang's opinion, the idea that "a child must not lose at the starting line" is "the greatest misconception" which has led to long hours of study at a young age and learning merely by reading and memorizing textbooks. This has had a tremendous impact on the mental status of students and brought on a number of problems.[25]

[25]Wang (2010).

Education has long been examination-oriented in China, and little has been done for the all-round development of students, especially their mental health. We are gradually seeing the consequences of such an approach. The all-round development of students and reducing their burden are now important tasks of primary and high school education in China during the process of social transformation. The over-burdening of primary and high school students has resulted in "sub-health" in a considerable number of young people.

### 2.1.1 Physical and Mental Health Issues Caused by Study-Related Stress

Physical health problems: The problems of overnutrition and nutritional imbalance are both seen among primary and high school students. It is common to see students with poor bodily constitutions, either too thin or too stocky. Parts of the students' bodies tend to be overused like never been before. For instance, their eyes have been overloaded, and myopia is highly prevalent. Sitting for too long is not conducive to the development of the spine, and heavy school bags can affect the height of the children. According to a study conducted by the Chinese Young Pioneers National Working Committee, 46.9% of primary and high school students do not get the recommended amount of sleep.[26] A study of the Guangzhou, Hong Kong, and Macau Youth Research Institute of Guangzhou also shows that 63.9% of the youths surveyed reported symptoms of "fatigue," 51.2% reported "poor quality of sleep/insomnia," 25.0% reported "bodily aches," and other symptoms of discomfort reported include "gastrointestinal discomfort/stomach pain" (23.8%) and dizziness (15.1%).[27]

Mental health problems: Pressure from families, schools, and peers to excel academically at the expense of everything else can take an enormous toll on young people. There is a widely held belief that doing well on tests is the only thing that matters. Such pressure can give rise to rebelliousness, learning fatigue, and the like, and affect the mental health of adolescents. Nearly, a quarter of primary and high school students present with a certain level of mental health issues and the prevalence of mental illness among these groups has increased due to social transformation, competitive pressures, the high expectations from parents, and the inability of the children to adapt.

Emotional health problems: Adolescence is a period of life that is full of hopes and dreams. Adolescents should have passion for life and be curious about the world. However, many of them are in fact indifferent to the outside world and cold and cruel to others. This has led to bullying and addiction to computer games and anime.

[26]Yang (2000a).

[27]Tan (2002).

Psychological health problems: Young people tend to think in simple and superficial ways and can be easily influenced by whatever is around them.

Behavioral problem: This is seen mostly in rigid daily routines specifying when to get up, when to have meals, when to do their homework, when to listen to English programs, etc. There is little time in such a schedule for leisure activities and can have deleterious consequences.

### 2.1.2 Suicides on the First Day of a School Term

February 8, 2000, was the first day of a new school term for primary school students in Zhengzhou, but two kids killed themselves on this day. A 12-year-old boy hanged himself from a ceiling light in his home, with a violin lying on the ground nearby. The other one is an eight-year-old boy, who jumped from the sixth floor of a building in order to avoid going to school. A local newspaper stated: "The dread of school is spreading in primary and high schools like a miasma."

On the first day of the spring term of 2000, three junior high school students (two in the first year and one in the third year) killed themselves in Jinfang City, Jiangsu Province. On the afternoon of February 2 of the same year, a 13-year-old sixth-grade boy in Nanjing was found hanging from the hanging rack inside a closet in his home. The boy had consistently ranked first in his class, but ended up in second place for the final exam in the previous semester. He committed suicide as he was afraid of seeing his teachers and classmates at school in the new semester. On February 26, 2002, when school opened after winter holiday in Yuxi, Yunnan, a fourth-grade girl who had just celebrated her tenth birthday hanged herself with two red scarfs on the anti-theft rail of her home. On the same day, an eight-year-old third-grade girl gone to school in Guiyang City on the first day of school but was asked to return when she had finished her homework for the winter. Returning home, she hanged herself in a closet. On September 19, 2011, three ten-year-old girls from a primary school in Jiujiang City, Jiangxi Province, jumped off a building holding hands together. The three did so as they would "no longer have to do any homework once dead."[28] A total of 16 primary and high school students killed themselves in Shenzhen between 2008 and 2010, and most of these cases occurred around the start of a new semester or around examinations.[29]

Why do so many children choose to end their lives on the first day of school? The first day of school should be a day when they would head to school happily to meet schoolmates and teachers after a long break, and to pick up new school supplies. However, some students would rather die than going back to school. This is a poignant reminder that we must wait no longer to address the problems with our school education.

---

[28]Wang (2011).

[29]Bao (2011).

### 2.1.3 Pressure from Teachers

Pressure from school teachers is also a reason for suicides among primary and high school students. Some teachers like to ask to speak with a student's parents as a way of admonishment. On October 27, 2000, a 14-year-old girl at a Sichuan high school poisoned herself to death. The act was explained in her suicide note: "I have decided to protest the act of asking to speak to my parents through my death." A first-year student at a junior high school in Jintan City, Jiangsu Province, was found by a teacher to have altered his result slip. The student later committed suicide by ingesting agrochemicals after his/her parents were summoned by the school.

On November 20, 2001, four third-year girls from a junior high school in Shihezi, Xinjiang Uighur autonomous region, attempted suicide by taking rat poison on the day their parents met with their teachers. Two of them died.

On the evening of May 8, 2000, a 12-year-old sixth-grade girl in Shenyang of Heilongjiang Province committed suicide by swallowing poison in her home. The girl had been made by her teacher to scribe four characters 3000 times each as punishment for having gotten them wrong earlier. She had completed a significant proportion of the task before resorting to suicide.

In June 1996, a fifth-grade boy in Jize County, Hebei Province, was asked by his teacher to pay a fine for failing an examination and subsequently committed suicide by taking pesticide. In June 1998, a third-grade girl from Changchun, Jilin Province, took her own life by lying across railway tracks after "the teacher compared her to hooligans." In February 2000, a boy in the second year of junior high school in Kunming committed suicide by taking agrochemicals as he was scolded by his teacher for failing to make it to the top three in his class in the previous semester. And in November 2001, a 14-year-old junior high school student from Hohhot, Inner Mongolia, killed himself/herself to "prove the veracity of his/her words" after being accused by a teacher of squirting ink on the teacher's clothes four times (instead of the one accidental instance that the child claimed).

In a survey involving 42 primary and high schools, 72.59% of the students clearly indicate that they had been subjected to corporal punishment, corporal punishment in disguise, and/or verbal insults by their teachers, and 38.78% of the parents reported that their children had experienced these. The study found that corporal punishment, disguised corporal punishment, and mental abuse were inflicted mainly by homeroom teachers, particularly younger ones.[30]

In 2002, Lao Shengkai and Sun Yunxiao led a study on the physical harm to children and adolescents in China. The team surveyed 6000 students from the fifth grade to the second year of junior high school across ten provinces and municipalities, and the results were as follows: Up to 30.8% of the children surveyed were most afraid of "criticism and corporal punishment by the teacher," 29.5% feared "being looked down upon" most, 19.4% feared "examinations" most, and 11.3% were most afraid of "being bullied by classmates." Meanwhile, for the following forms of punishment,

[30]Li (2001, p. 215).

17.1% of the students surveyed reported having received them "often," while another 24.1% reported having experienced them "occasionally." These include: being made to stand or run as punishment by the teacher, being detained at school after classes were over, being scorned, taunted, or rebuked, being prohibited from entering the classroom to attend class, being made to scribe text or homework multiple times, and being hit by teachers. Also, 19.9% of children said that they had opted to tell no one or had no one to confide in when such things happened to them.[31]

According to a survey of 2000 primary school students conducted by the Nanjing Research Center of Education Science, 40.1% of the surveyed said they had uttered the words "I would be better off dead" and around 40% responded "No" or "Not really" when asked if they thought their homeroom teacher liked them. However, more than 90% of the teachers surveyed answered affirmatively and then were asked if they liked the students in their class.[32]

Schools are where children are educated and teachers should be role models who teach by doing. However, in recent years, unbelievable things have happened in schools: Students were made to eat feces, to slap each other, and to endure carvings of words on their faces and even the cutting off of a finger. Sexual assault has also occurred. All these were committed, astoundingly, by teachers who were to educate and to nurture their students. In these cases—admittedly involving a tiny minority of teachers—the teachers, who are compared to gardeners who nurture and care for young flowers, have mutilated or even killed those under their care. These infuriating incidents have occurred in part due to the poor legal awareness and the lack of a moral code among some teachers, but mental distortions are also an important factor that cannot be ignored.

According to study results released by the Shanghai Primary School Teacher Mental Health Research Group, mental health issues have been detected in 48% of primary school teachers in Shanghai. In particular, 12% presented with clear signs of poor mental health, and 2% showed serious symptoms.[33] We can hence deduce the general mental health status of primary school teachers in China at present. The National Primary and Secondary School Mental Health Education Research Group conducted a study of 2292 teachers working in 168 urban and rural schools in the Province of Liaoning, and the result showed that 51.23% of the teachers had mental problems, with 32.18% presenting with mild symptoms, 16.56% with moderate symptoms, and 2.49% with symptoms that can be classified as mental illness.[34] A 1998 survey of the health status of 1000 urban and rural school teachers showed that 88% of high school teachers and 77.84% of primary school teachers presented with fairly serious symptoms of depression and anxiety, feeling more "frustration" than "joy."[35] In fact, mental problems are present among teachers in general,

[31]Liu (2003).
[32]Xi (2001).
[33]Yi (2000).
[34]Qian (2003).
[35]Yu (2001).

including those at any level or type of school, though such problems may differ in terms of seriousness and prevalence.

In the course of social transformation, competition mechanisms were introduced into schools and pressure from society, school authorities, and families increased for teachers. To make things worse, teachers in China are generally overloaded and may have nowhere to vent their feelings. Some have thus chosen to vent on the relatively weak (i.e., students) to achieve some kind of mental balance. This represents a somewhat deviated and distorted mind-set of some teachers. Mandated to educate, teachers interact directly with students with pure and innocent minds. How can we expect students to be mentally healthy if teachers are not? How can we expect students to have balanced minds and normal moods if teachers are neurotic and emotionally erratic, employ excessive punishment with students, and act coldly to them? Students who feel helpless in the face of attacks from their teachers may turn toward themselves. Thus, the harm caused to students by teachers with poor mental health is no less than the impact of poor teaching ability on students' academic performance. To ensure mental health of students, teachers must first have a healthy mind as mentally unhealthy teachers are likely to "produce" a constant stream of students with unfit mental statuses. While society in general is paying more attention to students' mental health, it is imperative that we start working on improving teachers' mental health.

### 2.1.4 Bullying and Youth Suicides

Bullying is a particular type of aggressive behavior that often occurs among children and adolescents, especially primary and high school students. Bullying poses great harm to the physical and mental health of the bullied. Frequent bullying often leads to depression, distraction, loneliness, truancy, deterioration in academic performance, and insomnia, and can even lead to suicide.[36] For the bully, the act of bullying others can also upgrade into violent crimes or behavioral disorders in the future. Bullying is common and one of the causes of youth suicides. Some helpless children who are bullied (especially in violent ways) may project the violence inward and kill themselves.

In primary and high schools, students are bullied less as they grow older, but boys tend to bully more as they grow while the opposite is true for girls. The most common form of violent bullying that boys adopt is physical attack. Among girls, the preferred methods are indirect ones such as verbal attacks and mental bullying. Peers play an important role in bullying among youths for bullying is more often than not a group behavior. Gang-like groups are common among students in China, and these groups often engage in fights or bully others.

[36]Sharp and Smith (1994).

## 2.2 *Suicide at a Lower Age and Mental Maladies*

Many cases of child suicide are caused by schizophrenia or depression, showing a close relationship between child suicides and depressive symptoms such as depression and low self-esteem. As early as a century ago, Sigmund Freud observed that almost all mental health issues traced back to traumatic experiences during childhood.

### 2.2.1 The Worrying State of Psychological Health Among China's Minors

In October 2001, Yin Dakui, then Vice Health Minister, stated: "A survey shows that about 30 million of the 340 million children and adolescents under the age of 17 in China are suffering from emotional disorders and mental and behavioral problems." The results of another survey show that 17–20% of children in major cities in China have various types of mental problems, including "test syndrome," social phobia, and personality disorders, which are manifested as varying degrees of insomnia, depression, anxiety, the dread of school, hypomnesia, and even hallucinations and psychiatric disorders.

Mental illness has already leapt to the top of the world's top ten diseases. Currently, among all patients with mental illness in China, one-third have the onset during childhood or adolescence. Statistics show that mental problems are present in 20–30% of households in China. Zheng Richang conducted a study in several large cities in the late 1980s and found that the older the students, the higher the frequency of mental problems: Students with mental problems accounted for about 13% of primary school students, 15% of junior high school students, 19% of senior high school students, and 25% of college students.[37]

Another survey shows that 35% of high school students in China currently have mental abnormalities and that 5.3% have depression, phobia, obsessive-compulsive disorder, or other mental disorders.[38] Patients under the age of 25 accounted for about 40% of the 40,000 patients seeking help at the Mental Health Hospital of China Medical University in 2000. The Beijing Huilongguan Hospital started a clinic for depression in May 2000, and more than half of the patients there during the half-month were under 16 years old, with the youngest patient being only two-and-a-half years old. A survey was conducted in Hefei, Anhui Province, with 3300 high school students aged 16–18 using the cluster sampling method and Symptom Checklist-90 (SCL-90) and the Family Environment Scale (Chinese version) (FES-CV). The data collected was analyzed using SPSS, and the results showed that 68.5% of youths with suicidal ideation had at least two mental symptoms.[39]

---

[37]Zheng (1994, p. 1).

[38]Qian (2003).

[39]Xu (2001).

A survey done by the research group for mental health nurturing of primary and high school students of the Institute of Developmental Psychology of Beijing Normal University in July 2005 shows that among the 16,472 primary and high school students surveyed in Beijing, Henan, Chongqing, Zhejiang, and Xinjiang, 20.6% of primary school students, 17.1% of junior high school students, and 17.3% of senior high school students presented with signs of mental abnormalities or serious mental and behavioral problems.[40] Respondents were measured against indicators in six dimensions of mental health, and the rate of those showing medium or higher levels of problems is ranked separately for primary school, junior high school, and senior high school students. The results are as follows: For primary school students, the ranking was interpersonal relationships, emotional state, self-control, motivation, self-concept, and evaluation of one's own learning abilities; for junior high school students, self-control, emotional state, evaluation of one's own learning abilities, self-concept, interpersonal relationships, and motivation; and for senior high school students, self-control, emotional state, evaluation of one's own learning abilities, self-concept, interpersonal relationships, and motivation.[41]

In November 2006, Guo Xianghui, et al. conducted a survey of 1405 junior high school students from Sanlitun Middle School of Beijing and used SPSS ver. 11.5 for data analysis and validation. The results are as follows: In the 12 months prior to the survey, 16.8% of the students experienced suicidal ideation, 5.9% had intentions of suicide, 2.0% attempted suicide, 23.3% thought about running away from home, and 2.8% left home.[42]

"Depression is felt within but originates externally." The impact of the external environment is a major cause of personality disorders in youths and children. Child personality disorders are a class of mental illnesses involving severe personality defects or pathological personality deviations or otherwise generally unsuitable personalities. These disorders manifest as disorders of emotions, will, and behavior. However, patients may still have clear thinking and normal intelligence. Patients generally have poor control over thoughts of suicide, and this makes them more prone to suicidal behavior. Most children today are the only child in their families and are doted on by their parents. They are well cared for and as a consequence develop stronger self-centeredness. When schooling starts, these children have to grapple with the stern faces of their teachers, heavy school pressures, the high hopes of their parents, as well as competition from their peers. On top of these may be long-term lack of social interactions, which, together, can make the kids solitary, autistic, socially isolated, and hence extremely prone to developing personality disorders. In recent years, teachers and parents have found themselves at a loss as to how to deal with increasingly fragile children.

---

[40] Xie (2005).

[41] Yu (2010).

[42] Guo (2008).

A total of 61 cases of suicide occurred between 1987 and 1991 among the young patients seeking help at Nanjing Child Mental Health Research Center. The oldest of these was 15, and the youngest, 7. The average age was 13.3.[43]

In 2006, Shanghai Ideological and Political Work Research Association and the Youth Research Institute of the Shanghai Academy of Social Sciences published the *Blue Book on Adolescent Mental Health.* According to it, emotional health among young people in Shanghai requires great concern. Around 24.7% of the individuals studied had emotional disorders, 21.1% presented with a certain degree of emotional problems, while only 55.2% maintained "normal levels" of emotional health. However, the mean score (15.68) was much higher than the general Chinese mean based on the Center for Epidemiologic Studies Depression Scale (CES-D), which was 11.52.

According to a survey conducted by the Shanghai Primary and Secondary School Psychological Counseling Association, mental problems among children aged 6–11 also call for attention. Various behavioral disorders are detected in 23.2% of children in this age group, which is much higher than the 13.9% of senior high school students and 9.1% of junior high school students. In particular, the incidence of attention deficit disorder (ADD) is the top problem.[44]

According to an adolescent mental problem survey of Shenzhen published by the Shenzhen Center for Disease Control and Prevention in 2008, 12.1% of the students surveyed had considered suicide and 2.2% had made attempts. Among the reasons cited for suicidal behavior, 24.4% mentioned school stress.[45]

A 2010 mental health survey conducted among students of district-level schools in Shanghai showed that 22.8% of the students were vexed by interpersonal problems, including their relationships with family members, teachers, and classmates; 3.8% of high school students reported very poor interpersonal relationships and difficulty in getting along with others. Up to 62.6% of the students surveyed felt heavy school pressure, and the rate for junior high school students was highest, at 66.8%, followed by senior high school students (60.4%) and primary school students (59.9%).[46]

### 2.2.2 Defects in Emotional, Personality, and Humanity Education for the Young

Sound emotional education is the basis for personality building. Mental state and character are important factors in the formation of personality, but they are usually neglected in our education today. Such negligence is, on the one hand, due to the difficulty of delivering such education effectively; on the other hand, it resulted

[43]Luo (1992).

[44]Liang (2006).

[45]Bao and Zhou (2011).

[46]Su (2011).

from the heavy workload in other fronts in schools and the lack of a direct connection between emotional education and academic performance. Moreover, current school education is highly uniform and the characteristics of individual students are often ignored and even rejected. As such, the strong competitive pressure in one single aspect (academic performance) at school, some students develop distorted and deviated personalities in varying degrees. However, what causes even more concern is that many people do not think this is a problem.

We can only talk about humanity education on the basis of normal personality. School and family education alike should be people-oriented. This means that each student should be truly regarded as a "person" so that their emotions and personality can be fully understood and respected. Every child has a "small world" that is peculiar to his or her age, and it is this diversity that determines the richness of man. Although it is impossible to have all the needs of every individual fully met, we should still seek to create a healthy atmosphere that supports every child as a unique person. We should first bring them up to be healthy persons. That comes before development in every other aspect. If not, our obsession with some utilitarian purposes may deprive the kids of their right to be "persons" without us even knowing.

Only with comprehensive and healthy development in all aspects of their emotions, personality, and humanity can young people feel for themselves the dignity of being a person, and appreciate and understand naturally the value of life. If schools, families, and society are highly critical and demanding of children under all circumstances, they will become highly demanding of themselves and of others under all conditions. Such individuals can be thrown off-kilter mentally by the smallest of disappointments and even commit suicide as a result.

It may be very confusing for many adults how a child, young as he/she is, can possibly cover the long and painful journey from life to death in the mind. Actually, young people (especially younger children) usually have not yet developed respect for life and do not have a clear understanding of what death means. Children have yet to obtain the cognitive ability to fully understand the logic of cause and effect, and they are not yet capable of a rational expectation of the outcome of self-harm or suicide. Generally, young children do not really understand the true meaning of death and it is usually not until they are about ten years old that they begin to feel some fear for the consequences of suicide. Children are emotionally immature, and the majority of those who commit suicide are prone to anxiety and depression. Impulsive suicidal behavior can be triggered by unexpected blows. Meanwhile, it is also worth noting that many cartoons from Japan and the USA tend to disseminate a highly unserious attitude toward life and death among children. In electronic games, a character can come back to life again and again after being killed. For example, in the Disney cartoon Tom and Jerry, which is highly popular among Chinese children, Tom the cat is blown up, thrown against hard surfaces, drowned, crushed, or becomes hole-ridden but it will always survive. Such plots may give viewers quite an unserious understanding of life and death, which brings nothing more than fun. In Japanese "pocket books" widely welcomed among children, the theme of death is played up in many stories. As such, children are induced into appreciating death from an aesthetic point of view. The playing up of death as a theme in television, films, and games has also had a subtle influence on children. In particular, direct shows of suicide provide curious children with something to imitate. Our young generation today has grown up immersed in television and online media, and such media forms an indispensable part of education for them in the process of socialization.

### 2.2.3 Family Factors for Child Suicide

Families are the cells of society, where individuals are brought up. One's home is the starting point of his/her socialization process, and parents serve as the first mentors of their kids. The home has a direct impact on how a child thinks, acts, and feels. Many child and youth suicides are caused by serious conflicts in the home.

The environment of the home is the sum of the material living conditions and social status of the family, relationships between family members, and what family members say, do, and feel. It bears direct influence on the mental development of children and adolescents and on the emergence and development of suicidal ideation. The environment of the home includes the physical environment, the verbal environment, the mental environment, and the interpersonal environment. Vast amounts of data show that children and youths who commit suicide are likely to come from families where members are not treated equal, where there is interpersonal tension, where affection is absent, where the parents educate the children in inappropriate ways, and where it is hard to make ends meet. This is especially true in rural families. Of course, the impact of the family environment involves multiple aspects, occurs on multiple levels, and thus cannot be generalized or neatly summarized.

The home is a major source of subjective experience, physical awakening, and external behavior for children and adolescents, and a lack of equality and harmony in the home tends to have profound influence on the physical and mental well-being of children and adolescents. Dislocated subjective experience starts a complex awakening process on the physiological front, which may in turn result in aberrant behavior. This is usually how the mental basis is laid for kids. Early education in the home has an impact, to one degree or another, on suicidal ideation and behavior in children and adolescents.

Parents are the most important teachers of their kids. They not only provide the first experience of education, but also have strong emotional bonds with the kids. Moreover, children are economically dependent on their parents. All these determine that the parents play a role in the course of the children's socialization that cannot be replaced by any social group. The home provides early experience, shapes the initial personality traits of the children, and lays the foundation for subsequent education and personality development. Further, even as a kid continues to develop, the home remains a central point of reference in the education process. The home plays an important role in the academic success and personality formation of young people. Similarly, family-related factors also play their roles in suicide cases.

## The Impact of Discipline in the Home

Chinese scholars identified and named various parenting styles such as "overindulgent parenting," the "authoritarian parenting," "inspiring parenting," and "laissez-faire parenting." Another classification includes "rejecting parenting," "strict parenting," "parenting of high expectations," "contradictory parenting," and "divergent parenting."[47]

There is a close relationship between parenting styles and child suicide. In Chinese tradition, the mother is responsible for caring for the child while the father is responsible for disciplining the child. The child is cared for mainly by the mother in his/her early years which has a greater impact on the child's personality. Mothers, who intervene too much, who are overprotective, rejective, and negative, who punishes heavily, or who are emotionally unstable or neurotic, may plant the seed of child suicide in their children. Fathers generally adopt a stricter parenting style (after the child's early years) and also tend to mete out more severe punishments. They have high expectations of their children and tend to reject more of the children's requests than mothers. Chinese parents tend to regard their children as part of their possessions and their subordinates rather than autonomous individuals. As such, they tend to control, manipulate, and punish their children more.[48] Parenting styles characterized by excessive refusal and denial are manifested as lack of respect for the child's will, ignoring the child's needs, the frequent denial of the child's abilities, or excessive criticism of the child's actions. These are likely to give rise to an indelible poor self-esteem in the child whenever he/she is in front of adults. Punitive actions may take the forms of corporal punishment, disguised corporal punishment, scolding and insults, etc. They may lead the child to internalize the parents excessively harsh and frequent punishments, chiding, and demands and form a superego with extremely high moral standards. Children with such superegos are typically overly demanding on themselves in regard to their personal behavior, attitudes, and desires, and easily develop a clear sense of guilt, shame, and self-blame, laying the ground for neurosis[49] as well as suicide. The majority of children who grow up in such homes face great mental pressure and tend to be stressed, vexed, irritable, and anxious. They will also probably experience a sense of emptiness and helplessness, and live in despair and pessimism about the world. Children who grow up under the authoritarian parenting style often pick up fights easily; are aggressive and arrogant; find it hard to cooperate with others, form meaningful relationships, or see things from in a different perspective than their own; and experience mood swings, lack self-motivation, and are indifferent toward incentives and punishments. Conversely, children who grow up in democratic homes are more compassionate, enjoy good relationships, understand others better, are emotionally stable, turn out to be better listeners, and are better

---

[47]Hu et al. (1999, 52).

[48]Yue et al. (1993).

[49]Hu et al. (1999, p. 54).

motivated. Children who grow up in overindulgent homes are generally poor at self-management and more likely to suffer setbacks in interpersonal relationships as they tend to grow up as "little tyrants" as a result of the all-encompassing care of their parents.

Many parents understand family education to have more to do with knowledge than anything else and focus only on academic performance. Some pay lip service to moral education in addition. This is why many young people today are indifferent, solitary, and emotionally ill-developed. Very few parents understand the importance of emotional education. Quite a number of parents even believe academic success to be the only thing that matters for their children and regard emotional development to be nothing important. What these parents fail to understand is that an individual who lacks love will be indifferent not only to people around him/her but also to himself/herself.

Currently, there is a saying that "five plus two equals minus one." It describes the phenomenon that as children go to school for five days and stay home for two each week, when the two days at home fail to play their due role, the final result may be negative rather than positive. Causes of such a failure may be one of the following two: Overly strict parents fill the kids' schedules with a variety of courses to brush up on their skills, such as piano, drawing, and English, while overly indulgent parents leave the kids unattended to while they themselves go for leisure activities such as mahjong or meeting up with friends. It seems, while reducing burdens for students, we should also make efforts to prevent this "minus one" phenomenon.

### The Impact of Interpersonal Relationships in the Home

Studies show that a sound and harmonious family environment is conducive to the healthy growth of children and adolescents and that three generations under one roof do not bring obvious drawbacks if the relationships are harmonious. The physical and mental health of children and adolescents from broken families or families where the parents quarrel a lot can be significantly affected. Such children are more likely to be lonely, indifferent, rude, and bored, and are more likely to tell lies, escape from home, be pessimistic about the world, and commit suicide.

It is normal for parents and children to have different mentalities given that they are born and raised in vastly different times and social backgrounds. As children grow up, they will likely experience a period of rebelliousness during which they may communicate less or even have conflicts with their parents. This kind of "intergenerational conflict" may become more acute as the child grows older and is very likely to cause children to become pessimistic about the world around them. On the contrary, in a harmonious family, the parent and the child get along well with no generation gap and they understand and respect one another. These are essential for the normal mental development of children and adolescents. Statistics from the USA show that poor relationship of the parents or misconduct by them is a direct cause of suicides by their children.[50]

US Psychologist Frederick Herzberg once conducted a survey on children and youths aged from eight to fourteen in more than 20 countries on all the five continents around the world and found that what children asked of their parents and what they were unhappy about were quite similar across countries, races, and societies. Children do not place that much emphasis on the economic conditions and social status of their families. Instead, whether they are happy depends on whether the family can give them a true sense of belonging and make them deeply loved and cared for. What children were most displeased with was quarreling between their parents.[51] Liu Jiucheng reports that among the fifteen cases of child suicide in Shuangliu County, Sichuan, seven were caused by family strife.[52] Taylor Stansfeld found through a study of the family backgrounds of children who committed suicide by poisoning that family quarrels occurred in 32.1% of the cases studied, 21.4% of the families involved had separated parents, serious mental illness occurred in 10.7% of the families, another 10.7% suffered from serious physical ailments of their members, and for 3.6% of the cases, death of the parent(s) was involved.[53]

### The Impact of Family Structure

The family structure in urban China has undergone tremendous changes in recent decades, and nuclear families have become the mainstay. With the transformation of our society, Chinese families, which used to be relatively stable based on the ties of marriage, have "loosened" in the past 20 years, with divorce rates rising. Family planning policies are another reason why the family structure has been changing. A higher divorce rate produced more single-parent families and remarried families, and more children are brought up in such families. In addition, it is also common for parents to remain married but live separate lives. Moreover, more than a hundred million young and middle-aged rural laborers now stay far from home to work in cities and rural family structure has thus also changed significantly. The weakening of family ties and the disintegration of families are key reasons for the rise in child suicide rate. When the family unit disintegrates, the biggest victims are the children. The rate of suicides among children and adolescents from single-parent families and remarried families is relatively higher.

The sudden changes in family structure can have a huge impact on children. A considerable number of children find themselves at a loss when changes in the

[50]Joffe and Offord (1983).
[51]Li (2001, p. 217).
[52]Liu et al. (1991).
[53]He (1997).

family environment occur, and they may experience much more mental stress than parents and teachers expect.

A survey of primary school students shows that more than 50% of students with mental disorders come from families with a history of divorce and some are from single-parent families. The consequences of mental disorders are manifested not only as learning disorders.[54] Parenting by divorced and remarried parents can often be problematic. In particular, "evil stepparents" can be a nightmare for many children. Remarried families are often unable to provide children with the care and love that they need, and the children may thus feel abandoned. Naturally, they can feel disappointed, lonely, and cynical, and these feelings in turn may trigger suicide ideation. Therefore, changes in the family structure can have a bearing on the current life of the child and, more importantly, have a decisive impact on how the child turns out in the future.

Children who live in desperation in a broken family do not enjoy a carefree and idyllic childhood.

"How would we act as fathers now?" This was a question that the writer Lu Xun posed with some pain in 1919. Lu also proposed the slogan of "The Young Front and Center." He wrote: Those who have awakened should first liberate their children, and "take up the heavy burden of treading the old ways again and again on their own two feet and carry the gates of darkness on their own shoulders, and let them out to a place that is expansive and filled with light [so that] they can henceforth live happily and live as reasonable persons."[55] The one cry that had pierced the darkness of those times was Lu's cry of "Save the children!" Nearly a century later, would we have to cry the same cry again?

## 3 The "Twitter Effect" and Youth Suicide

In Emile Durkheim's opinion, the influence of a role model is sufficient to trigger imitative or copycat suicide. D. P. Phillips termed this the Werther effect, while in Japan this is known as the Okada Yukiko syndrome.[56]

Many studies have shown that detailed reports of suicide cases in movies, television, radio, newspapers and magazines, and especially the ubiquitous "fourth media," i.e., the Internet, in recent years, have directly led to a sharp increase in the number of suicide or attempted suicide cases.

Some scholars also believe that both reports of real and fictitious suicide cases can lead to an increase in suicide rate.[57]

---

[54]Ma (1999).

[55]Lu (1919).

[56]*Liberation Daily* (1986, December 23), 3.

[57]Liu and Xiao (2007).

## 3.1 Media Influence and the "Celebrity Effect"

News reports that are most likely to cause imitative suicides are those that contain detailed descriptions of how the suicide was committed but give no account of the physical disabilities caused, the suffering of committing suicides, or the horrible scene. Such reports usually give no mention to the long-term mental problems suffered by the suicide victims in their lifetimes; simplify and romanticize the causes of suicide; and render suicides for love in a "lyrical" or "poetic" manner. People who receive such information can be misled into thinking that committing suicide can free them from their pain in the real world and send them along the way to "the kingdom of heaven," "paradise," or the "afterlife." Or, they may be lured into thinking that committing suicide can make them "famous." For example, suicide bombings by Palestinians in the Palestinian–Israeli conflict have occurred in waves in what is known as the "CNN phenomenon."[58] Between 1973 and 1979, due to excessive reporting of suicides on television, the average annual suicide rate in the USA increased by 13.0% among women and 5.5% among men.[59]

The Australian Sociologist Riaz Hassan analyzed 19,425 cases of suicide that occurred in Australia between 1981 and 1990 and found that the number of men killing themselves, especially young men, would spike in the three days following each report of a suicide case in local newspapers. Over the decade covered by this study, an average of 4.13 men committed suicide in Australia every day. In comparison, the average of the three days following each newspaper report on suicide cases was 4.62 per day.[60]

Television programs about suicide offer examples for young people to follow. When an idol or popular media character (such as those in television programs or films) commits suicide or shows signs of suicidal ideation, or dies, the number of youth suicides may increase. Young people may resort to imitative suicide because they have limited experience of life and lack a fully developed personality and a clear understanding of the relatively abstract concepts of life and death. These factors can lead to the so-called targeted seeking behavior,[61] wherein one imitates what someone similar to him/her does in real life, in art, in television, in films, or even in computer games. Thus, young people take the extreme path and pay the price with their lives.

In November 1998, the first ever case of charcoal-burning suicide was reported in Hong Kong. Local media romanticized and simplified the event, claiming the method to cause no pain and lead to no disfigurement. As a result, suicide by burning charcoal soon went rampant. By 2001, 25% of the suicide cases in Hong

---

[58]"CNN" stands for the Cable News Network. It is generally believed that the network's sustained reporting of suicide bombings has played a role in inducing and fueling further suicide bombings.

[59]http://health.fan8.com/data/200279/1995508074.htm. Accessed: 10 August 2009.

[60]News of suicides lead to chains of suicides. *The Elite Reference*, May 24, 1996, 3.

[61]Cui, Xinjia and Zhou, Dasheng. New developments in overseas studies of the problem of youth suicide. *Foreign Medical Sciences*, 4(4), 207.

Kong had involved charcoal-burning, and the method replaced hanging as the second most frequently used method of suicide in Hong Kong. This trend even spread to the Chinese mainland, Macau, and the overseas Chinese communities.[62]

Famed Hong Kong Singer and Actor Leslie Cheung leapt to his death on the evening of April 1, 2003, and the event was widely covered in the media. Six people followed suit within only 9 h. The Hong Kong SAR Government and a number of local psychologists therefore made an urgent call that fans of Cheung with the tendency of committing suicide should be watched closely and not be left alone to listen to Cheung's music.[63]

In the days immediately following Cheung's suicide, a number of cases of suicide and attempted suicide occurred among young people in Beijing as well. Although we cannot assert that Leslie Cheung's suicide triggered a mental health crisis among his fans, and even induced suicide in some, what we can be certain of given Cheung's status as a star with great appeal, is that his suicide provided a negative prompt to social psychology, a prompt that, amplified by the media, had an impact on the mental world of many young people.

It is indisputable that how celebrities behave has a demonstrative effect especially on youths. While providing information and entertainment, modern media also serves up the values of public figures as "models" to the world. This is termed as the "marketing character" by experts. Regrettably, despite the dazzling aura surrounding celebrities, these public figures are but humans and also bear tremendous amounts of pressure unbeknownst to the general public. This is why problems such as drug abuse, alcoholism, and suicide are common among celebrities. Of course, what is truly odd is not the abnormal behavior of the celebrities but the fact that such behavior is worshipped and emulated by ordinary people. The media often portrays the suicide of celebrities in a romantic fashion, creating serious imbalance in the mental world of some individuals as a result. On April 5, 1994, Kurt Cobain, Lead Singer of Nirvana, shot himself. His death brought on a massive outpouring of praise in the culture and entertainment circles. All of a sudden, suicide became fashionable.

Such advocacy of celebrities by giving poetic accounts to whatever they do can easily causes youngsters, especially celebrity chasers, to fall under delusion. Suicide has already become the main cause of death among young people in China. Under such circumstances, don't we need to pay more attention to the non-poetic consequences of the "poetic pursuit" of death?[64]

---

[62]Hong Kong media cause spate of charcoal-burning suicides worldwide. *Yahoo! News Hong Kong*. http://hk.news.yahoo.com/030303/12/qf74.html. Accessed: 10 May 2010.

[63]Leslie Cheung suicide leads to wave of tragedies in Hong Kong. *Southern Metropolis Daily*, April 4, 2003.

[64]Cai (2003).

## 3.2 Idol Worship and Suicides by Fans

Idol worship is defined as a social identification with, and emotional attachment to, a personality. According to Sigmund Freud, idol worship represents standard sexual development of adolescents as adolescents cannot direct their enhanced sexual drive solely at their parents and peers. They must also direct it toward idols, who are at a greater distance. Erich Fromm believes that idol worship is an attachment to an outstanding figure in one's imagination or fantasies, and such fantasies are often overenhanced or overidealized. E. H. Erikson understands idol worship as an expression of the shift from attachment to his/her parents in childhood to a romantic attachment to the opposite sex.

As part of the mental changes in adolescence, idol worship is an important way for adolescents to explore and better understand themselves. Sometimes, adolescents have to take certain risks before they can find themselves and complete the identification process.

The majority of idols for young people in China are movie stars and singers. In the late 1980s, many young students took rock stars like Cui Jian as their "absolute heroes." There are commonly two types of attachment to idols: romantic attachment (the hope of becoming the "lover" of the idol) and identificatory attachment (the hope of becoming someone like the idol). A detailed survey of 2500 young people in Hong Kong in 1997 showed that teenagers who base their moral judgments on their idols' are more likely to perform erroneous behavior and are less likely to accept positive ethics. They are also more likely to lack confidence when solving problems.[65] Compared to non-celebrity chasers, the celebrity chasers among Hong Kong's secondary school students show significantly lower self-confidence.

Adolescents are generally attached to, and learn from the social behavior of, specific personalities, such as famous singers, movie stars, or sports stars. Such attachment is likely to be intuitive, emotional, and extreme.[66] One manifestation is what is known as direct modeling, which means that an individual simply copies the worldview, mannerisms, and even appearance and hobbies of his/her idol. This can be seen among the fans of Elvis Presley, Michael Jackson, Madonna Louise Veronica Ciccone, and the late Diana Spencer in the West and among chasers of Faye Wong, Nicholas Tse, Jay Chou, and Andy Lau in China. The second manifestation is "total acceptance," where an individual identifies with and worships the idol's behavior and values without question. That is, when a person takes someone as an idol, he or she will unconditionally accept all qualities associated with the idol no matter if these qualities are worthy. In such cases, the person also willingly rejects other people's identification with, and reliance on, other idols, such as in the case of feuds between fans of different celebrities and fights between fans of different sporting teams. The third manifestation is "preoccupied attachment," which is when attachment is built upon the negative assessment of the self. Studies show

[65]Chan et al. (1997).

[66]Yue (1999).

that preoccupied attachment can easily lead to reliance on, and reverence for, others, and such reliance and reverence are used as indicators of self-confidence. For many celebrity chasers, the attachment to an idol is based on self-censure, and the more one worships the idol, the more negative the person feels about himself/herself. Therefore, a simple rumor that a certain famous singer or movie star died can easily sink some of his/her fans into despair and even cause them to commit suicide.

Personage-centered social learning and attachment can lead to an intuitive, irrational, and mystical approach to one's idols and role models, and cause adolescents to be overly obsessed with the appearance of their idols. This can be highly detrimental to their growth.

## 3.3 *Instigation of Publications Such as* the Complete Manual of Suicide

In 1993, *The Complete Manual of Suicide* by Tsurumi Wataru was published by Ohta Books in Japan to great sensation. Some 500,000 copies of the book were distributed between July 1993 and February 1994, which was a rarity for the Japanese publishing world. In February 1994, Tsurumi published another book, *Our Opinion on "The Complete Manual of Suicide*," which made things worse.

*The Complete Manual of Suicide* is indeed an "encyclopedia of suicide methods," introducing in detail 11 main approaches such as poisoning (including types of poisons, dosages, method of consumption, and expected post-consumption sensations), hanging, jumping from heights, slitting the carotid or wrist artery, motor vehicle crashes, gas poisoning, electrocution, drowning, self-immolation, freezing to death, etc. The book also details other aspects of suicide, such as the choice of method, timing, location, how long it takes, how much pain to expect, what preparations are required, and how the corpse looks with a liberal use of photographic illustrations. At the same time, a number of "case studies" are also included. All these made the book the most convenient "suicide textbook" for young people.

The launch of the book caused a great furor, but the book still sold extremely well. It was soon published in a number of other languages. What is quite worrisome is that the full text of the Chinese version can still be found online using domestic Chinese search engines. Translated by Ding Shen, it was released in Taiwan on December 1, 1994, by Jasmine Publishing, but was soon banned in both Taiwan and Hong Kong. In particular, the work was categorized by the Hong Kong authorities as a Class III book, meaning that any publishing, sales, and dissemination of the work are prohibited. In Japan, local governments at various levels began issuing bans on the book in 1997. In recent years, the Chinese language version of the book has been widespread online and has drawn the attention of the police in the Chinese mainland, Hong Kong, and Taiwan alike.

In 2003, a Japanese film company made a horror film under the same name starring Morishita Chisato, Mizuhashi Kenji, Nakamura Yûko, and Maeda Ayaka. The film, which is based on Tsurumi's book, caused a sensation in Japan, as well as in the Greater China region.

The Ministry of Public Security of the People's Republic of China made its first official statement concerning the Chinese version of *The Complete Manual of Suicide*, which is available online, on March 30, 2005: In the case that harmful information that helps others commit suicide is disseminated online and it constitutes a crime, criminal responsibility shall be investigated in accordance with the law, and punishments shall be meted out where public security regulations and cyberspace administration rules are violated.[67]

On April 11, 2005, a female high school student in Taiwan and a friend she had made online were found to have killed themselves by burning charcoal in a hotel room in Fengshan City. The computer crime task force of the police department found to two to have joined an online community focused on suicide, and the full text of *The Complete Manual of Suicide* was seen in their e-mail boxes. It is suspected that they planned their suicide by referring to the book. On December 30, 2007, a young man from Taoyuan County, Taiwan, whose wedding was scheduled for the next day, was found by his father to have hung himself with a piece of electrical wire strung from the window pane in his new home. There were also several cuts on the man's wrist and a pool of blood on the ground. Police investigation revealed that the man had left his computer on showing the online text of *The Complete Manual of Suicide*.

## 3.4 The Influence of Unsavory Animation Content

Over the past twenty years, a large quantity of comic book content (printed and online versions, mainly from Japan) have quietly gained ground among Chinese children. Except for a small number of formal publications, most of them are illegal pocket books that are bundled with anime content, online videos, and video games. The influence of online comic content has grown significantly in the last few years. Such content generally focuses on campus life, romance, martial arts, and violence, and some are of a comedic nature. Death is a perennial topic. Many Japanese anime stories combine violence, sex, and death (including suicide). Such content exerts a great influence on children who are inundated by image-dominated content before they are fully capable of choosing what to read for themselves.

Japanese anime has become popular among a large number of Chinese youths. These young readers have become increasingly fascinated by certain animated titles to the extent that they identify with and imitate the characters in these works. Thus, their mind-set and behavior are likely to be changed. "What kind of behavior people

[67] He (2005).

adopt in time and space depends on the 'customs' or 'rules' (code) of a certain culture that exists behind them. These 'codes' restrict one's behavior in various situations."[68]

In 2005, with the spread of the Japanese manga *Densha Otoko* to China, the term "otaku" (*yuzhai*)[69] became popular in China. It was even used to refer to those who have a superlative knowledge of the manga/anime culture or who are otherwise highly regarded within the circle. To these anime fans, there are two worlds: One is the real world known to adults, and the other is the world of manga/anime that exists on television and online. In the real world, these fans are subjected to various arrangements, attempts at shaping them, and manipulation; in the world of manga/anime, however, they are the true masters of themselves and have their own homes.

Young people have a strong desire to imitate others and express themselves. However, when they imitate, create, and be part of a certain fashion, they may not be able to see the cultural and ideological connotations that lie beyond the surface. Former Japanese Foreign Minister Aso Taro has spoken highly of the country's animation industry, saying: "What you have done is to capture the hearts of young people in many countries, including China. This is something that our Ministry of Foreign Affairs can never do." In real life, many young people in China are deeply influenced by Japanese anime. They follow Japanese fashion, enjoy Japanese cuisine, and are eager consumers of Japanese goods, which has made a dent on their cultural identity as Chinese.[70]

## 4 Negative Impact of the Internet

In the era of computer and the Internet, pregnant with both benefits and hidden risks, the World Wide Web plays an increasingly important role in shaping the way people think, live, and interact. Adolescents form a major part of the cyber community, and they can be strongly affected by what is available to them online due to their distinctive psychological characteristics. Around the world, the Internet has greatly increased the quantity of information available and the speed it is disseminated, and changed the ways in which young people live and interact with one another. The Internet has provided young people with new concepts, the spirit of innovation, a wealth of knowledge, an awareness of efficiency and equality, a global vision, and respect for diversity. However, just like all the previous technological revolutions, the revolutionary Internet has also brought to us, in addition

---

[68]Ikegami (1985).

[69]*Otaku* is a Japanese term that is known as *yuzhai* in Chinese (based on the Chinese characters used) or "Aotaku" when transliterated. In Japanese, the term means "your home." While originally not a pejorative term, as otakus are generally known to be absorbed in the world of manga/anime are spend long periods of time at home alone, the term has also become shorthand for someone with poor interpersonal skills, who is unkempt, introverted, and solitary.

[70]Dong (2011).

to great convenience, ethical and moral confusions. For youths, what the Internet brings along is not only positive influences, but also hazards.

According to CNNIC, there were a total of 137 million Internet users in China as of December 2006, up to 23.4% over 2005. Over more than ten years since China connected to the Internet in 1994, the country has seen the number of its Internet users rocketed to the top of the world. At the same time, the number of Chinese domain names has also soared. In particular, .cn domain names have grown by 64.4% over the same period of 2005. China also topped the world in 2006 in terms of the average amount of time spent online by its Internet users. According to Ipsos Insight, a US-based survey company, Chinese netizens spent an average of 17.9 h online per week, the highest of the world; in comparison, the figure was 13.9 h for Japanese, that for 12.7 h for South Korean users, 12.3 h for Canadians, 11.4 h for Americans, and 9.2 h for Mexican users (see Fig. 10). CNNIC's research also shows that Chinese netizens were spending increasing amounts of time online, 92% of them use search engines frequently, and 45% chat online often.[71] Different studies may have produced results that differ here and there, but they all share one point: The 18–25 age group is the mainstay of Internet users. According to the National Internet Survey, 76.2% of Internet users are 21–25 years old, and 62–85% of users have completed junior college or higher-level education.[72] The Internet will surely play a growing role in the lives of young people and have a tremendous and far-reaching impact on their minds and lifestyles. On July 16, 2009, CNNIC released its *24th Statistical Report on the Development of the Internet in China* in Beijing. It shows that as of June 30, 2009, the number of Internet users in China had reached 338 million, including 320 million, or 94.7% of the total, broadband Internet users, and 155 million mobile Internet users had amounted to. China topped the world in terms of the numbers of its Internet users, broadband Internet users, and top-level domain names (12.9 million). The advent of 3G mobile Internet services has pushed the number of mobile Internet users up to 155 million or 46% of all Internet users, up to 32.1% within merely six months. The number of young Internet users stood at 175 million, or 51.8% of the total. Specifically, 0.9% of all Internet users were aged under 10, 33.0% between 10 and 29, and 29.8% between 20 and 29.[73] China is the world's largest market of Internet services in the twenty-first century.

On June 18, 2010, in the city of Beijing, the Youth Research Center of the Chinese Academy of Social Sciences and the Social Sciences Academic Press jointly released the first blue book of teenagers of China, the *Annual Report on the Internet User by Minors in China (2009–2010)*. According to the report, minors made up an important part of Internet users. By the end of 2009, there were a total of 384 million Internet users in China, of which 31.8% were aged 10–19. Also according to the report, this amounted to a total of approximately 122 million

[71]Jones (2007).

[72]Yang (2000b).

[73]China Internet Network Information Center (2011).

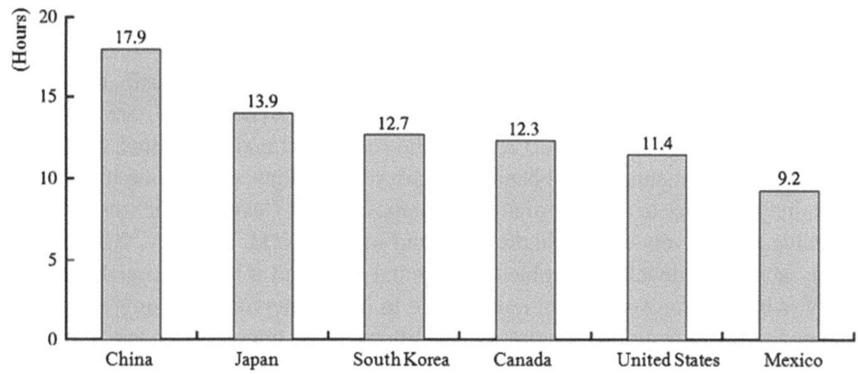


**Fig. 10** Average time spent online per week by Internet users

persons. If Internet users under the age of 10 are included, the total number will amount to 126 million.[74]

On January 16, 2012, CNNIC released the *29th Statistical Report on the Development of the Internet in China* in Beijing and it shows that by the end of 2011, the number of Internet users in China had surpassed the 500 million mark to hit 513 million, an increase of 55.58 million from the previous year. The Internet penetration rate had risen to 38.3%, and the number of mobile Internet users totaled 356 million.[75]As of June 2017, the number of Internet users in China reached 751 million, and the number of mobile Internet users reached 724 million.

## 4.1 Negative Impact of the Internet on Youth

First, the Internet hinders the development of a healthy personality in adolescents. It may produce "digital persons" who are aloof and alienated without much interpersonal interaction and show a lack of morality.

The Internet has a decentralized structure and does not have any central control mechanism. In the virtual world of the Internet, youths indulge in a colorful labyrinth of digital content and highly stimulating entertainment and games. Over the long term, obsession with the virtual environment which is novel, exciting, and challenging is bound to have an influence on their personalities and personality disorders such as "narcissistic personality," "paranoid personality," "dramatic personality," and "borderline personality" may develop. In the Internet age, individuals are easily submerged in the vast ocean of information online and become "digital persons" as a result. They tend to respond quickly to advances in

[74]Li (2010).

[75]China Internet Network Information Center (2012).

technology, but stay out of reality, live in isolation, and become indifferent to others. They prefer facing the computer screen to real-life interpersonal relationships. They interact with others only over the Internet, and individualism becomes widespread. Young Internet addicts, immersed in the cyber world, are unable to effectively switch between their roles in the real world and the virtual world, and show dislocated mentality and behavioral disorders. Reliance on online media, over time, may give rise to an "information suprematism" and leave the victims unable to perceive and actively engage in the brick-and-mortar world. It is easy, therefore, for these victims to develop a problematic mental state and a lack of social responsibility, which features isolation, indifference to others, nervousness, aggressiveness, and engagement in fraud. According to Clifford Stoll, Internet users sit in front of their Internet-enabled terminals, interact with "socially impoverished" media and anonymous strangers, and cut off from society and from real interpersonal relationships.[76] All these are potential drivers of suicidal behavior in youths and are not conducive to the development of sound personalities.

Second, the Internet delays the emotional socialization process for young people.

Adolescence is a time when emotional experience is the most intense and a person transitions toward maturity. During this period, social emotions gradually dominate people's emotional life as they gradually have more experience in social life. Addiction to and over-reliance on the Internet, however, can trap adolescents in a cycle of feeling guilty but unable to stay away, becoming frustrated, confused, lonely, pessimistic, and disappointed in real life. The Internet becomes a substitute for social activities for such young people and at the same time also causes an overload of information for them. The overload of information can destroy the balance of adolescents' somatosensory information and have serious adverse effects on their bodies, resulting in their feeling of "indifference" to the world.[77] Dependence on the Internet can turn people toward "machines" of emotional indifference in the course of solely human–machine interaction. Internet addiction blocks the normal channels of adolescents' social–emotional experience, and these individuals are torn between wanting to express their emotional experiences and the inability to face the evaluation of others and society. For example, in Japan today there are an increasing number of "otaku"—those who hide in a corner of the classroom or at home all day long to play computer games or to read/watch manga/anime. The existence of these individuals, who do not interact with others, has already drawn social attention. In a relatively closed environment like that of "man–machine–man" interactions, a number of Internet-dependent youths have become solitary and are unable to interact with their real-world peers because for them, social interaction with people has been replaced by reliance on the Internet. Japanese scholars refer to teenagers who have grown up in front of computers as "beetle-type" individuals who use the computer screen as their "compound eyes" to look at the world and use the communication antenna as the "tentacles" for contact

[76]Stoll (1995).

[77]Peng (2001).

with society. This will inevitably lead to emotional alienation and eventually erode their memories and awareness of their nation, traditions, or arts, and ethics.

Third, Internet-related mental disorders can easily develop among youths.

Individuals suffering from Internet-related mental disorders often spend a lot of time and energy on the Internet in an unrestrained manner for no specific reason, damaging their health in the process. In real life, these individuals also usually present with various personality disorders, partial dysfunction of the sympathetic nervous system, and behavioral abnormalities. In 2002, among over two hundred million users of the Internet around the globe, around 11.4 million, or 6% of the total, had some sort of Internet-related mental order.[78] Unquestioned beliefs in technology and the admiration of speed make one even more desirous of Internet use. This is the driving force for a group of Internet users. Disillusionment with the world and secluding themselves from the real-world online have become a means for many people to escape from reality. For individuals with Internet-related mental disorders, their reliance on the Internet grows by the day, and they are unable to stop themselves. They spend increasingly long hours online, and their dependency grows. According to Sigmund Freud's theory of psychoanalysis, the causes of Internet-mental disorders go back to the oral stage of psychosexual development. In this stage, a child is mentally satisfied by breast-feeding and retains positive memories and thoughts of the warm feelings, sense of care and security, and other good feelings that represent mother's love. Through Internet use, the individual regains such satisfaction which seems to have disappeared as the oral stage ended but is actually still hidden in subconsciousness. In adulthood, the individual seeks liberation from setbacks at school, at work, in social life, in relationships, etc., through immersion in the online world. Typical manifestations of obsession with the Internet include poor mood, loss of interest, sleep disorder, circadian rhythm disorder, loss of appetite and weight loss, lack of energy, psychomotor retardation and irritability, low self-esteem, the deterioration of various abilities, slow thinking, suicidal ideation and behavior, reduced social activity, heavy smoking, alcohol abuse, and drug abuse.

Fourth, information can appear and vanish online instantly and this may make young people pessimistic and live only in the moment.

On the Internet, millions of websites appear every day, while hundreds of thousands of them disappear at the same time. Information of all kinds is overwhelmingly proliferated. Everyone can be the source of information, and how to tell the correctness and completeness of available information becomes a great challenge. Young people no longer have to worry about the lack of information, but they are concerned about not being able to digest and make choices on the breathtakingly vast amount of information that is available. The overproliferation of information has overwhelmed young Internet users left them at a loss. Young people are deeply impressed by the rapid changes that occur in online life. Everything that exists on the Internet can be transient and gone too soon. Young

---

[78]Wei (2002).

people can be fatigued by such an ever-changing cyber world. Many of them feel that the world is changing too fast, and they are not sure about what would happen the next moment. As such, the attitude of "you only live once" is becoming popular among young netizens. The impermanence of online information has made short-term behavior prevalent among young people. In addition, online information is all-encompassing, and vast amounts of poor-quality information also serve to play an inducing or abetting role in this regard.

Fifth, the Internet has, to a certain extent, delayed the development of young people's thinking.

Web pages contain images, texts, and sounds, which together constitute a multidimensional form of communication that is highly appealing to the young. Online games have also proven very alluring to them. The Internet gives young people great opportunities to reach out to the outside world with each click leading to a great amount of new knowledge to help them know more and build a better knowledge structure. However, the Internet can also be a hindrance, to a certain extent, to the development of adolescents' thinking, especially abstract and logical thinking.[79] Adolescents are at a critical stage in the development of their thinking, which is the result of interactions between the subject and the object. In the cyber world, with the blind perusal of a chaotic array of information storming out of the Internet, young people no longer need to work to actively process and summarize content or reflect on and explore the essence of things as they do in reality. Youths who are addicted to the Internet tend to have more developed visual thinking skills, but their logical thinking is poor and they tend to rely heavily on perception rather than rationality. They react to matters in an emotional and superficial way. The Internet weakens young people's ability to think deeply about things and gives rise to a group of young people that approach issues in a simplistic, "flattened," and mono-dimensional manner. Online, the knowledge structure, and way of thinking of young people are assimilated by machines, and their wisdom is reduced to no more than ones and zeros. The overarching culture of the young population group has been homogenized.[80]

Sixth, young people are heavily influenced by pornographic and violent online content.

Eight out of the top ten keywords used on the AltaVista search engine were related to the subject of sex.[81] Back in 1998, a study showed that 47% of non-academic information on the Internet was related to pornography, with about twenty thousand pornographic images coming online each day.[82] By 2007, there were more than 370 million pornographic websites on the Internet.[83] Over half of Chinese Internet users come from the young population. By the end of 2009,

---

[79]Yang and Li (2002a).

[80]Zhong and Su (2002).

[81]Yang (2000b).

[82]Chu (2000).

[83]Zhang (2007a).

126 million users were under the age of 18. Half of these were frequent visitors of pornographic sites. Some young persons have gone on to commit crimes because of their addiction to online pornography. More astonishingly, data of 2007 revealed that there were tens of thousands of Web pages related to pornography in China.[84] On May 27, 2007, the Ministry of Public Security announced that as of May 15, more than ninety thousand pieces of online pornographic information were detected from around the country, and more than 4800 illegal websites were closed down in accordance with the law. However, Zhang Xinfeng, then Vice Minister of Public Security, said frankly: "Although we have significantly reduced the amount of obscene materials on Chinese websites with the current campaign, we have not yet stopped the "yellow wind" on the Internet, as online pornographic information has not been fully cleared and we have not yet prevented more such information from entering China from overseas sources."[85] In 2010, more than seven hundred pornographic websites, including more than eighty mobile porn websites, were closed down in Beijing alone. A total of 131 overseas pornographic websites were also blocked, and more than forty-four thousand pieces of pornographic information were removed.[86] At present, due to the high levels of pressure at home, Chinese pornographic websites have moved their servers overseas, making it difficult for the police to work on these sites. A study shows that 60% of young people encounter online pornographic information inadvertently, and that more than 90% of those who are exposed to online pornography develop the motivation to commit, or have committed, sex crimes.[87]

## 4.2 *Internet-Related Mental Disorders and Suicide*

As more and more people get onto the Internet, a new category of mental disorders —Internet-related mental disorders—has been seen in a large number of Internet users, attracting attention from the global medical and psychiatric circles. Individuals suffering from Internet-related mental disorders often spend a lot of time and energy on the Internet in an unrestrained manner for no specific reason, playing games, chatting, Web browsing, etc. Such behavior has a severe impact on their health. In real life, these individuals are also present with abnormal behavior, mental disorders, personality disorders, partial dysfunction of the sympathetic nervous system, high rates of suicidal ideation, as well as suicidal behavior.

On February 1, 2010, China Youth Association for Network Development and the Survey and Statistics Institute of Communication University of China released the *2009 Report on the Survey of Youth Addiction to the Internet* in Beijing.

[84]Zhang (2007b).

[85]He (2007).

[86]Zhang (2011).

[87]Yang and Li (2002b).

According to the report, at present, around 24.042 million Chinese youths are addicted to the Internet, accounting for 14.1% of all young Internet users, and nearly double the figure of 2005 and 2007. Addiction to online games is the mainstay, and second on the list is addiction to online relationships. Nearly, half of all youths addicted to the Internet (47.9%) regard "playing online games" as their main purpose of getting online and the activity they spent the most amount of time doing while online. This falls under the category of "addiction to online games." In addition, 13.2% of the addicted spend the most of their time online "chatting or making friends." This belongs to "addiction to online relationships."[88] When asked why they get online, a much higher percentage (47.9%) of the addicted cites playing online games as the main reason, compared to 21.1% among non-addicted youths, while a much larger proportion (45.5%) of non-addicted youths choose "learning or working" as the main reason, compared to 31.5% among the addicted. Survey shows that 67.7% of young Internet users have their personal Web pages and 58.4% have personal spaces associated with instant messaging tools. A total of 28.1% of young Internet users have their own blogs, and 20.8% have social media account(s).[89]

In the early stages of Internet-related mental disorders, an individual experiences endless fun when surfing the Internet. Then, as he/she spends more time online, he/she begins to suffer from a lack of concentration and memory loss. Some cannot help turning on their computer to go online even late at night. The initial mental dependence then gradually develops into physical dependence which is manifested in inexplicably poor moods in the mornings, slowness of thinking, dizziness, trembling hands, fatigue, and loss of appetite. The individual's mental state can only return to normal after spending time online again. In the advanced stage of the disorder, the patient loses weight with no physiological reason and appears wan and sallow. Once he or she stops surfing the Internet, acute withdrawal syndrome ensues, and the symptoms can even include self-harm or suicide. Studies show that long time of Internet use raises the level dopamine, an adrenaline-like substance that gives a boost to the mood in the short term, yet the "up" is soon followed by a "down" that leaves one unmotivated.

Robert Kraut and others found in their extended studies of Internet users that Internet use reduces the "social involvement" and "psychological well-being" of the users, which are manifested in increased loneliness and depression. Kraut explains that those suffering from Internet-related mental disorders have lower psychological well-being levels because of "displacing social activity" and "displacing strong ties." The former means that Internet users spend the time that could be spent on face-to-face interaction staying online, leading to reduced social involvement. The latter means that low-quality online relationships take the place of high-quality

[88]China Youth Network Association and Institute of Survey and Statistics of the Communication University of China (2011).

[89]Lan (2010).

real-life relationships.[90] Research on Internet dependence has also led to conclusions that it may lead to suicidal behavior.

Patients of Internet-related psychological disorder are mostly aged between 15 and 45. Up to 98.5% of all patients are male, and the disorder is especially common among single men aged 20–30.[91] Separating the patient from the Internet is the first step of the treatment. Patients are put under control to ensure that they spend no more than two hours online per day, and are also encouraged to actively participate in social activities and gradually wean off the Internet. Antidepressants such as imipramine hydrochloride or doxepin, as well as psychotherapy, are also used.

## 4.3 *Websites Dedicated to Suicide and "Online" Suicide*

The Internet is the most influential mass media ever in human history, and suicide-focused websites are among the most shocking and incredible legacies of the information age for mankind. Just type the word "suicide" into any online search engine, and you will see a number of suicide-themed websites. There are numerous Chinese sites, too.

"Are you thinking about committing suicide? Here are the most commonly-used, convenient, and quick methods!" This is the slogan of a Taiwanese website called "Jack's Three-Dimensional Space." In some Taiwanese online communities, a rumor goes that Panadol (acetaminophen) offers painless death, and many young people have made attempts. Suicide has been among the top causes of death for Taiwanese youths in recent years, and the cybercrime division of Taiwan's "Criminal Investigation Bureau" has launched an investigation into suicide-focused websites. On its homepage, Jack's Three-Dimensional Space features "suicide manual" as a selling point. On the site is the Chinese language version of *The Complete Manual of Suicide*, with images. The content of the site is divided into five sections: clothing, food, accommodation, travel, and others. Within these sections are detailed instructions on how to find the most convenient way to commit suicide in daily life. All of a sudden, suicide by means of jumping off buildings, drowning, drug overdoses, wrist-slitting, and hanging became popular and death became the ignorant romance of the young. In the first two days of July 2000, Taipei Veterans General Hospital treated five patients who tried to take their own lives with the same method and all were youngsters.

The homepage of another Chinese language website named "Paradise for Those Seeking Suicide" reads: "Are you feeling tired? Are you exhausted by all that this world has to offer?" "Do you think that being alive is even more painful than dying?" "Welcome to our community. We will help you experience what is a

[90] Kraut et al. (1998).

[91] Wei (2002).

once-in-a-lifetime joy!" Information on the various ways of committing suicide is easily available on this website.

The homepage of another website called "The Angel of Death" straightforwardly states the site's mission as to facilitate the discussion on and introduction of methods of suicide. It even welcomes all "to join the Angel of Death!"

A classic suicide-themed website is alt.suicide.holiday (also known as "ASH"). On the site are discussion threads, chat rooms, and guides to various forms of suicide, from the use of aspirin and rat poison to road and boating accidents, and jumping off from heights, and more. ASH was established in 1991 as a bulletin board on Usenet (a global newsgroup system). However, today, it has become a large-scale website with its own chat rooms and newsgroups. Apart from the main newsgroup, there is also an online comment thread on ASH where visitors can share their issues and experience related to suicide, and their suicide plans. Here, visitors can also comment on the suicide plans of others and offer suggestions. In addition, the website also carries detailed information on various forms of suicide and ranks each method by the degree of pain normally experienced. The site also offers suggestions on how to organize one's funeral, samples of suicidal notes, etc. The ASH site even provides studies of a number of "successful" cases for the reference of readers. The site has directly led to a number of suicidal cases with an extremely high success rate.

In recent years, a number of websites that seek to bring together individuals seeking to commit suicide have appeared in China. Some of these carry copious amounts of information on the various ways of committing suicide as well as mail order services for drugs to be used, while others seek to establish groups of "suicide buddies" among users. Members put up posts anonymously to create suicide plans together and put them into practice collectively once conditions are ripe. Online mass suicide incidents are a new form of suicide that has emerged in recent years to the surprise and helplessness of suicide prevention organizations and police authorities.

Someone who has attempted suicide on multiple occasions once said, "I have cut my wrists, taken sleeping pills, but never succeeded. I do not wish to die alone. Clicking on 'suicide matching' sites everyday has become a part of my life." Although this individual has tried psychiatric counseling, he still feels excited and envious when he encounters successful cases of mass suicides. He said, "I would probably be dead by now had I found people with the same inclinations." About this, a psychologist said this: "Those who would not have opted for suicide in the past may choose this option if they encounter postings calling for 'fellow' suicidal individuals. The herd mentality and group consciousness can lead those who have been wavering to decide on mass suicide." According to Itakura Hiroshi, a Japanese Professor of criminal law, although from the perspective of Japanese criminal law the provision of drugs meant for suicide to others is a crime, in Japan there have yet to be any laws targeting those who deliberately provide those who intend to commit suicide with help or those who propagate their intentions of suicide online.[92]

[92]http://www.chinanews.com/n/2003-02-14/26/272807.html. Accessed: 11 September 2008.

At one o'clock in the morning on January 27, 2010, an Internet user nicknamed "yecengzouguo" (literally "been there, done that") posted a suicide "livecast" on Tianya.cn. The user was a 26-year-old woman who lived in Ya'an, Sichuan. The title of her post was: Aconitine: record of a toxicity self-test—that is more or less how it feels like!" She wrote: "I am unable to move on from parts of my past, and the pain in my heart grows with age." She started taking aconitine at nine o'clock in the evening and finished the drug by midnight. She then posted how her body reacted to the poison on the site. Between 1:11 am and 2:55 am, she put up a total of six posts and the last one read: "My scalp feels like it is being torn apart, and the pain in the neck is getting worse. My head hurts a lot, and I feel extremely giddy. My vision is abnormal, and my breathing is less cumbered. I need to go lie down for a while..." She then went offline. The thread drew a massive response soon, with over seven hundred thousand readers in a few hours. Internet users from all over the country tried seeking help from the police and emergency services for this girl who "lived in a city never heard of." Despite complaining about the hard-to-understand local Sichuan dialect, these users still looked up the telephone numbers of the local police, telecommunications authorities, and even the Sichuan Provincial Traffic Radio Station (as it operated round the clock) in order to secure assistance. Some users tried looking up the IP address of this woman from her posts and previous visits. The person was located after nearly four hours of work, and the website's administrators then got in touch with woman's father through a registered fixed-line phone number. Eventually, the person was found by her family members and saved.[93]

Suicide is never merely a metaphysical issue but rather a problem involving physical practices. However, those who commit it are unable to see whether such "practice" is correct as he or she would no longer be alive. Today, in the Internet age, this problem that has plagued mankind for millennia is still here. Suicide-focused websites are but a projection of it on the Internet. These sites bring together suicidal individuals from all over the world. Some find ways to kill themselves on these sites, while others eventually come around meditating on all possibilities. Are such sites a blessing or a curse for those who seek to kill themselves? Whatever the answer, one thing is for sure: These sites are becoming "accomplices" that push the suicidal further toward death.

## 4.4 Addiction to Online Games

As computer and the Internet spread wider, Internet cafés that mainly cater to youths have come out in large numbers all over the Chinese mainland. For minors whose personalities are not yet fully developed, addictions to the Internet and video games can easily lead to personality disorders or defects. More than half of patients

[93]Zhang (2010).

with Internet addiction syndrome are minors. As minors tend to be highly curious, lack of self-restraint, and not fully able to tell right from wrong, Internet access can make it extremely easy for them to indulge in games, chatting, and various negative online contents. According to a survey conducted by the telecommunications authorities in 2001, pornography sites and columns accounted for 75% of online cultural content, "decadent content" accounted for 66, and 47 and 45% [of users] engaged in flame wars on bulletin boards and "making friends in an irresponsible manner" in chat rooms, respectively.[94] Some Internet café owners allow minors to spend long hours online playing video games or browsing pornographic materials for economic gains or due to neglect. A number of minors have suddenly gone blind after spending dozens of hours at a stretch in an Internet café. In a bid to help his/her child who was a student at a key high school) wean off the Internet, one parent brought the child on a number of holiday tours within only six months; parents have also been known to take the keyboard of their family computer with them to work as they feared that their children would be misled by online content at home when they are not there. No wonder, then, at the turn of the century the issues of video games and Internet café management had become hot topics of discussion among National People's Congress deputies and members of the Chinese People's Political Consultative Conference (CPPCC). Such discussions have in turn given rise to "Proposal No. 1" that aims to strengthen management over games, machines, and Internet cafés.

At the 2002 CPPCC meeting, Member Wen Kegang made a strong call for actions so that "Internet cafés would not enmesh our children." According to Wen, there were 1900 Internet cafés in Beijing and nearly half were illegal; among the 1.71 million primary and high school students in the city, three hundred thousand had used the Internet, about half of them used Internet cafés, and a hundred thousand often play games and chat online. Many children were addicted to Internet cafés, but these places were often poorly equipped and with unhealthy environments, probably with fire hazards. There was a tragic case of a fire at an Internet café in Beijing with heavy casualties. As such, Internet cafés can be very detrimental to the healthy growth of young people. What Wen mentioned was only an incomplete list of the harms that Internet cafés can bring. There are numerous cases of youth suicide related to long periods of time spent at Internet cafés and arcades.

Since the 1980s, video games have become popular among children and youths in advanced nations and the same occurred to China over the past decade. Some Chinese youths have even become addicted to these games. They spend the majority of their time in front of the computer playing video games, online or offline, in Internet cafés, and some also visit arcades frequently. Addiction to video games makes young people susceptible to the negative influence of game content, which play up themes such as violence, killing, death, and destruction. In particular, in most violent games the deaths of the key and auxiliary characters are but transitory. They die in an instant and are back to life the next moment. There are even

[94]Zhang (2002a).

some games (such as those created in Japan) that deal directly with the topic of suicide. Such content can easily mislead youths, especially those of a younger age, toward a “gaming attitude,” life and death, and inappropriate behavior. Some children have not yet attained psychological and cognitive maturity and may try bringing the violence they see in video games into real life.

As children who are addicted to video games place a large part of their energy, emotions, and minds on video games, they naturally become distant from their parents and other persons around them and are thus prone to developing resistance toward interpersonal relationships. In addition, as youths seek to satisfy their personal gaming needs, they may run into conflicts with their parents, and school or workplace superiors over various issues. Suicides caused by such conflicts are also numerous.

Overseas research on the psychological impact of video games on children and adolescents generally finds that while both positive and negative impacts are present, the negative part outweighs the positive part, especially in children. In particular, violent video games are very harmful, and the addictive nature of video games cannot be ignored.[95]

## 5 Mental Illness and Youth Suicide

WHO experts have predicted that by the mid-twenty-first century psychological crises will be the top cause of sustained and profound agony to mankind, causing far more pain than any disaster.

Suicide can be caused by myriads of complex factors, but whatever the reasons, mental mechanisms are always at play. Social, biological, and pathological factors can only play a role through the “prism” of psychological factors. What we must be aware of is that although suicidal behavior among youths does show clear psychological patterns to some extent, it is indeed unique in some ways because of the special mental characteristics of youths. Mental illness is a key cause of youth suicide.

Since the launch of the reform and opening-up policy in 1978, China has attained major, unprecedented achievements. Its great economic success, in particular, has caught the attention of the whole world. However, we must be soberly aware of the heavy costs that we have paid for the rapid growth, including pollution to the environment, waste of resources, and various social issues. “Change entails great psychological costs, in addition to economic and social costs.”[96] On the whole, the mental health of Chinese youth has been on the decline as society undergoes a dramatic transformation. Whether we should regard psychological changes, the direct result of social changes is up for debate, but what we can be sure

[95]Liu and Su (2002).

[96]Vago (2007).

of is that the two often coexist and occur in tandem. That psychological problems exist among the young is clear to see. Of course, this is not unique to China. Similar situations have been seen in a number of advanced nations in the West during rapid economic development.[97]

Some experts are of the opinion that the suicide rate among those with mental illness to be ten to ninety times that of the rate among ordinary population. At least 74% or so of those who commit suicide have been found to have mental disorders.[98] The levels found by those who study mental illness are even higher. For instance, E. Robins estimates that mental illness is present in 93% of those who commit suicide, and Brown came out with the figure of 94%. Murphy is of the opinion that only a tiny minority of those who commit suicide do not have mental illness.[99] The suicide rate is also very high in mental hospitals though such locations are usually closely monitored. According to He Zhaoxiong, the suicide rate among patients with mental illness in China stands at 0.22–6%.[100] Data obtained from Japan shows that among individuals who had committed suicide in Tokyo, 13.2% were warded patients, 19.4% were outpatients, and the status of 67.4% was unknown.[101]

Young people have become a high-risk group for mental ailments. It was noted at the recent annual World Psychiatric Association Congress that mankind is shifting from the "age of physical illness" to the "age of mental illness."

With rapid economic development, growing competition and pressure, and quickened pace of everyday life, the incidence of mental illness is rising among Chinese. According to the WHO, currently five out of the top ten diseases leading to physical disabilities, mental disabilities, and the loss of the ability to engage in labor and everyday life are mental disorders. Specifically, these are severe depression, severe schizophrenia, bipolar affective disorder, alcohol dependency, and obsessive-compulsive disorder. Mental disorders are now a relatively severe class of diseases in the world. The WHO designated the year 2001 as World Mental Health Year. As mental illnesses are highly debilitating, they (primarily schizophrenia) have been included in programs designed to take care of disabled persons in China.

According to data released by the Center for Mental Health at the Chinese Center for Disease Control and Prevention in early 2009, the total number of people with various mental illnesses in China was over a hundred million. That is to say, mental illnesses afflict one in every 13 people in China. The report also stated that according to international standard, mental illness is at the top based on the total disease burden caused in China, taking a larger share than cardiovascular diseases, respiratory diseases, and malignant tumors. Mental problems of various kinds

[97]Xin and Chi (2008).

[98]He (1997).

[99]Zhai (1997, p. 223).

[100]He (1997).

[101]Inamura (1977).

accounted for about one-fifth of the total burden, and this share is expected to rise to a quarter by 2020.[102]

Currently, behavioral problems among children, mental health problems among high school and college students, alcohol and narcotics abuse, and the problem of suicide arising from them have all on the rise in China.

China has included the prevention and treatment of mental illnesses in children and adolescents in its national basic public health service program in 2009. The Mental Health Law of the People's Republic of China was promulgated in October 2012 and officially took effect on May 1, 2013.

## *5.1 Poor Mental Health Conditions Among Chinese Youths*

By the end of 2010, there were a total of three hundred and sixty million children and adolescents in China. The incidence of mental illnesses in this group has been high, and the general mental health condition is worth of great concern. Each day, the various clinical facilities of the Children's Medical Research Center of China see an average of more than five hundred children with mental illnesses. The annual total is around one hundred and sixty thousand.[103]

Data presented at the 19th World Congress of the International Association for Child and Adolescent Psychiatry and Allied Professions-cum-the 6th Congress of the Asian Society for Child and Adolescent Psychiatry and Allied Professions held in Beijing between June 2 and 6, 2010, showed that the prevalence of mental illness in children and adolescents in China had exceeded the international average of 15–20% and that at least thirty million children and adolescents under the age of 17 were suffering from various affective disorders. The mental and behavioral problems of the so-called left-behind children, children from single-parent families, and only children were particularly prominent. The event was attended by more than fifteen hundred delegates from sixty-eight countries and regions. Then-Chinese Health Minister Chen Zhu said at the event that the children and youths of China are the future of the country and the protection of their mental health is a shared responsibility.[104]

A survey shows that there are around thirty million adolescents with mental problems across the country. In particular, the incidence of mental disorders is between 21.6 and 32% among primary and high school students, and between 16 and 25.4% in college students, both on the rise.[105] Up to seven hundred and fifty thousand individuals in Shanghai suffer from various mental disorders, out of a total population of over thirteen million. The vast majority of these patients are young

---

[102]Lü (2010).

[103]Jing (2011).

[104]Fan and Hai (2010)..

[105]Ge and Qu (2011).

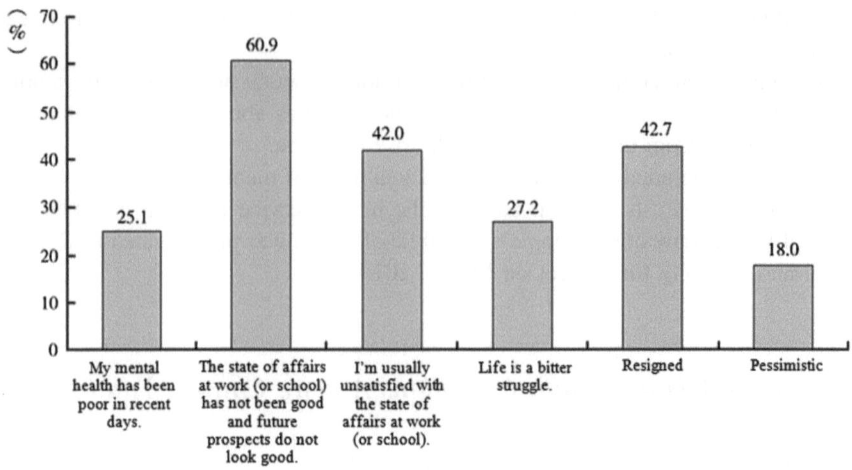


**Fig. 11** Mental health conditions among Chinese youths, 1997

people who work, study, and live under pressure, and who are overloaded all year round. The incidence of mental disorders among college students is especially high.[106] According to a survey conducted by the Social Survey Center of *China Youth Daily*, 25.1% of the young people surveyed believed that their "mental state has been unhealthy recently," and 60.9% felt that "the state of affairs at work (or school) has not been good and future prospects do not look good." Meanwhile, 42.0% of those surveyed reported that they were "often dissatisfied with the state of affairs at work, school, or in life"; 27.2% believed that "life is a bitter struggle." Also, 42.7% of individuals felt "resigned," and 18.0% felt "pessimistic" (see Fig. 11).[107]

Despite the grim reality concerning children's and adolescents' mental health conditions, related research and practices are still at an early stage, of low quality, with limited specialization level, inadequate coverage, and almost no relevant care service available. Crisis intervention mechanisms for children and adolescents in public emergencies are also in the initial stage, and the awareness levels regarding mental health issues among children and adolescents in China remain low among both the general public and the medical professionals who do not work in psychiatry. Many children and adolescents with mental disorders and mental and behavioral problems are not diagnosed in a timely manner or treated properly.

The former National Education Commission conducted a survey of 126,000 studies across the country in 1988. The results show that the incidence of mental ailments among Chinese college students was 20.33%. This has a grave impact on the academic performance of these students and constitutes a key cause of suicide.

[106]Social Survey Center of China Youth Daily (1997a).

[107]Social Survey Center of China Youth Daily (1997b).

Statistics from sixteen higher education institutions in Beijing show that between 1985 and 1987, a total of 293 students dropped out of school or suspended their studies due to mental health issues. Specifically, 37.9% suspended their studies and 64.4% dropped out of school. Between 1978 and 1988, a total of twenty-one students at Renmin University of China passed away. Seven of these students were confirmed to have been suffering from schizophrenia. Five out of the seven committed suicide.[108] Two students (including one foreign student) at a certain comprehensive university in Guizhou had killed themselves in the first two weeks of the spring term of 2007 by jumping off from a height. Both cases were deemed to have been caused by depression.

Many primary and high school as well as college students experience mental disorders such as anxiety, phobia, neurological depression, and emotional crisis. In the decade between 1977 and 1986, 74.6% of dropouts from three key universities in southwest China left school because of health problems and 42.2% suffered from neurasthenia or schizophrenia. In 1988, the Shanghai Municipal Education Bureau and some other institutions studied the mental health status of students in seven high schools. The results showed that 30.0% of the students had poor mental health, with 17.0% presenting with "mental flaws" and 13.0%, mental illness. In 1993, a health research institute conducted a three-year-long study with more than 40,000 individuals and found 16.8% of the young students to have serious mental problems and the incidence of mental problems to grow with age. The study also revealed that, respectively, 13.8, 18.8, and 25.4% junior high school students, senior high school students, and college students had mental problems.[109]

In some colleges and universities, nearly 50% of the dropouts were for mental health reasons, and suicide caused 26.5% unnatural deaths of their students. According to an extended study of the basic mental health conditions of students matriculated in a certain university in southern China in 1991, 48.6% of the students reported feeling lonely (compared to 6.4% from a year prior when they had just entered college), 17.8% often suffered from insomnia, 21.2% experienced headaches, and 25.6% reported to have little appetite.[110] Zheng Richang, et al. conducted a study of 3000 junior and senior high school students and college students across China and found that 42.73% reported that they "feel nervous easily," 55.92% reported that they "worry too much about trivial things," 47.41% felt that "people are cold to one another," 67.26% reported "having no friend to talk to when feeling vexed," and 48.63% reported that they tended to be "overly-nervous and are somewhat overwhelmed during exams."[111] Xinghai Conservatory of Music conducted a mental health survey among its freshmen in 1999 and 2000, and the results showed that 6.93% of the students had "very poor" mental health and fell into Class I in terms of the care required. Eleven of these

[108]Shangguan (1995).
[109]Yu et al. (2001, p. 51).
[110]Yu et al. (2001).
[111]Zheng (1994, p. 121).

students had clearly stated that they had thoughts of suicide. Meanwhile, 16.40% had "poor" mental health and fell in Class II for the care they needed. Yunnan Province administered the Symptom Checklist-90 (SCL-90) self-assessment instrument with 4421 college students and found the overall mental health conditions of college students to be poorer than among the general public.[112] In 2000, Chongqing Education College Student Union and the College Students' Psychology Association conducted a survey on the mental states of female students and found that 52% of them depended on others; 48% feared failure; 43% felt incompetent and unattractive though they had not been told so; 43% did not like a competitive environment; 48% often suppressed their feelings; and 29% believed what others demanded of them to be more important than what they wanted for themselves.[113] A survey conducted by the Ministry of Education in 2006 showed that around half of all college students who had dropped out of school or suspended their studies had done so due to mental problems, and that mental problems were present in 30% of college students and disorders in 16–25.4% of college students.[114]

Even more astounding is that a number of young radio show hosts of "psychological helpline" programs committed suicides in succession, which were widely reported in the media. People involved in such cases of suicide include Teng Jia of a Shanghai radio station; Wen Da of a Beijing radio station in May 1994; Shang Neng of Hunan Financial Radio in August 1997; and Chen Yunqing who was the founder and person in charge of China's first private suicide prevention organization and a pioneer of suicide prevention research and practice. Their suicides drew attention from around the nation. Although these hosts helped countless others work through their problems and saved lives, for some reason, they still chose to kill themselves. According to another report, between 1980 and 2000, over 1200 entrepreneurs committed suicide in China. Entrepreneurs had become a high-risk group for depression. An extended study of entrepreneurs in the Yangtze River Delta found that a considerable number of them were at risk of a mental breakdown.[115]

Young people today are the future of China. Sound mental health is a must for them to pursue successful careers. Mental health is an important indicator of the overall competence of a person. As China is building and improving its market economy, urbanization and industrialization speed up, and competition is everywhere in society. Young people, not yet fully socialized, are more likely to suffer setbacks when they encounter conflicts and increased stress in terms of morals and ethics, personal values, behavior, interpersonal relations, etc. The number of individuals with mental disorders will grow, and suicide will also probably increase.

[112]Zhao and Zhong (2002).
[113]Li (2000).
[114]Ouyang and Wu (2011).
[115]Lü (2005).

With family planning established as a basic national policy in China, the proportion of only children is increasing and family structures are changing. Mental health problems have been detected in a high proportion of China's only children, which is worrisome and requires close attention from all walks of life.

The mental health status of Chinese college students—once known as the "ones favored by heaven"—is significantly poorer than the average level of the country, which is worrying. Ji Jianlin, et al. conducted a study of 547 college students using SCL-90 and found more than 10% of the respondents experienced "mental agony," and that the proportions of people having various mental health issues such as obsessive-compulsive disorder, interpersonal issues, and depression were also higher.[116] Ji Jianlin, et al. also diagnosed 83 college students undergoing psychological counseling using the third edition of the *Diagnostic and Statistical Manual of Mental Disorders* (DSM-III), and they found that anxiety (in 43.36% of the students studied), affective disorders (30.12%), and adjustment disorder (19.28%) were the most common among the college students studied.[117] The results of Li Fan's survey on the incidence of neurasthenia among 4868 college students in Lanzhou, Gansu Province, showed an incidence of 8.4% in the surveyed group and an incidence of 7.37% in students from minority ethnic groups.[118] Fu Jingchun and Li Ruijun et al. conducted a survey on the mental health status of 2001 students of Mongolian and Han "nationality" from eight colleges in the Inner Mongolia Autonomous Region. The results showed that 26.14% of the students had mental problems, and that Mongolian students were had worse conditions than their Han peers. Han boys were found to be more emotionally unstable than Mongolian boys and tended to shrink from challenges more; Mongolian girls were found to be more optimistic and sociable than Han girls. The overall incidence of neurasthenia was 12.64, 12.12% for Mongolian students, and 13.24% for Han students.[119] Wang Xiaogang et al.'s survey on the state of mental health among college students found that the common mental problems among college students were anxiety (9.8%), obsessive-compulsive disorder (8.6%), psychosis (8.6%), hostility (7.2%), and somatization (6.5%).[120] Zhao Jingping et al. studied a group of junior medical students using SCL-90 and found that 21–35% of the medical students sampled suffered varying levels of mental problems, with obsessive-compulsive disorder, interpersonal sensitivity, depression, and paranoia being the more common.[121] A survey of medical college students by Cui Xinjia et al. found about 20% of the students to have depression.[122] A survey of 1127 college students from minority ethnic groups in the 1990s by Xie Yaning and Gong Yaoxian showed that around

---

[116]Ji et al. (1990a).

[117]Ji et al. (1990b).

[118]Li (1988).

[119]Fu et al. (1998).

[120]Wang et al. (1992).

[121]Zhao et al. (1991).

[122]Cui et al. (1990).

10% suffered from various types of mental problems, with the more common ones being obsessive-compulsive disorder, interpersonal sensitivity, and paranoia.[123]

Hu Qixian, Yi Fajian, Yuan Yuqiang, and others amassed a sample of 3500 students randomly selected from 47 colleges and universities in 15 provinces and municipalities across six regions of the country and did a survey using SCL-90. The sample covered an unprecedented 18 ethnic groups. The results of the self-assessment show that the average value for SCL-90 factors was higher than the norm of China, and that among these students the scores for symptoms of obsessive-compulsive disorder, interpersonal sensitivity, depression, paranoia, and hostility have already reached, or approached, the "mildly painful" levels. The scores were highly dispersed, and when the standard deviation of 1.96 was added to the average score all respondents scored 3.00 points or higher, meaning that they were at least at the "moderate pain" level. This is a clear reflection of the gravity of the mental health issues plaguing college students today.[124] This survey reveals to us that the mental health conditions of Chinese college students were significantly poorer than the national average, with 18.58% of students presenting with mental abnormalities. The more common types of mental problems found include obsessive-compulsive symptoms, interpersonal sensitivity, depression, paranoia, and hostility. Gender differences were found, with men less healthy than women on the whole, mainly in the areas of somatic disorders, obsessive-compulsive symptoms, anxiety, hostility, paranoia, and psychosis (significant differences were found). Mental health conditions also varied across different cohorts of students, with sophomores having the poorest conditions, followed by freshmen, then juniors and seniors. There were no significant differences between juniors and seniors, and in general the freshmen and sophomores had more problems. No significant differences were found in terms of the incidence of abnormal psychological reactions between men and women, between students in different departments, and different cohorts.[125]

The above-mentioned domestic studies tell us that about 10% to 30% of college students suffer from mental disorders, and the more common types of mental disorders include depression, anxiety, obsessive-compulsive disorder, interpersonal issues, maladaptation, and personality disorders. Personality factors such as one's approach to dignity, temperament, and attributional style also have an impact on the mental health of youths.

The gross enrollment rate of higher education in China reached 15% in 2010 in accordance with the state's Action Plan for the Revitalization of Education for the twenty-first Century. The National Mid- and Long-Term Plan for Education Reform and Development (2010–2020) introduced in July 2010 required the gross enrollment in senior high-level education to reach 90% by the year 2000, and higher education to become more accessible, with the gross enrollment rate set to reach

[123] Xie and Gong (1993).

[124] Hu et al. (1999, p. 243).

[125] Hu et al. (1999, p. 255).

40%. In 2016, the gross enrollment rate of higher education in China has reached 42.7%, thus the expected target has been achieved ahead of schedule.

Enrollment in higher education expanded dramatically from 1999 to bring higher education to more people, but it has had tremendous impact on various aspects of the existing system of education. Challenges are grave. First, the number of college students increased dramatically as a result of such an expansion, and there have been insufficient resources (faculty, material resources, management measures, etc.) to meet students' needs in the areas of learning, day-to-day life, and development as such needs have soared. Second, as society becomes more complex and social relationships become more intertwined, students experience more pressure on the development front because of job market conditions, employment policies, and the overall environment development. After the 1980s, mental ailments became the main reason why college students dropped out of school, suspending their studies, or even committing suicide. Mental sub-health has become a common phenomenon among college students today, and mental problems are more diverse and complex. College students appear to be the disadvantaged group when it comes to mental health. The first batch of college graduates that had benefited from the expanded enrollment graduated in 2003. Competition in society had become more intense, and the resulting employment issues drew wide public attention. Some scholars who disagree with the expansion believe that if the employment problems of graduates are not solved there will be serious consequences.

## 5.2 *Psychological Characteristics of Youth Suicides*

The mental ailments that are more closely related to suicide in adolescents are affective disorders, schizophrenia, neurosis, personality disorders, organic mental disorders, and toxic psychosis. Statistics show that one out of every four to five individuals with manic depression exhibits suicidal behavior, and that the suicide rate of individuals with depression is ten times higher than that of the general population. Moreover, these individuals are highly motivated and often do not give up on their attempts at suicide. Those with families or lovers produce even more destructive suicidal ideas due to their evil delusions and often first murder their spouse, children, and other relatives out of "pity" before committing suicide. This type of murder-cum-suicide is common among China's youth.

To understand the motivation is the first step toward identifying suicide. Many scholars studied individual suicide attempts and came up with some targeted recommendations. According to Hawton, adolescents thinking of committing suicide usually do the following thirteen things:

(1) Seeking help from others; (2) expressing hopes of escaping from what frustrates them; (3) expressing horrifying ideas; (4) trying to influence others or trying to make others change their minds; (5) suddenly expressing love for others; (6) apologizing to someone for what they have done in the past; (7) doing something good for others; (8) expressing the fear of repeating the path that others have

traveled; (9) expressing the hope that others understand their feelings; (10) asking if they are really loved; (11) expressing the sentiment that the current situation is unbearable, and that they will have to do something to change the situation but not knowing how to go about it; (12) losing control of their lives but not knowing how to get back on the right track; and (13) expressing wish to die.

Danuta Wasserman proposed the psychodynamic theory of youth suicide. This theory assumes that people may believe on the subconscious level that their bodies do not belong to themselves and such beliefs may manifest as narcissistic injuries. These individuals issue "cries for help" as a way to attract everyone's attention rather than as a sincere expression of wishing to die. In this stage, it is necessary to carefully identify the motivation behind the suicide threat and to seek out a plan to help.

Shneidman also identified six common traits among people who commit suicide: The first is a situational characteristic, where the individual suffers unbearable mental pain and his/her mental needs are thwarted; the second is an ideation, in which they see suicide as a solution to a problem/problems; the third one is emotional, where the individual experiences despair and helplessness, and feels torn inside; the fourth is cognitive, where the individual is narrow-minded and extremely stubborn; the fifth is interpersonal, where the individual hopes to communicate with others and find a way out; the sixth pertains to continuity, where the individual uses suicide as the only way to solve the problems of his/her life.

There are still debates about the psychological profile of suicides. Studies on suicides (mainly those who attempt suicide and those with suicidal ideation) have shed light on some common characteristics in terms of cognitive function, emotions, interpersonal relationships, and response to stress.[126]

### 5.2.1 Cognitive Function

Suicides generally have "tunnel vision" and a dichotomous way of thinking when it comes to matters of right and wrong. As such, they are unable to effectively solve complex problems or to make a more objective assessment of themselves and the surrounding environment when setbacks and difficulties occur.

Suicides tend to be stubborn and passive when assessing and analyzing the problems they encounter, and simply attribute their problems to fate, luck, or the environment. They tend to believe that their difficulties or problems are intolerable, painful, interminable, and inescapable.

In the face of difficulties, suicide attempters are either unable to do anything and lack the ability and methods to solve problems, or cannot correctly assess their ability to solve problems. The outcome is the same: They often end up choosing solutions inappropriate for their problems.

---

[126]Xiao (2009).

Individuals who attempt suicides often lack patience and seek to achieve immediate results. If a certain way of solving a problem does not achieve direct and quick success, the individual quickly changes course or gives up halfway. As such, these individuals are rarely successful in tackling problems. Even more importantly, they tend to regard suicide as a last resort. Studies have shown that this is closely related to the intensity of one's suicidal tendencies.

Individuals who attempt suicide tend to be wary of, or belligerent against, others and the world as a whole, and emotionally distance themselves from others and society. They lack confidence in themselves, in others, and in society, and do not believe that individuals and the society can change. They are also filled with hopelessness about the future. Their pessimism can lead to depression, which in turn leads to suicidal thoughts. Adolescent depression is a psychological phenomenon unique to the period of adolescence. Many of the ideals and fantasies formed at this stage of life cannot be realized in the real world. So, some resort to suicide in the face of a failed pursuit.

In real life, those who attempt suicide are often indecisive but tend to take action impulsively.

### 5.2.2 Emotions

Individuals who attempt suicide often have had painful experiences, and anxiety, depression, anger, boredom, or guilt is usually the dominant emotion they hold. They often detest these negative emotions and find them hard to accept. Some young people may lack the ability to control their emotions. An analysis of the psychologies of patients with depression reveals that they usually resent themselves and try to direct aggressive impulses toward themselves. Suicide may occur when such an impulse is highly intense. The main function of the ego is to help the individual adapt to the environment he/she lives in, and disorders in this aspect mainly stem from resentment and attacks and destructive tendencies, and can lead to poor ability to adapt, disputes, alienation, suspicion, paranoia, etc. The destructive impulse that should have been targeted at an external object is directed internally toward the self because of the lack of an appropriate object or frustration in trying to direct the impulse at an object. Suicide may then occur.

Suicides are often emotionally very unstable and tend toward neuroticism. They often try to vent their emotions in impulsive ways and deliberately harm themselves in various ways, such as alcohol abuse, drug abuse, binge eating, and deliberate self-injury.

### 5.2.3 Interpersonal Relationships

Those who commit suicide often have problems interacting with other people. They are often embroiled in conflict with family members, neighbors, co-workers, and friends, and at the same time they are also afraid of rejection. Those who commit suicide generally lack effective social support and assistance, and find it difficult to establish new tie relationships. They typically are unable to adjust to new social environments, thus are prone to social anxiety and tend to avoid social activities.

### 5.2.4 Stressful Event

Individuals who commit suicide often meet frequent stressful events prior to their suicide, especially negative ones. Apart from having to deal with difficulties that have long been bothering them in life, these individuals may have, prior to their suicide, experienced unsettling occurrences of harassment or hassle, which may not worth much attention if they had occurred to other people. Studies show that a very high proportion of suicide cases occur within 24 h after a stressful event or relationship loss.

Young suicides often turn inward and attack themselves when facing difficulties and frustrations. These young people are very concerned about their appearances and tend to amplify their flaws. Subtle changes in their appearance, skin color, height, weight, breast size, and genital size can cause great concern. Melancholy, a deep sense of inferiority and even suicide may result when their appearance does not match their standards about what is ideal. In China, cases of youth suicide by individuals unhappy with their single eyelids, body shape, height, and genital size (in males) are common. Such individuals also tend to lack self-confidence on the academic front. They also lack patience and focus, and tend to be less responsive.[127]

Due to the influence of media, young suicide attempters can easily romanticize the notion of suicide and believe that death is a temporary, effective solution to all problems as well as the means to winning sympathy and forgiveness from others. Some even believe they would be saved by someone anyway, or that suicide attempts do not necessarily result in death. Some people even regard suicide as the best means of revenge against others or society in the belief that by hurting themselves directly, they can hurt others indirectly. In particular, in conflicts related to romantic relationships, when the couple cannot get what they want, the one who believes himself/herself to be the "weaker party" in the relationship often resorts to suicide as a means of "revenge" "waking up" the other party. The reasoning here is that the suicide would create a deep sense of guilt in the other party, who would then remember the protagonist for life. Some individuals who feel that they have not been treated fairly in the relationship also use suicide as a means of protest.

[127]Chen (2011).

### 5.2.5 Impulsive Suicide and Rational Suicide

Based on how a case of suicide occurs, suicides can be divided into two categories. The first is impulsive suicide, which is an impulsive behavior caused by the outburst of emotion such as anger, remorse, guilt, and shame caused by a stressful event. This type of suicide is characterized by its sudden occurrence, rapid progress, and short development period. The second is rational suicide, where the thought of suicide develops over a long period time, and is put into practice after full reasoning. It is a purposeful and well-planned action with careful preparation. This type of suicide is characterized by a slower process, a longer development cycle, and complex inner struggles.

In terms of the consequences of suicide, impulsive suicide occurs suddenly and is difficult to predict and prevent. As such, the mortality rate is high. In comparison, the long cycle of rational suicide and the inner struggles which may give some hint make it possible for others to discover the intention and prevent the attempt. Intervention is therefore more likely for the latter type. However, the extended duration of the decision-making process and the thorough preparation made by the individual can also pose difficulties for intervention.

## *5.3 Psychological Conflicts in Youths at a Time of Social Transformation*

The mix of new and old systems, the rapid restructuring of, and proliferation within, the social structure, the dramatic changes in economic life, and the rapid widening of the gap between the rich and the poor at a time of social transformation, as well as the rapid loss of balance in terms of moral values, lifestyles, and emotional patterns, have had a tremendous impact on collective psychology. This is a time when multiple social problems can crop up at the same time and a time of prominent social conflicts, which often have the following characteristics.[128]

First, old conflicts show new characteristics. Examples include "internal conflicts among the people," the four new characteristics of which are: (a) an increase in the incidence of mass incidents; (b) greater resistance; (c) prominent interest-based conflicts; and (d) more complex causes.

Second, new conflicts arise within existing relationships, such as in interpersonal relationships, relationships within social groups and organizations, and the relationships between different classes and social status.

Third, new conflicts arise alongside new relationships. Many new social relationships and new conflicts have emerged in tandem with social transformation, such as the conflict between migrant workers and urban residents.

---

[128]He (2003).

### 5.3.1 Psychological Conflicts in Response to Social Change

First, as China's reform deepens, the various conflicts in society have become increasingly prominent and complicated. At the same time, social values have undergone profound changes, and people tend to pursue more diverse values. Young people are sensitive and open to new things. However, their abilities to analyze, make judgements, control themselves, and make adjustments are not yet fully developed. When faced with a plethora of value choices that may sometimes be contradictory, they may feel at loss and conflicts may take shape inside.

Second, the reform has given young people more freedom and opportunities on the one hand, but brought tremendous mental pressure on them on the other hand. Such pressure may come from competition for study opportunities, a changed employment system and increased difficulties in finding a job, a changed labor relation system, a reformed housing system, high prices, etc., It can be very stressful for the young, causing anxiety and tension for them.

Third, social problems have emerged amid the reform. These problems include corruption, a growing wealth gap, unfair distribution, the depreciation of knowledge, employment pressures, inflation, and rising prices. Adolescents may not be able to understand these correctly and find it hard to balance between what is ideal and what is realistic. When their desires come into conflict with reality, psychological conflicts arise and they can feel confused, suspicious pessimistic, and disappointed, and then become indifferent.

In *The Trap of Modernity*, He Qinglian, Economist, wrote: An overly large wealth gap has led to the broad intensification of social disquiet, while intense employment pressures and the rise of the crime wave as well as the "disorganization" of China's basic-level organizations (the revitalization of patriarchal organizations and the rise of local vicious powers) have led to distortions in China's social control mechanisms. The emergence of underworld organizations, as well as the presence of local vicious forces at the local level in a small number of towns and villages, have led to an exploitative control of the people.[129] While this "dark side" is clearly not the mainstream of contemporary Chinese society, it has exerted tremendous negative impact on the collective psychology of the disadvantaged across the country.[130] Unable to vent, some members of society turn their anger inward. It is generally believed that social conflicts would become prominent when the per capita GDP of a country falls in the USD 1000–3000 range.

### 5.3.2 Psychological Conflicts Amid Socialization Process of the Young

Socialization is an important part of adolescent life. Poor socialization is a common problem among Chinese youths, especially those who are only children.

---

[129] He (1998).

[130] He (2006).

E. Douvan regards adolescence as a period of "self-exploration." In his famed work *The Eight Stages of Man*, Psychologist E. H. Erikson stated that the most critical stage in adolescence was that featured by "identity vs role confusion." He also believed that identity is possible only when an individual's understanding is truly consistent with reality. Adolescents are enthusiastic and emotional. However, their understanding of life is clearly idealistic, mainly due to their lack of experience. When they truly step into society, they will probably find a significant gap between ideals and reality, which is hard to bridge. Their original identity may be incompatible with the demand of society, and it is necessary to "reconstruct" this identity. Socialization is the process where adolescents adjust their way of thinking and doing to fit into the norms of reality and fit into society as a whole.

The process of socialization is actually the initial exploration of life by adolescents under realistic conditions. It is a fierce collision between ideals and reality and an encounter of the two sides of a conflict. Psychological conflicts abound in this process, mainly manifested in: (1) a wide gap between one's ideals and the reality, which leads to various difficulties in all aspects of life (negative psychological traits such as loneliness, sense of inferiority and proclivity to retreat, self-destructive tendencies, spiritual sorrow, and extreme behavior may arise); (2) a temporarily smooth period of life when the individual is unable to control himself/herself to prevent conceited behavior such as self-important, arrogant, and dominant bearing (interpersonal tension may ensue and bring attacks and negative feelings such as guilt, remorse, and loneliness); (3) pessimism about reality which may lead to negative mental states such as poor mood, depression, dejection, suspicion, and emotional numbness; and (4) frustration because of failure to achieve his/her ambitions, which, if not processed properly, can result in negative mental traits such as a decline in self-confidence, self-deprecation, and self-blame.

### 5.3.3 Psychological Conflicts Arising from Interpersonal Interactions

For youths, interpersonal interaction is an important component of social life. Interaction is a way in which information is communicated and exchanged. It requires not only the skills and means of communication but also psychological alignment between the two parties. Social, historical, and environmental factors; personal subjective factors; and the objective environment experienced by individuals have caused many interpersonal problems among young people. The psychological contradictions caused by communication problems can affect the overall mood of adolescents and affect how young people learn, how they work, as well as their physical and mental health, etc.

This is mainly manifested as follows: (1) Some youths, having suffered failures in their interactions with other people, close themselves off from others and lose the desire to communicate and interact. They can also be suspicious or distrustful of others and develop anxiety and fear. In severe cases, social phobia may be the result. A typical example is phobia of the opposite gender which can be caused by the emotions generated from prior failures in dealing with members of the opposite gender. (2) Interpersonal problems due to poor personality traits. Some adolescents have certain personality traits that may be unaccepted or intolerable by others. Examples are absolute self-centeredness, disrespect for others, inability to understand others and to think in his/her shoes, vanity, boastfulness, insincerity, jealousy, suspicion, extreme reactions and attitudes, excessive self-esteem, stubbornness, arrogance, an inconsiderate lack of tact, excessive ambition, and excessive demands of others. Such qualities can hamper interactions with others and hinder sustained communication. This can also cause psychological conflicts. (3) Problems in interacting with others arising from the attitude of "self-rejection" due to insufficient self-knowledge in the course of self-assessment. Some young people feel inferior due to a perceived lack of attractiveness on their part; some tend to retreat as they feel inferior to others. Others do not dare to communicate with others as they believe that they know too little to do so. These are all manifestations of psychological conflicts.

### 5.3.4 Psychological Conflicts Arising from Encounters with an Unfamiliar Environment

Population movement has been growing continuously since the launch of the reform and opening-up policy in China. Youth make up a large proportion of this population movement. This is aligned with their curious nature, their willingness to try new things, and their refusal to be content with what they already have. In addition, young people also meet new environments at school and in their career. One can only adapt to a new environment by changing one's attitude toward life, way of life, behaviors, and way of thinking. One forms his/her own habits in a previous environment, and a change to that is not easy to complete instantly. Thus, psychological conflicts can form in the course of adjustment. For instance, psychological conflicts are common among college freshmen, who find that unlike in high school, they are no longer cared for every moment of the day and as closely as ever by their family. As a result, they may feel helpless, lonely, and with no one to turn to. The lack of familiarity in the new environment makes the adjustment process challenging. They suddenly begin to miss homeland. In high school, these students enjoy the care of their parents and the close supervision of their teachers. They compete with their classmates and help each other at the same time. Often, their lives are hectic but poetic nevertheless. In college, lecturers appear only at the lectern and are no longer as readily available as high school teachers. Classmates in college usually come from all over the country and bring with them different habits. Obstacles to interaction are commonplace, and relationships with classmates are not as close as in high school. Praise no longer comes from teachers or parents, no classmate envies good academic performance anymore, and the sense of superiority enjoyed by top students simply vanishes. Here, unlike in high school, one will have to deal with one's spare time on one's own on top of heading to classes. This can be a challenge for many college freshmen, who are not used to, and do not know how to, deal with their spare time. They end up just loafing about, and a sense of boredom, emptiness, and even dejection emerges.

The psychological conflicts that arise in young people who are facing new environments that are swiftly changing are mainly manifested as a lack of mental balance amidst adjustments to this new environment. If such conflicts are not resolved over time, in the milder cases negative emotions, personality traits, and behaviors can arise; while in more severe cases, serious mental disorders and mental illness can develop and even cause suicide and/or criminal behavior.

Many empirical studies or clinical cases show that when people are highly accustomed to the environment they are in and highly satisfied with themselves and the environment, their suicidal tendency decreases or even disappears. In a converse situation, the tendency grows. From an ecological point of view, people's satisfaction with themselves and the environment depends on mutual adaptation between the people and the environment. People's behavior can align to the environment when the interactions between the people and the environment are good. On the contrary, individuals whose behaviors are not well received by the environment will not be able to adjust well to live comfortably in the environment. As a person has less control over the environment, he or she may feel disappointed or dissatisfied with themselves. The person then becomes emotionally resistant to the environment and feels the pressure of life getting heavier on them. If everything stays the same and as the vicious cycle continues, the adaptation will become worse. Suicide may then come up as an option as one seeks to completely avoid the heavy pressure coming from the environment. It can be said that suicidal behavior is a manifestation of poor adaptation.

## 5.4 *Depression, Personality Disorders, and Suicidal Behavior*

### 5.4.1 Depression and Youth Suicides

Among individuals with mental illness, those with depression are at a greatest risk of suicide. About 25% of patients with severe depression have attempted suicide at one point or another, and 15% eventually succeed.[131] The suicide mortality rate in this group is 650 per 100,000 individuals, fifty times higher than in the general population. Women with severe depression are around five hundred times more likely to commit suicide compared to people with no mental ailment.[132]

According to a recent report of the WHO, nearly 130 million people in the world are currently dealing with mental health issues. The same report also reveals that depression is set to become one of the top three diseases plaguing mankind in the

---

[131]Fawcett et al. (1987).

[132]Zhai (1997, p. 224).

twenty-first century. In the year 2010, around 30% of the global population is suffering from different levels of depression. WHO also has it that depression has become the second contributor to China's disease burden.[133] By the year 2020, depression may cause the second largest economic burden to mankind following cardiovascular diseases and the No. 1 mental illness for mankind as recognized by the global medical community. In Beijing, China, three persons out of every thousand were diagnosed with depression as of 2000.[134]

Psychiatrist Zhang Mingyuan once observed that depression has become a common disease in general hospitals in China. A survey conducted in Shanghai concluded that depression is the top problem among various kinds of mental problems among Shanghai residents. Zhang also noted that in China, many signs of depression are not detected in time and the patients not treated as they should be as many doctors, patients, and families do not have sufficient understanding of the disease.

Based on the conditions of patients who have sought medical help, we see that depression, particularly masked depression, is growing. It is easy to misdiagnose patients of depression as the disease is often masked by somatic symptoms. Once it develops into repeated depression, it will likely push up the risk of myocardial infarction, stroke, and other severe diseases, speeding up physical decline; more severely, it may increase the possibility of self-harm and suicide. According to some surveys, between 50 and 70% of people who have attempted suicide or have succeeded doing so have depression.[135] Famous figures who were direct victims of depression include Painter Vincent van Gogh; Former British Prime Minister Winston Churchill; Writer San Mao; Head of Guangzhou Pei'ai Suicide Prevent Center Chen Yunqing; Poet Xu Chi; Former General Manager of SAIC Volkswagen Fang Hong; Singer Xie Jin; Radio Host Shang Neng; Movie Star Leslie Cheung; and young American Chinese Writer Zhang Chunru. The same tragedy has happened to numerous high school and college students. In fact, depression is often accompanied by physical ailments. More than one-third of patients with Parkinson's disease, coronary heart disease, myocardial infarction, and diabetes also suffer from depression, and more than 20% of patients with malignant tumor, those who have had cerebrovascular accidents, post-surgery patients, patients with Alzheimer's disease, and sufferers of emphysema are also present with depression.

Depression is also known as a "mental cold," meaning that it is as common and easy to pick up as a cold. Around 60–70% of adults experience varying degrees of depression or spells of blue during their lifetime. While usually these emotions gradually fade over time, in some cases, which are more serious depression, it exacerbates to affect daily life and physical conditions. Specific manifestations include sleep disorders, self-blame or the loss of confidence, fatigue, loss of

---

[133]Hu (2002, p. 84).

[134]Wang (2000).

[135]Liu (2000).

appetite, loss of energy, sexual hypoactivity, slow speech, difficulty to focus, and suicidal ideation or behavior. Depressive neurosis, also known as neuropathic depression, is a neurosis characterized by persistent low mood. It is often accompanied by anxiety, physical ailment, and/or sleep disorder, with no obvious motor inhibition or psychotic symptoms. The proportion of neurotic depression in adolescents is higher. Patients who meet the criteria for neurosis can be diagnosed with depressive neurosis if they show three or more of the following symptoms:[136] (1) loss of interest (but not completely); (2) pessimism or disappointment toward the future, but not in complete despair; (3) self-reported fatigue; (4) lack of energy; (5) decline in outcomes of self-assessments, but willing to accept encouragement and praise; (6) no inclination to actively interact with others, but able to engage in passive contact and accept sympathy; (7) wanting to die, though with a number of "buts"; and (8) feeling his/her condition is grave but willing to receive treatment in the hope of a cure. Onset of the disease usually occurs at 18 years old or older, and the disease often strikes on the basis of a depressive personality. The course of the disease spans at least two years. During this period, poor mood is present for more than half of the time; normal intervals, if any, last for no more than two months each time.

Suicidal ideation and behavior are the most dangerous and common symptoms of depression. These can occur when the disease is severe, in the early stage, or when the patient is getting better. Patients often plan the suicide carefully in advance and conceal their actions to avoid the attention of medical personnel and families for they fell dejection and guilt and believe it is themselves that are to blame and deserve to die. As their conditions worsen, patients tend to become sluggish, indifferent, in lack of spontaneity, and passive; they retreat from social contact. Suicide is an extreme action taken by a depressed patient who wants to escape reality. They believe that life is full of pain and improvements are impossible. Suicide becomes, then, a way out: The patients believe that suicide can end the pain and relieve the burden on their families. At the same time, they may also experience a series of somatic symptoms: They may look wan, gave a stupefied gaze, have poor appetite, lose weight, experience decreased sweat and saliva secretion, constipate, become unable to fall asleep, and stay asleep. Often, they wake up two to three hours earlier than usual and have difficulty going back to sleep. Patients' mood is the poorest after such an early wake-up. Sadness wells up, and they may feel it impossible to endure the coming day or the pain that hovers around. This is why most cases of suicide committed by patients with depression occur between three and five o'clock in the early morning. Therefore, medical personnel and families of these patients should be especially vigilant during this period of the day.

Studies show that depression is not caused solely by biological and genetic factors but is the result of a combination of biological, psychological, and social factors.[137] The reasons for the recent rise in China's depression incidence are quite

---

[136]Hu et al. (1999, p. 6).

[137]Yang et al. (2010).

complex. However, the following aspects are particularly worthy of attention: First, the diagnosis rate for depression is not high (especially among adolescent patients). As the early symptoms of mild depression are usually fatigue and anxiety, patients are often sent to internal medicine instead. Second, patients often have concerns about seeing a psychologist or a psychiatrist for fear of being despised or considered "insane." Statistics show that as many as 82% of patients with mental illness visit internal medicine clinics instead, while only 18% seek help from the psychiatry department. Third, depression is often mingled with mental disorders, and primary depression may even be treated as secondary to some other disease.

In China, there has always been misunderstanding about mental illness. This is also an important reason for the increase in adolescent depression.

For one thing, mental symptoms may be covered up by somatic symptoms. Many people believe that physical illnesses are "real" diseases while mental illness and depression are not. Even after a full recovery, patients who have had mental illness are still likely to face enormous social pressure. This kind of social prejudice has caused many patients to shy away from psychiatric treatment even when their condition is very serious. Moreover, influenced by the traditional Chinese social psychology, many individuals hew to the model of emotional restraint and self-control and do not have healthy channels for venting. Data shows that individuals suffering from depression in China generally have the tendency to cover up their mental illness with physical symptoms. As they are often reluctant to receive psychological counseling and treatment, they seek medical help from a physician instead. As such, they are often misdiagnosed or not diagnosed at all, and proper treatment is delayed. Their conditions thus aggravate, and some even commit suicide as the disease gets worse.

For another thing, patients with mental disorders may not know where to go for help. Traditionally in China, when one has a headache, he gets the headache treated; when there is pain in the foot, treatment is focused on the foot. Many people lack the awareness that a medical condition may derive from mental problems, and do not know that a "mental cold" can strike as easily as a cold at any time. They may not be able to tell the difference or understand the connections between physical and mental symptoms. When they suffer mental distress or mild mental problems, they do not dare to seek medical advice, and nor do they confide in others. Instead, they take and swallow the pain quietly, until some resort to suicide for a relief.

Furthermore, there is a widespread lack of awareness about mental health issues, and many people lack sympathy or understanding for patients with mental problems. There is much prejudice and discrimination against patients instead, which makes it difficult for mentally ill persons to fit back into society. In China's colleges and universities, students with mental illness are generally required to suspend their studies or quit school. Thus, patients and their families, even if they have relevant knowledge, would prefer to quietly endure the pain rather than actively seeking help from a psychiatrist for fear that they will be excluded from society and discriminated against. Social discrimination against mental illness seriously hinders the effective use of mental health resources, impairs the recovery of patients' social function, and delays effective treatment for patients. Moreover, due to the serious shortage of mental health resources in China, not all patients with mental illness can be treated (even if they take actions to seek medical help). Even more embarrassingly, the pool of Chinese psychologists is stretched and is far from sufficient to meet the needs of society in terms of both the sheer size of the pool and the competence. In the USA, there are 550 psychologists for every million people, and more than 87% of these professionals have a doctor's degree in psychology or philosophy. In China, in comparison, there are only 2.4 psychologists for every million people, and less than 2% of these professionals have a master's degree or higher.[138] In China' vast rural areas, many people do not go to the hospital for medical advice when they have mental illness. Instead, they pray to various gods and deities for the elimination of the disease.[139]

On October 26, 2012, at the 29th Meeting of the Standing Committee of the Eleventh National People's Congress, China's first Mental Health Law was officially adopted after a rare legislative process that lasted twenty-seven years.

According to Article 16 of the law:

Schools of all types and at all levels are to educate students about mental health issues and to avail themselves of, or hire, mental health education teachers and counselors, and set up a mental health counseling room to provide mental health education for students. Educational institutions at the preschool level are to carry out mental health education compatible with the characteristics of young children. In the event of natural disasters, accidental injuries, public safety incidents, etc., that may affect the mental health of students, schools are to promptly arrange for professionals to provide psychological assistance to students.

Teachers are to master mental health-related knowledge, pay attention to students' mental health status, and guide and motivate students in the correct manner. Education departments of the people's governments at various levels, as well as school authorities, are to pay attention to the mental health of teachers.

Schools and teachers are to communicate with students' parents or other guardians and close relatives about students' mental health conditions.

According to statistics from the Guangdong Provincial Health Department, in 2001, there were more than one million people with mental illness in the province. More than seven hundred thousand patients were classified as seriously ill, and 72% of the mentally ill were disabled. Between 1998 and 1999, as many as 426 individuals were killed by perpetrators with mental illness and another 463 were debilitated. The Communist Youth League Guangzhou Municipal Youth Rights Protection Center has, since the launch of its psychological counseling hotline in 1996, seen the number of young people seeking help increase from some five hundred per year to 12,560 in 2000. More than one-fifth of patients with mental

[138]Zeng and Cai (2001).

[139]Hu (2002).

illness who commit suicide in Guangzhou are young people under the age of twenty-five.

Women patients are taking a larger share in all patients with depression. A study shows that the majority of depression patients are urban women around thirty years old. Women are usually more emotional and sensitive, and tend to worry more. In addition, the increase of divorce, extramarital affairs, sexual harassment, and other similar issues in recent years has also made depression more likely for some vulnerable women. A study finds that relationship issues increased the probability of depressive symptoms in young women by around a third. Available statistics also suggest that women are twice as likely as men to suffer from depression. Suicide attempts are more common in women patients with depression than in men patients. Individuals suffering from depression who have a family history of suicide are thrice as likely to commit suicide as those without such a history.[140]

For young women, postpartum depression also takes many lives. Studies show that between 50 and 75% of women experience "baby blues" after giving birth. They have mood swings, crying or feeling low for no specific reason. This is related to the sharp decline of hormone levels postpartum and can be serious in 10–15% of new mothers. Levels of estrogen and progesterone[141] rise by tenfold during pregnancy and then plummet after giving birth, getting back to prepregnancy levels within three days. The incidence of postpartum depression, which is the result of a combination of physical, emotional, and behavioral changes, is on the rise in China. Under normal circumstances, young women will start to develop undetectable anxiety and depressive symptoms when they are thirty-two to thirty-six weeks pregnant. A real onset occurs two to three weeks after delivery, and symptoms intensify four to six weeks after childbirth. For women who can adjustment themselves effectively, such symptoms usually disappear in two to three weeks after the onset, and in severe cases, the symptoms fade away naturally in about three months. Manifestations of postpartum depression can take the following three forms.

The first is postpartum bad mood. Often, new moms feel sad for no specific reason and may sob quietly. Such bad mood usually wears off naturally after some time. This occurs to around 50% of women. Clinical data from Japan shows that 70% of women experience poor mood after childbirth, which is known as "three days of sulking."

The second, known as postpartum depression, can last from a few weeks to one or two years. The incidence is about 10%. Symptoms include poor mood, tiredness, headaches, and body aches. It makes people feel frustrated for things that would normally not bother them, as well as sorrowful, tearful, uninterested in dressing up

[140]Zhai (1997, p. 225).

[141]A natural progestogen is secreted by the corpus luteum of the ovary. It has a significant effect on the endometrium that has been previously stimulated by estrogen. It is needed to maintain a pregnancy.

or having meals, and even reluctant to take care of the child. In severe cases, the patient may try to kill herself. Of course, many still recover naturally.

The third and most serious manifestation is postpartum psychosis, a typical symptom of which is delusion. The patient believes that she or her child is being harmed by someone, and has suicidal tendencies. Postpartum psychosis occurs only in less than 1% of postpartum women.

On January 20, 2002, a 25-year-old young woman from Beijing committed suicide in Chegongzhuang subway station. Afterward, it was confirmed that the direct cause of this tragedy was severe postpartum depression. On February 7 of the same year, a 28-year-old woman from Shenzhen suffering from severe postpartum depression suspected that she and her child were in great danger, and turned on the gas and killed herself and her two-week-old baby while hiding out in the bathroom.[142] Also in the same year, famous Hong Kong Movie Star Pauline Chan jumped from a high building in Shanghai due to postpartum depression. On May 18, 2011, a 30-year-old woman living in Chengdu jumped off from the tenth floor, leaving her six-month-old baby behind. Postpartum depression set in only one month after this woman gave birth to her baby. Prior to her death, she had said repeatedly that she heard voices in her head, calling her to jump off a building.[143]

There is a certain correlation between suicide rates among patients with depression and the time of the year. According to foreign reports, there are two peak periods: the absolute peak in April and May, with a second and minor peak in October. The first coincides with the peak season for the hospitalization of patients with depression, and the latter coincides with the wave of depression cases that occurs following summer mania. Such depression is called suicidal manic depression.[144] Reports in China show that suicide rates in those with depression peak in the winter and summer, especially in winter.[145] Whenever the weather changes, especially when the weather is poor or gloomy, patients with depression are the first to react. One patient once said: "I feel horrible once a cloudy day hits. Winter is the worst: it is as if my mood, too, is gray." Studies show that one reason for depression is less exposure to the sun. The pineal gland in human brain is very sensitive to sunlight. When in bright sunlight, the pineal gland is stimulated and secretes more of a hormone that has the effect of regulating the levels of other hormones in the body. When less of this hormone is available, the secretion of thyroxine and adrenaline is reduced. Lower blood concentrations of these two hormones which can stimulate cells can lead to reduced cell excitability and activity, leaving the person in bad mood and a constant feeling of exhaustion. Human emotions are influenced by three major factors: mental state, the environment, and cognitive state. In the winter, the sun is up for a less time, and it is more often windy. The expressions on individuals' faces are more severe in winter than

[142]Chen (2002).

[143]Lu (2011).

[144]Zhai (1997, p. 230).

[145]Tong (2002).

in the other three seasons. Studies also show that in the summer, the scorching sun (and the showers that follow) is also a cause of depression. Excessively plentiful and burning sunshine as well as persistent rain can make people more irritable, hence leading to suicide by depressed patients.

### 5.4.2 Personality Disorders and Youth Suicide

The word "personality" is derived from the Latin word "persona," which originally referred to the special masks worn by on stage. Such a mask signals the identity, temperament, and features of the stage character represented. From the source of this word, we can see that personality involves two aspects: the behaviors that people display in life, and the true self that lies under. As Liang Qichao, a famous modern Chinese thinker, wrote in *The New Citizen Theory*: "Loyalty and filiality are key elements of personality." To equate "loyalty and filiality" with "personality" and to discuss personality from the perspective of virtue and ethics are typical in traditional Chinese culture.

"Personality" is a compound concept that encompasses a person's physical, psychological, and social behavior. It is the sum of one's inner qualities and external behaviors, and is a unique self one forms through socialization. It involves all kinds of mental processes, cognitive ability, behavioral motivation, emotional responses, interpersonal relationships, religious beliefs, moral values, aesthetic taste, and many other traits of a person.

Personality disorders are persistent and stubborn forms of maladaptation. They are a type of mental disorder, wherein social or occupational impairment or inner pain is caused by deviations in terms of behavior and inner experiences from the social and cultural expectations associated with the environment one is in. Such disorders tend to become milder in later stages of life as one's personality continues to develop and mature over time. Therefore, personality disorders are an important category of mental disorder more frequently seen in adolescents.

According to one study, about 9.0% of those who committed suicide were "mainly diagnosed with personality disorder," while as many as 30% were diagnosed with "abnormal personality." Another study reveals that as many as 34% of individuals who committed suicides were "mainly diagnosed with personality disorder," while 70% were diagnosed with "abnormal personality."[146]

Patients with personality disorder are at higher risk of suicide in the following situations: (1) where the disorder is accompanied by depression, alcoholism, or substance abuse; (2) where there are problems with interpersonal communication and social adjustment; (3) where there has been a stressful life event; (4) where the individual does not have the ability to cope with his/her mental and physical illness;

[146]Isometsä et al. (1996).

and (5) where there is a conflict with others (including family members and medical personnel).[147]

Different types of personality disorders carry different risks of suicide, and the resulted suicide, when it does occur, takes different forms. Generally, failed suicide attempts are the majority.[148] Personality disorders can be accompanied by other mental disorders, and different types of personality disorders can coexist. For example, antisocial personality disorder and histrionic personality disorder can overlap. According to Danuta Wasserman, Head of the WHO's Center for Collaborative Research on Suicide and the Prevention of Mental Disorders, around 9% of individuals with borderline personality disorder would kill themselves. Individuals with borderline personality disorder typically are present with clear problems with empathy, a persistent sense of emptiness, instability, and difficulty to establish intimate relationships with others. Individuals with antisocial personality disorder often lack moral values and compassion, are self-centered, are contemptuous of others, and place an excessive emphasis on self-perception. They often put their impulses and aggressive illusions into action without hesitation, arbitrarily indulging their actions and venting their inner dissatisfaction onto others or themselves. Very often, they commit suicide impulsively in an outburst of rage.[149]

In adolescents, personality disorders may interact with emotional disorders. Emotional disorders often lead to personality disorders, while personality disorders are reflective of emotional disorders. The manifestations can be diverse and complex, including sense of inferiority, depression, isolation, pessimism, recklessness, impatience, shame, suspiciousness, narrow mindedness, and anxiety though not every single form is very likely to directly lead to suicide. Suicidal behavior is often the result of interactions between multiple factors.

At present, there are few community studies on personality disorders in China. Huang Yueqin and Li Liming, et al. conducted a survey of personality disorders and discussed the risk factors for 2205 freshmen in a key university in Beijing (1785 male and 420 female) using the personality diagnostic questionnaire (revised edition). The results show that the prevalence of personality disorders was 2.49% (OCD type, 1.09%; emotional instability, 0.63%; anxious and avoidant, 0.54%; overly dependent, 0.27%; paranoid type, 0.14%; split personality type; 0.14%, histrionic type, 0.09%; and mixed-type, 0.05%). The incidence in women is 1.9 times that in men, and the incidence among those from single-parent families was 5.9 times that among those from two-parent families; those from families where relationships between the parents are not good are present with personality disorders at a rate that is 2.5 times that of the others.[150] The prevalence among college students, especially

[147]Zhai (1997, pp. 244–255).

[148]Zhai (1997, pp. 244–255).

[149]Wasserman (2003).

[150]Huang et al. (2000).

those from single-parent families, is significantly higher than the general prevalence revealed by a survey across seven regions of China (0.10‰).[151]

All relevant studies show that parenting style has a critical impact on children's personality development and mental health. Improper parenting styles can lead to negative personality traits in children and make it difficult for the children to adapt to society, thus pushing up the risk of mental illness. S. Benjiaminsen et al. are of the opinion that the personalities of those who attempt suicide are directly related to how they are raised and to the familial bereavement they experience in their early years. Individuals whose parents have attempted suicide are more likely to experience parental rejection and denial and are less likely to receive encouragement and recognition. A larger proportion of those who have attempted suicide have divorced parents or have been separated from their parents.[152] Qian Mingyi et al. also found from their study that poor parenting skills such as severe punishment, rejection, denial, excessive interference, and overprotection may be important factors for the formation of certain negative personality traits in children.[153]

Parental rejection refers to punishment, blame, humiliation, public reprimand, and corporal punishment by parents. Such behaviors tend to make children feel inferior, helpless, and insecure. They end up worrying too much about their behavior in social interactions and having excessively high demands for themselves. They become overly cautious and indecisive, and fear rejection by others. This way, certain negative personality traits form, placing the child at high risk of developing personality disorders.

Similarly, overprotective and doting parents can also hinder children's independence and social skills, resulting in a lack of self-confidence as well as excessive self-discipline and overdependence. In addition, negative personality traits such as waywardness, self-centeredness, and a lack of resilience can also form. As most children in China today are only children, they are more pampered and cared for. This hinders the formation of a healthy personality to a certain extent. Studies show that only children tend to be selfish, lonely, and unsociable. Some even think that the one-child policy has its drawbacks in terms of the overall mental health conditions of the generation. Domestic studies reveal that only children are more likely to show certain negative behaviors compared to children from multiple-child households.[154]

Family environment has a direct impact on the psychological and behavioral development of adolescents. A lack of harmony in family life and broken families is positively related to mental illness in adolescents. Wang Yufeng et al. surveyed 2432 school-age children in Beijing and found behavioral problems in 7.7% of children from harmonious families; 17.5% of children whose parents quarrel a lot;

[151]Zhang et al. (1998).
[152]Benjiaminsen et al. (1990).
[153]Qian et al. (1996).
[154]Shanghai Preschool Education Research Group (1980).

and 17.7% of children with divorced parents. The prevalence of behavioral problems was twice as high in children whose parents had lower educational attainment and lower poorer social and economic status as in children whose parents were better-educated and had higher social and economic status.[155]

Factors such as poor relationships between one's parents, hailing from a single-parent family, and poor family economic conditions are risk factors for personality disorders in adolescents, for these factors are likely to make children feel insecurity, incomplete, sensitive and suspicious, inferior, hostile, paranoid, and anxious, thus placing them at higher risk of personality disorders and suicide. Low family income can deprive children of better material support and affect parenting styles (and thus become a risk factor for personality disorder).[156]

A survey shows that 78% of adolescents believe that suicide is the biggest punishment for one's parents.[157] Willful, arrogant, solitary, closed-off emotional, and uncooperative… Our young generation today is quite worrisome as such. Extreme behaviors such as truancy, running away from home, hunger strikes, and even self-harm and suicide have become the means by which they can strike fear into the hearts of adults. Behind the growing extreme behavior on the part of adolescents are not only improper education styles adopted by adults and the irritability that arises in a time of social transformation, but also the "gaming" attitude toward life that is gradually being formed in adults and minors alike, together with a kind of indifference to life. This is a trend that requires heightened attention.

However, what have the parents, as adults, done in the face of all these social problems? In September 2004, a China Central Television channel was widely condemned by the public after it asked its audience to guess the casualty of a hostage-taking incident in Beslan, North Ossetia, southern Russia. In the same month, a young man on the streets of Beijing produced a price list in the hope of raising money to save his sick wife: He would eat part of a finger of his for RMB5,000, chop off of his left hand for RMB50,000, etc. Clearly, extreme behavior among the young is not just a problem of the young.

Pathological factors are also an important cause of personality disorders in adolescents. According to statistics released by the Ministry of Civil Affairs in December 2007, there were 82.96 million people with physical disabilities in China, which was 6.34% of the total population. That means more than seventy million families, involving some 260 million individuals, have at least one disabled person in the household.[158] In the mid-1990s, 8.17 million Chinese children under 14 were disabled. The suffering of children with disabilities occurs on both the mental and the physical fronts, both of which have a serious impact on the

[155]Wang et al. (1988).

[156]Liu et al. (2000).

[157]Sun (2004).

[158]Zhao (2008).

development of their personalities.[159] Studies reveal a high prevalence of personality disorders among disabled children.

As the times progress, the pace of life quickens and people become affluent in material terms. Spiritual needs thus grow and diversify. The young generation is in the midst of significant social changes. The diversification of values and the transformation of lifestyles have brought about alienation, loneliness, and inability to adapt with regard to interpersonal relationships. Many people find it hard to see their own value and lack a sense of security. With more and more choices to make, many young people have become confused about where to head in life. Although they now enjoy more freedom, they find themselves unable to take control of their own lives. While old values gradually dissolve, new values have yet to be established; while there are now more opportunities, assistance is rare when one finds it difficult to make a choice.

Growing competition in society has brought more pressure for survival. Population movements are accelerating, and the structures of the population and of families are constantly changing. Original social support networks have been undermined, and new ones are not yet strong enough. As a result, stress factors in society have increased dramatically, and mental health problems have become increasingly prominent. There has been a significant increase in behavioral problems in children, mental health problems among high school and college students (especially Internet-related mental disorders), as well as drug abuse (of narcotics), alcohol abuse, and suicide.

## 5.5 *Psychosexual Problems in Youth and Suicide*

### 5.5.1 Delayed Sex Education and Prominent Sex-Related Issues

For a long time, sex education for adolescents has been kept at the minimum in the entire school education system in China. As a taboo in our culture, sex is something that many people avoid wherever possible. However, sex education for adolescents has become a grave challenge in recent years as premarital sexual behavior increases, sex-related errors and crimes grow, sexually transmitted diseases and HIV/AIDS spread to younger population, teenage pregnancy becomes more common, and adolescent suicide caused by sexual issues increases.

Today, our young generation is physiologically better developed than their peers in the past. However, the reality is that sex education for adolescents lags far behind their physical precocity. Data shows that about half of the women who underwent midterm labor induction at Beijing Obstetrics and Gynecology Hospital between 1998 and 2000 were unmarried, and 14% of them were under twenty years of age.[160]

---

[159]Piao and Zhang (1996).

[160]Beijing Obstetrics and Gynecology Hospital (2007).

During the NPC and CPPCC sessions in 2001, 150 CPPCC members jointly submitted a shocking report on sexual health issues among adolescents. According to the report, minors in Beijing showed a severe lack of scientific sexual health knowledge: Specifically, 48.8% of high school students expressed positive attitude about premarital sex, and 9.9% even approved of sex on the first encounter; 32.8% thought that they would be despised by their schoolmates if, past the second year of high school, they did not have friends of the opposite sex; 34.5% of boys and 40.5% of girls did not know that gonorrhea is a sexually transmitted disease; many of them did not even know what menstrual onset or spermatorrhea meant. It is worth noting that 11.2% of the boys and 3.0% of the girls surveyed admitted to having gained sex-related information from pornographic materials.[161] According to another survey of more than 3000 high school students in Beijing, Shanghai, and Guangzhou, 46.9% of the students did not know or denied that fertility is possible once girls start to menstruate and boys start to experience nocturnal emissions; 49.7% obtained their knowledge on sex-related issues from the mass media, 22.4% from their teachers, 17.2% from their classmates, and only 4.1% from their parents (see Fig. 12). The acquisition of sex-related knowledge through the media is the most worrying. Such knowledge obtained from the Internet and pornographic websites can be largely detrimental and hamper the formation of healthy sexual awareness. The survey also showed that the students were having their first romantic relationship at a younger age: Specifically, 24.4% of high school students reported to "have been in a relationship" or "be in a relationship," 10% were "very interested in a relationship," and 64.4% had not had a relationship. Among the students with romantic experiences, the peak in the age distribution of their first relationships occurs during high school, but also quite a number of them started the journey while in primary school. Students are experiencing their first romantic experiences at a younger age. Among the students surveyed, 14% experienced their first romantic relationship while in primary school, 62.3% in junior high school, and 19.5% in senior high school.[162] Starting a relationship at an increasingly younger age is clearly detrimental to the healthy physical and mental development of adolescents.

In comparison with the situation described above, sex education in China is severely late and insufficient, and challenges are grave if improvements are to be made. First of all, we are looking at a large population. There are more than three hundred million young individuals from ten to twenty years old, and around twenty million mature sexually each year. Second, in the past fifty years, the age of sexual maturity among adolescents in China has moved, on average, two years ahead, resulting in an interval of more than ten years from sexual maturity to marriage. This has thus led to greater uncertainty of adolescents' sexual experience. Third, the way people view and understand marriage, family, and sexual behavior has changed

---

[161]Wang (2002).

[162]Wu (1999).

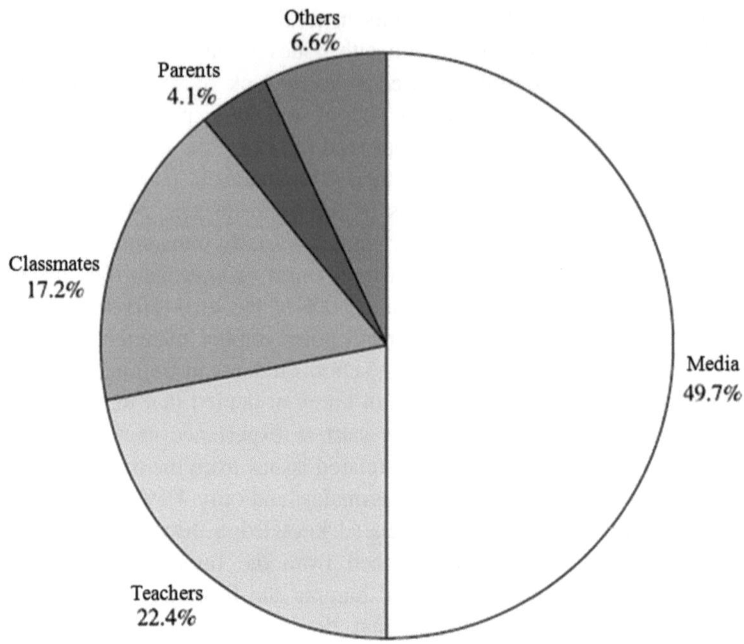


**Fig. 12** Where students obtain sex-related knowledge

dramatically over the years, and people tend to be more open and individualistic in this regard. Frustration has become more likely in this front for the young.

Relationship and marriage are sensitive topics for young people, and a large number of youth suicide cases are caused by issues related to premarital sex or relationship. In 160 cases of suicide by poison, 31.9% was caused by these two types of issues, and the number of women within this share is 4.1 times that of men. In 290 other cases of suicide by poison, 12.4% was due to these reasons, mostly premarital or non-marital sexual relations.[163]

In the past twenty years, Chinese adolescents have shown significantly different features in their puberty. While physiological changes occur at a significantly younger age, the development of cognitive ability and mental endurance has not sped up. This relative delay in psychosocial growth has been termed by E.H. Erikson as the "great extension of puberty." At this stage, young people have to rise gradually to the pressures of marriage, childbirth, and career. Some will try to evade sex or follow a different trail, such as homosexuality, bisexuality, and sexual crimes. According to Erikson, this kind of social psychological lag is an inevitable outcome of industrialization, a process that goes at the expense of the lasting and stable psychological identity of the young.[164] In contemporary China, where

[163]Wen (1998).

[164]Erikson (1980).

tradition and modernity collide, the maladjustment of adolescents' sexual psychology is also manifested in the conflicts between sexual impulses and sexual repression, and disorders in one's sexual psychology.

### 5.5.2 Sexual Inversion and Suicide

Sexual inversion usually takes the following forms and is closely related to suicidal behavior among adolescents.

Homosexuality refers to sexual attraction between persons of the same sex. Existing moral and legal restraints leave homosexuals in anxiety in most cases. If one party in a homosexual relationship shifts his/her affection to another person, which is especially likely when the one is bisexual, the other party will suffer and fall into despair. This may lead to depression or suicide. Studies show that most homosexuals are relatively lonely, have low self-acceptance, are neurotic and depressed, and have a high suicidal ideation rate. These individuals, regardless of their gender, are more likely to have a history of suicide attempts and seeking help for relevant reasons.[165]

Gao Li and Zhang Hong, both from Xinjiang, had been in a lesbian relationship for years when, in 2001, Gao began a "romantic relationship" with another woman surnamed Sun. On the night of July 10, the three women were in the same home and Zhang killed herself by taking poison. On August 6, 2000 ("Ghost Festival" in the Chinese lunar calendar), two girls surnamed Yip and Lam (aged fourteen and thirteen, respectively) in Hong Kong killed themselves by burning charcoal in a Cheung Chau villa after facing objections to their homosexual relationship. The two were found in each other's embrace.

Sex-associated asphyxia is a form of self-destructive abnormal sexual behavior in which an individual tries to obtain feelings of satisfaction and pleasure by self-stimulation that results in cerebral hypoxia, i.e., oxygen deprivation in the brain. Among forensic scholars in other countries, this is referred to as "adolescent self-destructive asphyxia," with a reported incidence of 0.25 per 100,000 individuals.[166] Most people who do this first accidentally find that they experience the greatest sexual pleasure when masturbating while half-suffocated, and thus indulge in this pathological masturbation habit. The purpose of applying pressure on the neck here is to deliberately cause hypoxia in the brain, not to kill oneself. However, often, excessive or extended pressure results in severe hypoxia of the brain and leads to the loss of consciousness. Or, improper methods of doing this lead to a loss of control. Both result in accidental death. Therefore, although sexual asphyxia is a special type of "pathological suicide," it is not suicide in the true sense. In overseas forensic circles, it is generally believed that sexual asphyxia causes only a kind of accidental death. Death from sexual asphyxia occurs mostly among male

---

[165] Zhai (1997, p. 248).

[166] Zhong (2000).

adolescents. All victims of the twenty-two cases of such deaths reported in China were male, with the youngest being only twelve years old, and the oldest, thirty-nine. The average age of the victims was 32.2 years old. Up to 13.64% received college education, 31.82% had senior high school education, 36.36% completed junior high school, and 18.18% attended only primary school.[167]

Transsexualism is a gender identity disorder and a manifestation of sexual psychopathy. The patient mentally denies his/her biological sex and has severe difficulties in reconciling with his/her physiological anatomy and gender identity. The patient also strongly and continuously believes that he/she is the same as the opposite sex, has no sexual interest in members of the opposite sex, and is eager to change his/her sexual organs through hormone therapies or surgery. Adolescents with a transsexual tendency start to experience growing dissonance with their sexual psychology, anatomy, and physiology from around fourteen or fifteen years of age, and feel pain and aversion toward their sexual anatomy and physiology. Girls would detest menstruation and growing breasts, while boys would detest their penises. Because of gender identity disorder, the patient would show interest in members of the same sex. Men believe themselves to be women and thus are attracted to men, while women regard themselves as men and are passionate, protective, and loving to women. In this way, homosexuality may develop by the time they are fifteen to sixteen years old. In adulthood, some transsexuals will demand firmly for the removal of anatomical features that mark their sex, and worry about not having the sexual organs and sexual characteristics of the opposite sex. Some have even tried to do it themselves. A man may cut off his penis or crush his testicles by their own hand. Some can eventually commit suicide out of despair. In recent years, some of the country's transsexuals with the financial means have chosen "sex reassignment surgery" to try to change their sex. In such surgeries, male patients undergo resection of the penis and testicles, artificial breast augmentation, and vaginoplasty. Female patients undergo removal of the ovaries and breasts, phalloplasty, and scrotoplasty. After the surgeries, the patient will have to receive hormone therapy in order to become a "real" woman or a man. However, sex reassignment surgery is not very likely to be completely successful. Though some patients have tried to love and marry in their new identities, the outcomes have mostly been unsatisfactory. This increases the risk of suicide. Studies prove transsexualism to be a form of sexual psychopathy, but there is currently no drug to treat the condition. Once formed, transsexualism is extremely difficult to treat, and drugs are of no avail for now.

Voyeurism is a kind of sexual deviation in which the individual obtains sexual pleasure by peeping at the naked bodies or genitals of the opposite sex, or at the process of sexual intercourse between others. Patients often use special means such as miniature video cameras, small cameras, high-powered telescopes, and mirror reflections in specific locations such as toilets and bathrooms to peek at, and sneak shots of, the opposite sex. Exhibitionism is a form of a deviation in which the

[167]Zhong (2000).

individual obtains sexual pleasure from the exposure of his/her genitals in the face of the opposite sex in an inappropriate environment, thus causing emotional reactions in the opposite sex. This is a fairly common form of sexual perversion, with patients mostly male and aged 25–35 years old. Female patients are rare, with a male-to-female ratio of around 14:1. Patients with voyeurism are always looking for opportunities to peep at others even at the risk of being caught, losing their reputations, and potentially losing their futures. Patients are often in a very conflicted state of mind and torn between the impulse to peep and the knowledge that one should restrain such impulses. This often results in a strong sense of uneasiness and agony as the individual finds himself/herself unable to stop, repeatedly. Patients with exhibitionism generally know what they are doing. They often regret the act afterward, especially when they are taken as "perverted" and "rogue" as a result. They then experience even more shame and regret. However, the exhibitionist impulse is difficult to control. Patients with the aforementioned behavior often see their reputations suffer when they are caught. They are condemned by society and blamed and resented by their families, but are unable to control themselves. Some people have no choice but to commit suicide at moments of extreme pain.

## *5.6 Drug Abuse by Youths and Borderline Suicide*

Drug abuse is a kind of borderline suicide. Borderline suicide is an antinomic activity that is centered on the pursuit of happiness or the reduction of physical pain but can result in death. Borderline suicide can be further classified into chronic suicide and disguised suicide. Forms of chronic suicide include drug abuse, smoking, alcoholism, and the deliberate decision by patients with diabetes not to control their diet,[168] while disguised suicide includes euthanasia (including both active and passive euthanasia).

From the mid-nineteenth century to the mid-twentieth century, China suffered from the scourge of opium and other narcotics. The memory of the two Opium Wars is still fresh. After the founding of the People's Republic of China, the government immediately launched a vigorous campaign against drugs. In the short span of a few years, drugs were eradicated in China in what was a miracle that led China to be known around the world as a "land of no drugs." However, since the 1980s, the drug problem has resurfaced in China as international drug cartels sought to open up the so-called Chinese channel for the "Golden Triangle" and "Golden Crescent." Drug abuse has spread and become increasingly rampant, and most drug users are quite young.

Figures from the Office of the National Narcotics Control Commission show that young people account for around 80% of all drug abusers in China in recent years. Available statistics also reveal an increase in the number of drug abusers under the

[168]He (1997, p. 653).

age of 16, and adolescents have become the "high-risk group" most vulnerable to drug abuse. By the end of 2001, the number of drug users known to China's public security organs totaled nine hundred thousand, of which 77% were under the age of 35. Statistics also have it that the number of drug abusers under the age of 16 has been on the rise since 2000. Even children only six or seven years old have appeared in the pool of first-time drug users. In addition, many young people lack an understanding of the addictiveness and serious consequences of amphetamines such as methamphetamine and ecstasy. As a result, the number of people using "ice" and ecstasy has increased significantly. Around 30% of theft, robbery, and similar common criminal cases are related to drug abuse. In areas where the drug problem is serious, this figure can be as high as 60%.[169]

A survey shows that the vast majority of drug users start using drugs between 20 and 25 years old. Statistics from developed Western countries show that one-third of Americans under the age of 25 have used drugs, 73% of Italian drug users are 18–20 years old, 80% of French drug users are young people, and up to 43,536 Japanese adolescents were put into detention facilities because of drug abuse. Among registered drug users in China in 1998, more than 65% were under the age of 25, and 83.6% under 35.[170] The number of registered drug users in the same year was nearly six hundred thousand, thrice the number of 1990. Analysts believe the actual number of drug users to be far greater. According to a survey of drug abusers in ten provinces and autonomous regions, drug users under the age of 25 accounted for 79.8% of the total; in Guangdong Province, young drug abusers accounted for 60–80% of the total, and in Bao'an County, in particular, the proportion was higher than 90%. In terms of the age structure of drug users, in Shenzhen, the proportion of under 25 bracket is relatively stable, while that of users in the 26–35 bracket surged, from an average of 28% between 1991 and 1997 to 38.3% in 1997, and 46% in 1998.[171] Drug abusers and drug traffickers in China are becoming younger. Take Chongqing's Shapingba District as an example. The drug rehabilitation center of the district was established in 1995, and 70 drug abusers were admitted in that year. By 1998, the number of people admitted was already over a thousand, representing an increase of thirteen times. Among these, 74% were under the age of 30. Worse than that, the number of high school students using drugs is also on the rise. In a certain district in Chongqing, more than fifty high school students aged between 14 and 16 were found to be abusing drugs, accounting for 1.7% of the total number of students in the district (including senior high students).[172]

According to data released by the Ministry of Public Security, the number of drug users registered in China reached one million in 2002, which was a year-on-year increase of 11%. The number of counties (cities, and districts) where drug use if found amounted to 2148, 97 more than the previous year. Young drug

[169]Zhang (2002b).

[170]Office of the National Narcotics Control Commission of the People's Republic of China (1998).

[171]Xu (2000).

[172]Song and Zhou (2000).

abusers accounted for 74% of the total. In recent years, the cumulative number of deaths from drug abuse in China has exceeded twenty-five thousand. Drug abuse is also a major channel of HIV transmission in China. In 2002, about two-thirds of the more than forty thousand HIV-infected persons reported nationwide were drug users. According to data released at the 2004 Anti-Drug Forum held in Beijing, by 2003, there were 1.05 million drug users registered in China, rehabilitation had been difficult, and the relapse rate was as high as over 90%. Each year, drug abuser spent up to RMB200 billion on drugs.[173] On February 1, 2010, the Office of the National Narcotics Control Commission announced that as of the end of 2009 there were 1335,920 registered drug users nationwide, which was an increase of 209,158 from the end of 2008. Among them, 84.6% were male, 15.4% were female, and 58.1% were under the age of 35. The proportion of users of heroin had dipped to 73.2% of the total (or 960,000), while the proportion of users of synthetic drugs such as ice and ketamine rose to 27% (360,000 users). The number of individuals using ice rose rapidly. In 2009, public security organs in various areas found a total of 75,505 persons using ice, accounting for 37.9% of all newly registered drug users.[174]

The following are the characteristics of drug abuse in China.

First, drug abuse is spreading fast. Since the late 1980s, drug abuse among youths has gradually spread to almost all provinces, municipalities, and autonomous regions, but still mainly concentrates in the southwest, southeast, and northwest. Statistics show that 70% of all counties and cities in China have a drug abuse problem.

Second, drug use starts at a younger age. It is no longer uncommon to see drug users who are only thirteen or fourteen years old.

Third, the number of girls using drugs is also on the rise. Prior to the mid-twentieth century, drug use among young women was rare. However, from the late 1980s on and especially since the 1990s, drug use among females has grown rapidly. According to statistics from a drug rehabilitation center in Guangzhou, twenty female drug users were admitted in 1989, and the figure rose to 834 in 1994, an increase of 40.7 times in five years. Female drug users make up the majority of female inmates in reeducation camps in Guangdong Province. According to a survey in Wuhan, female drug users accounted for 30% of all drug users, and most were under 25 years old.[175]

Fourth, drug abuse is primarily a group activity. Along with the sharp increase in the number of drug abusers among young people comes the shift from drug use alone and secretly to drug use in groups at regular haunts and even in public places. Statistics show that among the young people arrested for drug abuse in Shenzhen in 1993, 82.6% engaged in group drug use. The majority of drug users arrested by

[173]He (2008).

[174]Office of the National Narcotics Control Commission (2011).

[175]Guo (1997).

Guangzhou authorities in 1994 had used drugs at regular haunts.[176] At the beginning, users would share a smoking implement, and after one or two months, they would start injection. Often, two or three people would share one syringe. The drug they use can also be the result of crowdfunding, which makes HIV/AIDS transmission a high possibility. When drugs are being consumed in groups, individuals are more likely to affect each other. With peer pressure, relapse is more likely for the young.

Fifth, drug users are mostly unemployed, and student drug users are also growing in number.

Sixth, more and stronger kinds of drugs are being used. While the drugs currently used by young abusers diversify, heroin is still the mainstay. According to statistics from Fujian authorities, the six main types of drugs in use are heroin, ice, dihydroetorphine hydrochloride, pethidine, marijuana, and caffeine. Among drug addicts in Guangxi, 99% are heroin abusers, 0.3% opium users, and 0.7% morphine and pethidine users. A survey of a random sample of 373 female drug abusers in Guangdong revealed that 77.7% used heroin, and 28.8% used at least two kinds of drugs such as heroin, marijuana, ice, cocaine, morphine, opium, and sedatives such as pethidine and midazolam.[177] In recent years, more young abusers have started taking amphetamines such as ice and ecstasy.

Seventh, drug abuse and trafficking do harm to social order and morale in society. Most young drug addicts eventually end up trafficking drugs in order to pay for their expensive habit. As they have to stump up large amounts of money for drugs, drug users engage in all kinds of other criminal activities, thus bringing great harm to society. Among the 1320 cases of juvenile crimes investigated in one certain district of Guangzhou in 1994, 1080 cases, or 80%, were caused by drug abuse.[178] According to statistics from a drug rehabilitation center, more than 80% of drug users also engaged in criminal activities such as theft, robbery, fraud, corruption, bribery, drug trafficking, murder, fornication, and the like; more than 90% of female drug users had prostituted themselves in order to pay for their habit.

Eighth, detoxification is difficult, and the relapse rate is high. Up to 90% of young drug users who return to society after detoxification, compulsory or voluntary, would relapse under the combined effect of various factors. Thus, a vicious circle of drug abuse–detoxification–relapse–labor rehabilitation is usually formed.

Ninth, the suicide rate among drug abusers is high. Scholars found the suicide rate of male drug users to be fifty times that of the average male population,[179] and the overall suicide rate among drug users is ten to fifteen times higher than that among the general population.

[176]Zhou (2000).

[177]Zhou (2000).

[178]Guo (1997).

[179]Bai (1983).

## *5.7 Drug Abuse and Youth Suicide*

In the past twenty-plus years, the problem of drug abuse has spread rapidly around the world. It has actually been more rampant in the world, especially among the young population than any plague that has ever occurred on the planet. Drug users are primarily young people who represent the future and hope of mankind. Therefore, drug abuse is one of the most serious medical and social problems that threaten human survival.

Once an adolescent becomes addicted to drugs, they can get seriously harmed mentally and physically. Physiologically, when drugs enter the human body, adaptive changes will take place, and a new equilibrium will be formed. This is how a person gets dependent on or addiction to drugs. Once drug use ceases, the equilibrium fails, and the body suffers. Symptoms may include uneasiness, anxiety, sudden chills and hot flashes, tears, night sweats, nausea, vomiting, abdominal pain, and diarrhea. Then comes memory loss, malnutrition, decreased immunity, and multiple diseases. Mentally, drugs exert their influence on the human nervous system, leading to a strong desire for more drugs. Drugs destroy the spirit and will of drug addicts, undermine their values and morality, and lead to personality disorders and mental perversion. Young people are not yet mature in either physical or mental terms. They have poor self-control and weak will power. Once they are addicted to drugs, they suffer even greater harm than adults both physically and mentally. For example, some young addicts may harm themselves, such as by cutting off their fingers, chopping off their hands, or burning themselves with cigarettes, when the urge for drugs strikes but they cannot get the substance. Some individuals commit suicide in a moment of delirium or despair.

In 1993, a total of 177 individuals died of drug abuse in an autonomous prefecture in Yunnan Province. Between 1992 and 1995, nearly a hundred young people died or committed suicide as a direct consequence of drug abuse in Guangxi. According to the United Nations Office on Drugs and Crime, each year, around the world, more than a hundred thousand people are killed by drugs.[180]

Data suggests that the average life expectancy of drug users is ten to fifteen years shorter than that of the general population. A quarter of drug addicts die within ten to twenty years after starting drug use. That is to say, about one in every four drug users dies from drug-related problems between the thirty and forty years of age, since most drug users start taking drugs around the age of twenty. In recent years, drug use has spread to people of a younger age group and is not uncommon among high school students in some developed nations.

The death rate among drug users is fifteen times higher than that of the general population. According to US estimates, heroin abusers account for less than 1% of the nation's population. However, as many as six thousand people die directly from heroin poisoning each year. In the UK, it is estimated that the annual death rate of heroin users is as high as 16–30%.

---

[180]Zhou (2000).

# References


Bai, Z. (1983). *Diseases of western society* (p. 126) (Z. Huilan, trans.). Beijing: SDX Joint Publishing Company, 126.

Bao, W. (2011). School stress main driver of suicide among primary and high school students. *Guangzhou Daily,* April 1.

Bao, W., & Zhou, W. (2011). School stress main driver of suicide among primary and high school students. *Guangzhou Daily*, April 1.

Beijing Obstetrics and Gynecology Hospital. (2007). *Half of women undergoing mid-term labor induction not married.* http://www.people.com.cn/GB/channel9/568/20000603/87836.html. Accessed September 13, 2007.

Benjiaminsen, S., Krarup, G., & Lauritsen, R. (1990). Personality, parental rearing behaviour and parental loss in attempted suicide: A comparative study. *Acta Psychiatr Scand, 82,* 389–397.

Cai, F. (2003). Guarding against the romanticization of celebrity suicides. *Beijing Youth Daily,* April 8.

Chan, W. T., et al. (1997). *Moral values of youth in Hong Kong.* Hong Kong: Department of Applied Social Studies, City University of Hong Kong.

Chen, D. (2002). Severe postpartum depression can easily lead to tragedy. *Southern Metropolis Daily,* February 8.

Chen, Y. (2011). *The relationships factor in youth suicide and means of prevention.* http://www.tces.chc.edu.tw/8709.12/1014.htm. Accessed July 17, 2011.

China Internet Network Information Center. (2011). *The 24th Statistical Report on the Development of China's Internet Network.* http://www.cnnic.net.cn/uploadfiles/doc/2009/7/16/125040.doc. Accessed May 10, 2011.

China Internet Network Information Center. (2012). *The 29th statistical report on the development of China's Internet network.* Retrieved from: http://www.cnnic.net.cn/research/bgxz/tjbg/201201/t20120116_23668.html. Date of retrieval March 16, 2012.

China Youth Network Association and Institute of Survey and Statistics of the Communication University of China. *2009 Report on the Survey of Youth Addiction to the Internet.* http://mat1.gtimg.com/edu/pdf/wangyinbaogao.pdf. Accessed May 12, 2011.

Chu, L. (2000). The shaping of youths' morals in online society. *Contemporary Youth Research, 2.*

Cui, X., et al. (1990). A study of the psychological health of college students studying medicine. *Chinese Journal of Social Medicine, 4,* 32–35.

Dong, X. (2011). Surviving, cartoon-like: The impact of Japanese animation on youth behavior. *Movie Literature, 8,* 39.

Durkheim, É. (1998). *Suicide: A study in sociology* (p. 18) (X. Zhong, L. Ma, & Q. Lin, Trans.). Hangzhou: Zhejiang People's Press.

Erikson, E. H. (1980). *Identity and the life cycle.* New York: WW Norton.

Fan, Y., & Hai, H. (2010). Incidence of mental illness among China's children and youth higher than international average. *Guangming* Daily, June 3.

Fang, J. (2010). Stream of suicides by students in mainland China. *Lianhe Zaobao*, January 10.

Fawcett, J., et al. (1987). Clinical predictors of suicide in patients with major affective disorders: A controlled prospective study. *American Journal of Psychiatry, 144*(1), 35–40.

Fu, J., & Ruijun, L., et al. (1998). A survey on the state of psychological health among college students in the Inner Mongolia Autonomous Region. *Chinese Journal of Psychiatry, 4.*

Ge, Q., & Qu, G. (2011). Urgent need for attention to issues of psychological health among China's Youth. *Xinhua News Online.* Retrieved from: http://www.54youth.com.cn/gb/paper419/1/classo41900003/htm. Date of retrieval June 15, 2011.

Guo, X. (1997). China's drug problem and countermeasures. *Academic Journal of Politics and Law, 4.*

Guo, X., et al. (2008). A study of the mental health of 1.344 junior high school students in Beijing. *Chinese Journal of School Health, 29*(4).

He, Z. (1997). *The pathology of suicide.* Beijing: China Traditional Chinese Medicine Press.

He, Q. (1998). *the trap of modernity: economic and social issues in contemporary China* (p. 98). Beijing: China Today Press.

He, S. (2003). *Social formations at a time of transformation in contemporary China* (pp. 45–48). Shanghai: Xuelin Publishing.

He, X. (2006). Destruction and the fear of life in antiquity: Reflections on the phenomenon of suicide in China. *Frontiers, 3,* 35.

He, C. (2005). Ministry of public security issues statement on online suicide manual: Criminal charges possible. *China Youth Daily*, March 31.

He, C. (2007). Ministry of public security: Over 4800 web sites and online bulletin boards shut due to "yellow" content. *China Youth Daily*, May 27.

He, C. (2008). Anti-drug efforts: as many as 1.05 million drug users registered in China. *China Population*. http://www.chinapop.gov.cn/rkkx/ztbd/t20040727.htm. Accessed March 11, 2008.

Hu, Y. (2002). Sociological reflections on depression. *Psychology, 1,* 84.

Hu, Q., Yi, F., et al. (1999). *The social and psychological problems of university students today, and countermeasures*. Nanchang: Jiangxi People's Press.

Huang, Y., Li, L., et al. (2000). The current state of personality disorders in first-year science and engineering students in college and risk factors. *Chinese Journal of Psychiatry, 33*(1).

Ikegami, Y. (1985). *Introduction to semiotics* (p. 16) (Z. Xiaoyun trans.). Beijing: China International Culture Publishing.

Inamura, H. (1977). *Suicide studies: For the treatment and prevention of suicide* (p. 89). Tokyo: University of Tokyo Press.

Isometsä, E. T., et al. (1996). Suicide among Subjects with personality disorders. *American Journal of Psychiatry, 153,* 667–673.

Ji, J., et al. (1990a). An analysis from the use of the SCL-90 instrument on college students from various majors. *Chinese Mental Health Journal, 4,* 123–125.

Ji, J., et al. (1990b). An analysis of 83 college students undergoing psychological health counseling. *Chinese Mental Health Journal, 4,* 34–35.

Jing, T. (2011). *An analysis of the current state of mental illness among Chinese children*. http://www.jk4006.com/detail.aspx?catid=2&id=163113. Accessed June 15, 2011.

Joffe, R. T., & Offord, D. R. (1983). Suicidal behaviour in childhood. *Canadian Journal of Psychiatry, 28*(1), 57–63.

Jones, D. (2007). *Study shows that number of Chinese netizens has grown to 68 million*. http://tech.sina.com.cn/i/c/2003-07-21/1831211895.shtml. Accessed May 12, 2007.

Kraut, R., et al. (1998). Internet paradox: A social technology that reduces the psychological well-being? *American Psychologist, 53*(9), 1017–1031.

Lan, T. (2010). 2009 report: 14.1% of China's young Internet users addicted to the Internet. *China Daily*, February 2.

Lester, D. (1994). The epidemiology of suicide in Chinese population in six regions of the world [*sic.*]. *Chinese Mental Health Journal, 7,* 25–36.

Li, F. (1988). A survey of 4868 college students with neurasthenia in the Lanzhou area. *Chinese Mental Health Journal, 5,* 229–233.

Li, H. (2001). *An interview on violence: A record of psychological harm on school campuses, and countermeasures*. Beijing: China Writers Publishing House.

Li, J. (2000). Survey: Relatively unhealthy personalities and psychologies among female college students at present. *Chongqing Morning New*, December 29.

Li, L. (2010). First-ever blue book on youth released, over 126 million minor netizens in China. *China Youth Daily,* June 19.

Liang, Y. (2006). Blue book on adolescent mental health. *Prosecutorial View, 8.*

Lin, J. (2002). Comparatively high suicide rate in China, severe lack of research and prevention institutions. *China Youth Daily,* December 11.

Liu, J., et al. (1991). *Unveiling the mystery behind suicide* (p. 93). Chengdu: Sichuan Science and Technology Press.

Liu, S. (2000). Depression: A topic that we cannot avoid in the 21st century. *Psychiatrist, 7,* 32.

Liu, H., & Li, X. (1996). The current state of research into suicide, and trends. *Foreign Medicine (Psychiatry volume), 23*(2), 125–126.

Liu, L., Huang, Y., & Li, L. (2000). A case-control study of personality disorders in college students. *Chinese Mental Health Journal, 14*(2), 88–92.

Liu, W. (2003). Paying attention to the hidden on-campus harms to individuals. *China Education Daily*, March 30.

Liu, X., & Su, L. (2002). The impact of video games on the behavior of children. *Chinese Mental Health Journal, 16*(1), 65.

Liu, Y., & Xiao, S. (2007). The impact of media reports of suicide incidents on suicide behavior in the community (an overview). *Chinese Mental Health Journal, 5,* 312.

Lu, J. (2011). 30-year-old mother with postpartum depression jumps off building, kills herself. *Huaxi Metropolis Daily*, May 19.

Lu, X. (1919). How would we act as fathers now? *Xin Qing Nian, 6*(6).

Luo, S. (1992). *61 cases of suicide behavior among children with mental illness*. Paper presented at the National Crisis Intervention and Suicide Prevention Conference.

Lü, Z. (2005). 1200 entrepreneurs commit suicide in two decades in China. *Corporate Culture and Management, 6,* 51–52.

Lü, L. (2010). China in "era of mental illness"? *China Comment*, June 3.

Ma, L. (1999). The reasons for imbalances in psychological health in children. *Population and Eugenics, 4.*

Ministry of Health Statistics and Information Center. (2004). 2004 *China Health Statistics Yearbook.* http://www.moh.gov.cn/publicfiles/business/htmlfiles/mohbgt/s8274/200805/35286.htm. Accessed March 13, 2008.

Ministry of Health Statistics Information Center. (2006). *2006 China Health Statistics Yearbook.* http://www.moh.gov.cn/publicfiles/business/htmlfiles/zwgkzt/ptjnj/year2006/index.htm. Accessed March 13, 2008.

Ministry of Health Statistics Information Center. (2007). 2007 *China Health Statistics Yearbook.* http://www.moh.gov.cn/publicfiles/business/htmlfiles/mohbgt/s8274/200807/37168.htm. Accessed March 13, 2008.

Ministry of Health Statistics Information Center. (2008). *2008 China Health Statistics Yearbook.* http://www.moh.gov.cn/publicfiles/business/htmlfiles/mohbgt/s8274/200809/37759.htm. Accessed October 12, 2011.

Ministry of Health Statistics Information Center. (2009). *2009 China Health Statistics Yearbook.* http://www.moh.gov.cn/publicfiles/business/htmlfiles/zwgkzt/ptjnj/200908/42635.htm. Accessed October 12, 2011.

Ministry of Health Statistics Information Center. (2010). *2010 China Health Statistics Yearbook.* http://www.moh.gov.cn/publicfiles/business/htmlfiles/zwgkzt/ptjnj/year2010/2010t10/sheet.htm Accessed October 12, 2011.

Office of the National Narcotics Control Commission. (2011). 1.335 million drug users currently registered in China. *Official web site of the Ministry of Public Security*. http://www.mps.gov.cn/n16/n1252/n1897/n2872/2327636.html. Accessed August 15, 2011.

Office of the National Narcotics Control Commission of the People's Republic of China. (1998). *Annual Report on China's Efforts Against Narcotics, 1998.*

Ouyang, L., & Wu, R. (2011). The issues present with psychological health work on college campuses in China, and countermeasures. *Examination Weekly, 22,* 211.

Peng, D. (Ed.). (2001). *General psychology* (revised ed., p. 74). Beijing: Beijing Normal University Press.

Piao, X., & Zhang, A. (1996). Obstacles to the socialization of personality in youth. *China Youth Study* [*sic*.], *2.*

Qian, L. (2003). Psychological reforms must be taken into account in education reforms. *China Education Daily*, January 13.

Qian, M., et al. (1996). A study on the relationship between youth personality and parenting methods. *Chinese Mental Health Journal, 10*(2).

Shangguan, Z. (1995). The "native" characteristics of suicide among the Chinese. *Sociological Studies*, no. 2.

Shanghai Preschool Education Research Group. (1980). Parenting with only children. *Women of China, 5.*

Sharp, S., & Smith, P. K. (1994). *Tackling bullying in your school: A practical handbook for teachers*. London: Routledge.

Social Survey Center of China Youth Daily. (1997). The worrying state of psychological health among China's youth (Part I). *China Youth Daily,* November 7.

Social Survey Center of China Youth Daily. (1997). The worrying state of psychological health among China's youth (Part II). *China Youth Daily,* November 7.

Song, S., & Zhou, X. (2000). Drug abuse among high school students shocking. *China Youth Study* [*sic.*], *1.*

Stoll, C. (1995). *Silicon snake oil: Second thoughts on the information highway* (pp. 78–90). New York: Doubleday.

Su, J. (2011). Suicide deaths among Shanghai's primary and high school students on the rise. *Wen Wei Po*, January 26.

Suen, K. J. (1996). *1996 statistics for suicide in Hong Kong*. http://www.sbhk.org.hk/statistic/suicide1996.htm. Accessed February 3, 2007.

Sun, D. (2004). An agonized lament: how can there be so much indifference to life? *Chengdu Evening News*, September 21.

Tan, Y. (2002). 1.9% of students have attempted suicide, youth feel overwhelming levels of stress. *Southern Metropolis Daily*, November 29.

Tong, T. (2002, December 28). Majority of suicides by depressed occur in winter. *Beijing Morning Post.*

Uchimura, H. (1978). *Child suicide* (p. 9). Tokyo: Tokyo University Press.

Vago, S. (2007). *Social change* (p. 274) (W. Xiaoli, et al., trans.). Beijing: Peking University Press.

Wang, D. (2000). Eight in ten individuals committing suicide have depression. *Beijing Evening News*, June 20.

Wang, M. (2010). Saddening! 73 cases of suicide by primary and high school students in China this year. *Chengdu Economic Daily*, November 28.

Wang, P. (2011, September 20). Too much homework leads three primary school girls to jump off building together. *Jiangnan Metropolis Daily.*

Wang, S. (2002). Sex education for youth: Currently weak and "thin", urgent need to do better. *People's Daily*, 7, May 12.

Wang, Y., et al. (1988). A survey of behavioral problems in 2432 children of school-going age in the Beijing area. *Chinese Mental Health Journal, 2*(3), 114–117.

Wang, X., et al. (1992). An assessment of the state of psychological health among students of the Hangzhou Medical College. *Chinese Mental Health Journal, 6,* 108.

WHO. (1990). *World Health Statistics Annual.*

Wasserman, D. (Ed.). (2003). *Suicide: An unnecessary death* (pp. 110–111) (L. Ming, et al., trans.). Beijing: China Light Industry Press.

Wei, X. (2002, June 12). Around 6% of netizens afflicted with online-related psychological disorder of one kind or another. *Jiangnan Times*, 26.

Wen, Z. (1998). *Transcending death: Prevention and control of suicidal behavior* (p. 68). Shanghai: Shanghai Medical University Press.

World Health Organization. (1989). *World Health Statistics Annual* (pp. 364–369).

Wu, Z. (1999). The confusion regarding sexual issues that senior high students face today. *Contemporary Youth Research (sic.), 4.*

Xi, Y. (2001). Overwhelmed by stress, 8-year-old child seeks suicide; attention needs to be paid to problem of psychological crisis growing among younger children. *Yangtse Evening News*, June 15.

Xiao, S. (2009). A psychological study of suicide. *Hunan Crisis Intervention Center*. Retrieved from: http://hncic.virtualave.net/suibook/chapter4.htm. Date of retrieval July 15, 2009.

Xie, Y., & Gong, Y. (1993). Comparing the psychological health of minority and Han students. *Chinese Journal of Clinical Psychology, 1,* 33.

Xie, Y. (2005). Psychological issues among primary and high school students need urgent attention. *China Youth Daily*, July 30.

Xin, Z., & Chi, L. (2008). *Youth in the midst of social change* (p. 331). Beijing: Beijing Normal University Press.

Xu, Y. (2001). A study of the psychological health and family environment factors of high school students with suicide ideation. *China Journal of School Health, 22*(5), 449.

Xu, X. (2000). A sociological analysis on drug abuse among youth and the prevention and control of such abuse. *Youth Studies, 3.*

Yang, X. (2000b). An evaluation of the impact of the Internet on Chinese youth. *Youth Studies, 4,* 7.

Yang, H., & Li, Z. (2002a). A preliminary analysis of the "ten Internet harms" to youth psychology. *Qing Nian Gong Zuo Lun Tan, 2002*(1), 27.

Yang, H., & Li, Z. (2002b). A preliminary analysis of the "ten Internet harms" to youth psychology. *Youth Work Forum, 1,* 28.

Yang, Y., Wang, L., et al. (2010). Update on the study on tryptophan hydroxylase and depression and suicide behavior. *Chinese Journal of Public Health, 26*(3), 371.

Yang, B. (2000a). Nearly half of primary and high school students do not sleep enough, according to state-recommended standards. *Southern Daily*, March 22.

Yi, R. (2000). Psychological health of teachers should not be neglected. *Life Times*, September 11.

Yin, D. (2002). United, with a practical mind, we promote mental health on all fronts in the new century: Report of the 3rd National Conference on Mental Health Work. *Chinese Mental Health Journal, 16*(1), 6.

Yu, Z., et al. (2001). *Reflections on issues related to education of youth* (p. 51). Hohhot: Inner Mongolia People's Press.

Yu, Y. (2010). *Data point one on the psychological health of minors: The general situation*. http://www.cycs.org/. Accessed February 10, 2010.

Yu, Z. (2001). *Reflections on issues related to education of the youth* (p. 141). Hohhot: Inner Mongolia People's Press.

Yue, D., et al. (1993). Methods of parental upbringing: the preliminary draft of the EMBU and the applications of the EMBU with patients with neurosis. *China Mental Health Journal, 7*(3).

Yue, X. (1999). A comparative analysis of idol worship and learning from one's models among youth. *Youth Studies, 7.*

Zeng, G., & Cai, Y. (2001). Guard against growing psychological indifference and pay attention to psychological issues among youth. *Guangming Daily*, February 12.

Zhai, S. (1997). *Crisis intervention and suicide prevention*. Beijing: People's Medical Publishing House.

Zhang, J. (2007a). 370 million lewd websites harming our youth, public looks forward to the beating back of the "yellow poison." *China Youth Daily*, May 25.

Zhang, Y. (2007b). The task to clean out the "three harms" of online pornography to minors cannot wait. *Legal Daily*, April 27.

Zhang, K. (2010). Netizens work overnight to rescue suicidal youth, limits of emergency rescue mechanisms clear. *China Youth Daily*, February 3.

Zhang, R. (2011). More than 700 lewd web sites shut by Beijing in cultural clean-up campaign last year. *Beijing Times*, January 28.

Zhang, Y. (2002a). Don't allow Internet cafes to "enmesh" our children. *China Police Daily*, May 7.

Zhang, Y. (2002b). Number of drug abusers on the rise in China, [need] to keep youth away from drugs. *People's Daily*, June 26.

Zhang, W., et al. (1998). An epidemiological survey of mental illness in seven regions of China. *Chinese Journal of Psychiatry, 31*(2), 69–71.

Zhao, E. (2008). Disabled services sector in China developing strongly, 82.96 million persons with disabilities all covered under social insurance. *People's Daily*, September 8.

Zhao, D., & Zhong, C. (2002). Crisis intervention mechanisms for, and the prevention of suicide among, students. In Student Work Committee of the Ideological and Political Education Research Association of Guangdong Province (Ed.), *The education and management of student following expanded enrollment* (p. 356). Guangzhou: Sun Yat-sen University Press.

Zhao, J., et al. (1991). The state of psychological health among junior medical students and the factors that affect [their psychological health]. *Chinese Mental Health Journal, 1,* 76–81.

Zheng, R. (1994). *Psychological diagnosis of high school students.* Jinan: Shandong Education Press.

Zhong, J. (2000). *Unveiling the mystery behind suicide* (p. 141). Beijing: China Procuratorial Press.

Zhong, X., & Su, X. (2002). The possible youth alienation caused by computer networks. *Youth Studies, 2.*

Zhou, Z. (2000). Drug abuse among the youth of China today. *Journal of China Youth University for Political Sciences, 1.*

# Chapter 4
# Elderly Suicide

Population aging is a global trend. China will surely become old before it gets rich as both the absolute number of old people and their proportion in the population are growing.

## 1 Elderly Suicide: A Serious Problem

### *1.1 Fast Population Aging in China*

According to international standards, China became an aging society in 1999, and this aging trend is developing fast as the average increase in elderly population has gone from 3.11 to 8 million people per year. Data provided by the China National Committee on Aging shows that China's elderly population reached 159 million, or 12% of the total population, in 2008.[1] This rate was 10.1% in 2000 and 11.1% in 2005. The rate then grew faster to 12.7% in 2010. After that, China entered a stage where the elderly population grew rapidly. In 2018, the elderly population reached 249 million, accounting for 17.9% of the total population. It is estimated that the share of the elderly population will double to 25% by 2032, an increase of 1 percentage point every two years over the next 22 years. Expectations are: by 2020, the elderly population will reach 240 million and account for 15.6% of the total population, the share will be up to 31% by 2050, and then, the elderly population will peak at 430 million in 2053.[2]

As the elderly population grow, the problems of old age become more prominent. Very soon, every couple in China will have to support four old people. People between the ages of 20 and 40 will account for only 20% of the population, and the Chinese economy will diminish in innovation and vibrancy. China's share of world

[1]Zhang (2010).
[2]Du (2006).



J. Li, *A Study on Suicide*,
https://doi.org/10.1007/978-981-13-9499-7_4

population will go down faster and faster. Population aging and the concomitant changes will rock China's society and economy, bringing huge challenges to the sustainability of social and economic development.[3]

## 1.2 Increase in Elderly Suicide

People tend to believe that youth is the peak period for suicide. After all, old age, the last stage of life, is the time when people are experienced in life, emotionally stable, and most likely fortified with a nest egg. This is especially true for rural people who have worked hard all their lives and raised children, and whose old age should be a time of leisure, safety, and the enjoyment of grandchildren. They know how to survive the vicissitudes of fortune and have no reason to end their lives by suicide. But elderly suicide has increased in recent years and it is more prevalent in the countryside. Statistics show that the suicide rate in the countryside, where 90% of the suicides take place, is three to four times that in the cities, and the elderly is the age group with the highest suicide rate. In fact, suicide rate increases with age, and this is the reason that elderly suicide has become a social problem and a public health issue. Since China has traditionally emphasized familial ethics and filial piety, elderly suicide has become an ethical issue as well.

As the Chinese economy and society develop, healthcare standards and life expectancy rise, and as a result, the pace of population aging has accelerated in the past twenty years. Elderly suicide is generally known to peak at in the age group of 65 and above. According to data from China's Ministry of Health in the early 1990s, the suicide rate of seniors between the ages of 64 and 75 is 47.18 per 100,000 individuals, ranking fourth among low-income countries. Studying and analyzing elderly suicides in the cities and the countryside is important to senior health. Some scholars have pointed out the unique characteristics of the relatively high suicide rate in China compared with other countries: suicides in the countryside are three times those in the cities and elderly suicides in the countryside are five times those in the cities. In China, 90% of the suicides happen in the countryside.[4]

Seniors commit suicide for many reasons, including loneliness, illness, poverty, uncaring children, and the empty nest syndrome. Due to the funeral reform of the countryside in recent years, many seniors commit suicide in order to "catch the last train" for traditional burial. They may have made this decision at a moment's notice, but for the children who have to deal with the guilt and pain later, it is a sad and nightmarish memory that will last long.

---

[3]Liang and Li (2012).

[4]Xiao (2010).

In an era of rapidly aging population, it is an urgent task to study elderly suicide, discover its pattern, prevent it from happening, and allow seniors to live out their golden years in happiness.

# 2 Current Situation of Elderly Suicide

## 2.1 *Suicidal Ideation, Suicidal Deaths, and Failed Suicide Attempts*

### 2.1.1 Suicidal Death Rates Are High

In 1987, the suicidal death rate was 26.40 per 100,000 individuals for men and 30.20 per 100,000 individuals for women in the 55–64 age group; 54.10 per 100,000 individuals for men and 50.60 per 100,000 individuals for women in the 65–74 age group; 79.10 per 100,000 individuals for men and 73.70 per 100,000 individuals for women in the 75-and-over age group. In 1989, the suicidal death rate for men was 27.40 per 100,000 individuals and 25.60 per 100,000 individuals for women in the 55–64 age group; 52.50 per 100,000 individuals for men and 43.40 per 100,000 individuals for women in the 65–74 age group; 93.30 per 100,000 individuals for men and 69.00 per 100,000 individuals for women in the 75-and-over age group (See Fig. 1). In 1994, the general suicidal death rate increased to 22.85 per 100,000 individuals, totaling 273,900 deaths. According to the 1991–1995 data of the National Disease Surveillance System, the general suicidal death rate was 19.85 per 100,000 individuals, with an urban rate of 6.50 and a rural rate of 22.89; and the male–female ratio was 0.82:1. The proportion of the 15–34 age group was 40.7% while that of the over 60 age group was 29.74%.[5] Dr. Michael R. Philips estimates that 100,000 seniors over the age of 55 die from suicide every year in China.[6]

We can see from Table 1 that China's elderly suicide rate is clearly higher than the general suicide rate. The urban elderly suicide rate was higher than the general urban suicide rate by 16.33 per 100,000 individuals in 1990, by 12.56 per 100,000 individuals in 1995, and by 9.60 per 100,000 individuals in 2000. Rural elderly suicide rate was higher than general rural suicide rate by 42.96 per 100,000 individuals in 1990, by 52.19 per 100,000 individuals in 1995, and by 53.85 per 100,000 individuals in 2000.

The suicidal death rates of the various age groups from 1987 to 1989 are shown in Fig. 2.

[5]Gonghuan et al. (1997).

[6]Proceedings of Ministry of Health/WHO Conference on Suicide Prevention. *Chinese Mental Health* (2000), 14(5), 295–298.

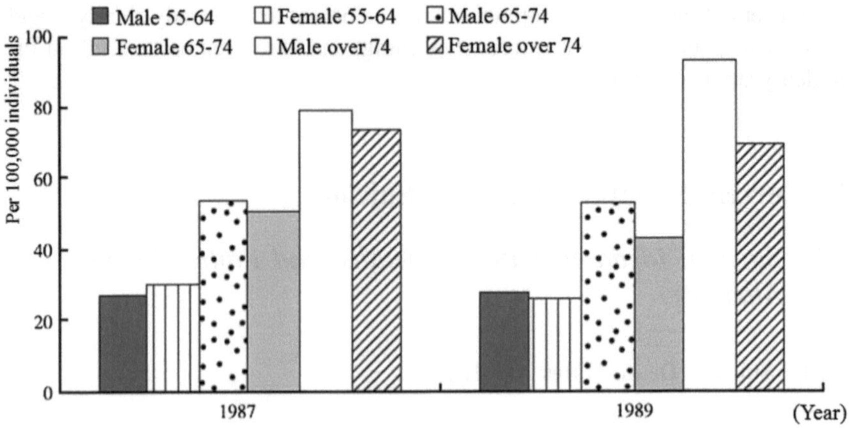


**Fig. 1** Elderly suicidal death rate of 1987 and 1989 in China

**Table 1** Elderly suicide rate versus general suicide rate, 1990–2000 unit: per 100,000 individuals

| | 1990 | | 1995 | | 2000 | |
|---|---|---|---|---|---|---|
| | Urban | Rural | Urban | Rural | Urban | Rural |
| Elderly | 24.90 | 65.42 | 19.98 | 76.24 | 15.56 | 74.73 |
| General | 8.57 | 22.46 | 7.42 | 24.05 | 5.96 | 20.88 |

*Source Health Yearbook of the People's Republic of China*, excerpted from Yan (2003)

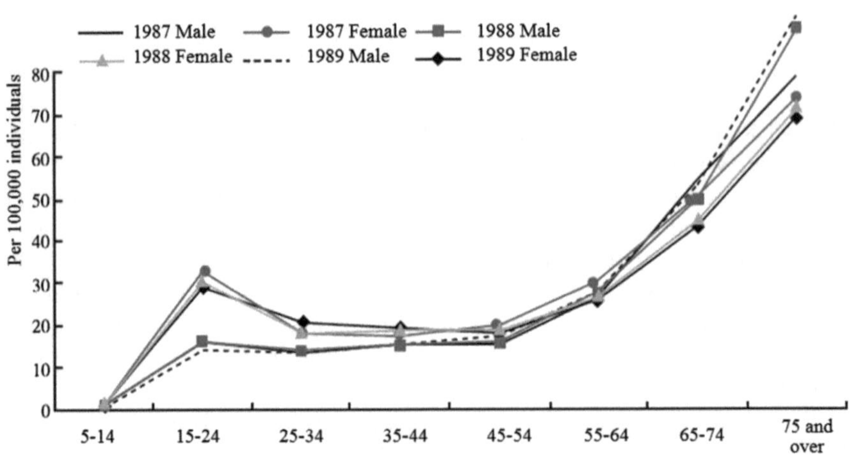


**Fig. 2** Suicide rate by age group, 1987–1989

According to the data of China Health Statistics Yearbook, in 2017, the suicide mortality rate in China reached 5.985/100,000, including 4.31/100,000 in urban

**Table 2** Suicide mortality rate of people of all ages in China (2015–2017) (1/100,000)

| Year | Gender | 5～14 | 15～24 | 25～34 | 35～44 | 45～54 | 55～64 | 65～74 | 75⁺ |
|---|---|---|---|---|---|---|---|---|---|
| 2015 | Male | 0.58 | 2.74 | 4.58 | 5.07 | 8.75 | 12.13 | 22.91 | 49.96 |
| | Female | 0.44 | 1.62 | 3.17 | 3.45 | 6.21 | 8.57 | 17.12 | 33.74 |
| 2016 | Male | 0.61 | 2.34 | 5.03 | 4.77 | 8.60 | 12.35 | 21.12 | 43.72 |
| | Female | 0.32 | 1.68 | 3.06 | 3.06 | 6.31 | 8.74 | 15.37 | 29.23 |
| 2017 | Male | 0.64 | 2.44 | 4.83 | 4.57 | 8.37 | 10.74 | 20.11 | 39.24 |
| | Female | 0.35 | 1.52 | 2.61 | 2.57 | 5.90 | 7.88 | 14.25 | 24.32 |

**Table 3** Comparison of suicide rates between the elderly and the total population (2015–2017) (1/100,000)

| | 2005 | | 2010 | | 2017 | |
|---|---|---|---|---|---|---|
| | urban | rural | urban | rural | urban | rural |
| The elderly | 78.91 | 58.43 | 20.71 | 37.41 | 15.62 | 30.57 |
| Total population | 12.89 | 10.08 | 5.07 | 8.39 | 4.31 | 7.66 |

*Sources* National Health Commission, *China Health Statistics Yearbook*
*Source Year Book of Health in the People's Republic of China* published by the National Health Commission of the PR, China

areas and 7.66/100,000 in rural areas. Among the suicide deaths, the elderly over 60 years old accounted for 23.09% (Tables 2 and 3).[7]

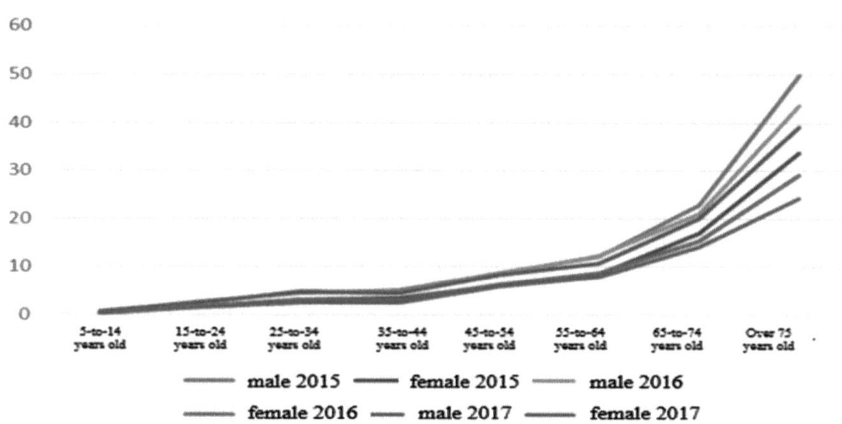


Suicide mortality rate of people of all ages in China (2015–2017) (1/100,000)

[7]Yang et al. (1997).

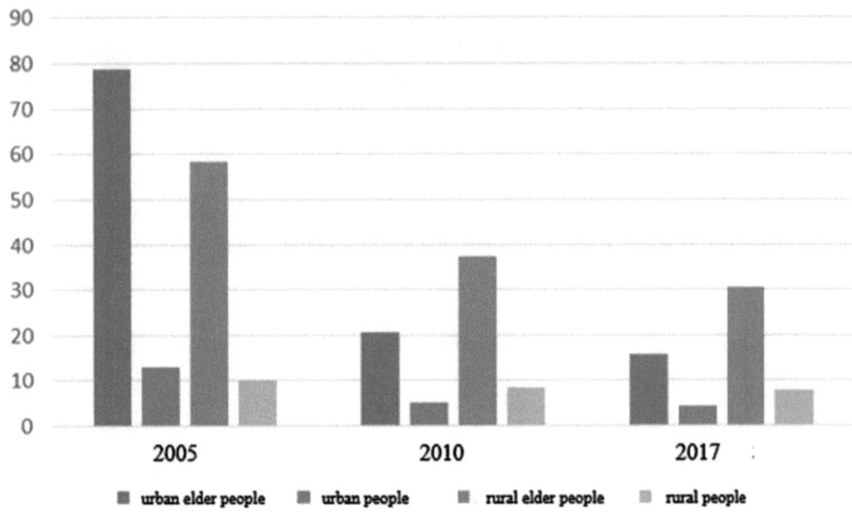


Comparison of suicide rates between the elderly and the total population (2005–2017) (1/100,000)

Data of the *2004 China Health Statistics Yearbook* indicates that, in 2003, the rural suicidal death rate reached 131.79 per 100,000 individuals in the 75–79 age group and 159.12 per 100,000 individuals in the 80–84 age group, 7.62 and 9.20 times the general rural suicide rates respectively, and 2.12 and 2.01 times the urban elderly suicide death rates, respectively.

According to the data of *China Health Statistics Yearbook 2018* published by the National Health Commission, in 2017, the suicide mortality rate for the 75–79 age group in rural China was as high as 31.57/100,000, that for the 80–84 age group was as high as 42.73/100,000, and that for the 85 and over age group was as high as 48.56/100,000, which was 4.12 times, 5.58 times and 6.34 times higher than the average rural suicide rate of 7.66/100,000, and 2.25 times, 1.98 times and 1.92 times higher than that of the same age group in urban areas.

We can see from Table 4 that the elderly suicidal death rate dropped somewhat in 2006 but the rural figure bounced back in 2007 and trended upward in 2009.

As China ages at a faster pace, elderly suicide has become a social problem which causes harm to seniors' well-being and quality of life; it has also become a prominent public health issue. Statistics show that 100,000 seniors 55 years and older commit suicide every year, representing 36% of all suicides. This is a huge increase from twenty years ago. Seniors have become a high-risk group for suicide.

Fan Peizhen, an associate professor of internal medicine and psychiatry at the Department of Medicine, School of Medicine, National Yang-Ming University of Taiwan, said that as the development of economy and the increasing urbanization rate, "China's suicide rate is declining sharply, especially for young women."

**Table 4** Urban versus rural elderly suicidal death rate, 2003–2009 unit: per 100,000 individuals

| Year | Category | 55–59 | 60–64 | 65–69 | 70–74 | 75–79 | 80–84 | 85 and over |
|---|---|---|---|---|---|---|---|---|
| 2003 | Urban | 18.03 | 23.55 | 31.19 | 41.73 | 62.28 | 79.24 | 75.59 |
| | Rural | 33.56 | 38.48 | 57.20 | 77.04 | 131.79 | 159.12 | 138.18 |
| 2005 | Urban | 21.70 | 32.68 | 41.49 | 70.70 | 96.82 | 128.10 | 103.67 |
| | Rural | 17.38 | 22.87 | 39.15 | 42.89 | 65.16 | 82.98 | 97.50 |
| 2006 | Urban | 7.67 | 9.22 | 9.62 | 14.38 | 18.59 | 27.67 | 39.22 |
| | Rural | 16.59 | 20.89 | 26.35 | 36.11 | 48.02 | 65.82 | 74.03 |
| 2007 | Urban | 6.25 | 7.37 | 8.35 | 14.16 | 14.83 | 23.13 | 22.70 |
| | Rural | 20.43 | 22.34 | 28.45 | 40.55 | 57.21 | 86.73 | 97.52 |
| 2008 | Urban | 4.63 | 4. 85 | 6.11 | 7.38 | 9.66 | 14.39 | 13.93 |
| | Rural | 17.72 | 18.52 | 20.51 | 26.93 | 41.18 | 51.87 | 62.48 |
| 2009 | Urban | 6.33 | 7.52 | 9.94 | 13.23 | 20.64 | 29.67 | 31.07 |
| | Rural | 14.96 | 19.83 | 23.68 | 35.10 | 53.00 | 81.16 | 104.92 |
| 2010 | urban | 7.94 | 11.54 | 15.54 | 24.88 | 32.77 | 57.37 | 89.46 |
| | rural | 13.71 | 17.67 | 27.02 | 44.25 | 68.78 | 108.13 | 191.74 |
| 2011 | urban | 6.62 | 8.34 | 9.85 | 13.97 | 24.1 | 37.13 | 38.91 |
| | rural | 17.39 | 17.82 | 25.59 | 35.23 | 46.36 | 78.5 | 93.46 |
| 2012 | urban | 5.34 | 7.5 | 10.51 | 14.88 | 22.06 | 28.63 | 32.36 |
| | rural | 13.23 | 15.49 | 19.79 | 26.58 | 43.47 | 53.08 | 71.17 |
| 2013 | urban | 7.25 | 9.04 | 11.67 | 14.69 | 18.98 | 29.52 | 29.23 |
| | rural | 11.83 | 15.56 | 22.06 | 30.96 | 43.95 | 59.18 | 72.4 |
| 2014 | urban | 5.53 | 9.81 | 12.86 | 15.85 | 19.48 | 25.69 | 41.19 |
| | rural | 11.24 | 15.16 | 21.44 | 30.99 | 42.02 | 55.83 | 70.29 |
| 2015 | urban | 6.09 | 9.7 | 13.17 | 15.32 | 18.16 | 26.81 | 41.09 |
| | rural | 10.71 | 14.94 | 21.99 | 29.58 | 39.85 | 52.48 | 65.6 |
| 2016 | urban | 5.83 | 10.67 | 11.91 | 13.62 | 16.96 | 24.26 | 37.05 |
| | rural | 9.65 | 16.05 | 19.77 | 25.295 | 34.145 | 45.16 | 59.31 |
| 2017 | urban | 4.55 | 9.11 | 10.58 | 13.07 | 14.03 | 21.6 | 25.31 |
| | rural | 8.12 | 15.52 | 20.51 | 24.5 | 31.57 | 42.73 | 48.56 |

*Note* 2004 data is missing from the official website of *China Health Statistics Yearbook*
*Source China Health Statistics Yearbooks* 2004–2010 accessed on the Ministry of Health website

However, the elderly suicide is still rising. According to the data of the annual report of National Health Commission of the People's Republic of China, the suicide rate of Chinese people over 60 years old is at least twice as high as the average level. In this regard, Fan Peizhen once said that in 2015, the suicide rate of Chinese people aged 65 to 85 was 2.75 to 7.08 times that of the general population. Among them, the rural suicide rate was significantly higher than that of the urban, and the male suicide rate was nearly 8 times higher than the average level.[8]

[8]The reasons why Asian old people commit suicide: Japanese elderly are mainly because of the big family, and the elderly in rural China are mostly because of helplessness. http://www.sohu.com/a/320257986_313392.

Fan Peizhen also pointed out that in rural areas, 21.99 per 100,000 elderly people at the age of 65 or over committed suicide, and this number increased with the age. For the people over 85 years old in rural areas, 65.60 per 100,000 individuals would choose to end their lives through suicide; and even in the urban areas, 41.09 per 100,000 individuals would commit suicide.

In early 2004, over four hundred experts from around the world gathered in Hong Kong for an interdisciplinary conference on elderly suicide prevention in the Asia-Pacific region. Wang Xun, head of Benefits Department of China National Committee on Aging, who was invited to the event told reporters that seniors 65 years old and over in the world commit suicide at a rate of 29 per 100,000 individuals, and this is according to data from the European Integrated Study Center of WHO. In East Asia, this figure is 34.5 per 100,000 individuals, 2.7 times the suicide rate of young people. Wang Xun pointed out that the more prevalent methods of elderly suicide included poisoning (pills or gas), hanging, and jumping from heights. The higher the age, the deadlier the method. In China's countryside, there are many incidents of people using pesticides for suicide; in Hong Kong, the elderly tend to use sleeping pills. A quarter of the people who commit suicide have had previous attempts.[9] Wang Xun said that old people face daunting difficulties in China, such as the empty nest syndrome, and the lack of care, social security, and psychological counseling. China does not have answers to these problems yet.

### 2.1.2 Seniors Have High Incidence of Suicidal Ideation and Failed Suicide Attempts

Contrary to popular thinking, suicide is not a continuous process starting with suicidal ideation, failed attempts, and finally death. People who have suicidal thoughts are at high risk for suicidal attempts which may succeed or fail, so there is an overlap of people who have suicidal thoughts and those who die from suicide.[10] We must understand the nature of suicidal ideation and suicidal attempts.

Suicidal ideation happens regularly with seniors; its intensity is also higher compared with other age groups. To reduce the incidence of elderly suicide, it is necessary to study elderly suicidal ideation and prescribe preventive measures. But this is a difficult task to undertake since suicidal ideation is concealed, random, and diverse. There is a dearth of research into this subject, with rare reports and little statistical information.

*Study of Elderly Suicidal Ideation and Risk Factors from Yuanjiang, Hunan*, authored by Qing Wenjing, is a good place to start. The study surveyed the elderly people of Yuanjiang, Hunan Province, using the stratified random sampling method through home visits and person-to-person interviews. The findings are as follows: First, the incidence of rural elderly suicidal ideation in Yuanjiang is 25%, up from

---

[9]Zhang (2005).

[10]Maris et al. (2000).

19.9% in the previous year, involving more women than men, and occurrences increase with age. Second, the main contributing events for suicidal ideation include death of child, untreatable illness, loneliness, financial difficulty, hospitalization, and death of spouse. Third, the main risk factors include negative life events, bad relations with neighbors, symptoms of depression, and feeling of despair.[11] From this, we see that the network of rural elderly care needs to be improved, familial interaction reestablished, and the ability to take care of oneself raised in order to prevent suicidal ideation and reduce the incidence of suicide in the countryside.

In contrast to the high incidence of elderly suicidal ideation, the incidence of failed attempts at suicide is lower with the elderly than with the young. Research shows that elderly attempts have a 4:1 failure to success ratio while the figure is 100–200:1 among young people. But, unfortunately, elderly suicidal attempts have been given short shrift as more attention is paid to youth suicidal attempts. It is wrong to ignore this issue because of a low incidence. Experts have pointed out that it is regrettable that the problem of elderly suicidal attempts has been ignored since suicidal attempts are very much linked to suicidal death; lower failure rate means higher death rate.

Research shows that the incidence of failed suicidal attempts in the 55–64 age group is twice that of the 65-and-over age group. The higher the age, the lower the rate failed attempts. In other words, the higher the age, the higher the successful attempts. There are more men with failed attempts than women in the 55–64 age group while no such gender difference exists in the 65-and-over age group. There are more men with successful suicide attempts than women in both age groups.[12] Elderly suicide is less impulsive, and the method taken is therefore deadlier, such as poison, hanging, and drowning. The elderly can conceal their suicidal intentions more easily, and they are less likely to be rescued.

There are two reasons why we should not ignore failed suicidal attempts of the elderly: First, if the elderly fail to receive psychological counseling after failed suicidal attempts, their intention of committing suicide grows stronger, and the likelihood of a subsequent successful attempt is greater. Second, the rural elderly has few opportunities for social interaction, and they are more likely to be negatively influenced by the suicidal attempts of people around them. In short, elderly people who have had failed suicidal attempts need more support and attention from society and their families in order to eliminate suicidal ideation and live out their golden years in happiness and safety.

[11]Qing (2007).

[12]Zhai (1997).

## 2.2 *Special Features of Elderly Suicide*

Elderly suicide differs naturally from that of other age groups. We will now attempt to describe the differences and similarities between rural and urban elderly suicide and between suicide committed by the elderly and by the young. We will also describe the telltale signs and causes for elderly suicide.

### 2.2.1 Elderly Suicide: Urban Versus Rural

Different Suicide Rates

According to *2004 China Health Statistics Yearbook*, the 2003 rural suicide rates climbed up with age for the age groups of 60–64, 65–69, 70–74, 75–79, 80–84, and 85 and over, respectively at 38.48, 57.20, 77.04, 131.79, 159.12, and 138.18 per 100,000 individuals; these numbers are far greater than those in the cities (23.55, 31.19, 41.73, 62.28, 79.24, and 75.59 per 100,000 individuals). This is especially the case for the 75–79 and 80–84 age groups for which the rates in the countryside are 2.12 and 2.01 times the rates in the cities (Fig. 3). Rural elderly suicide rate is much higher than the national average suicide rates, too.

As the above figure shows, in 2003, the elderly suicide rate is higher in the countryside than in the cities, and the gap keeps widening. The elderly suicide rate in the countryside is 2.63 times that of the cities in 1990, 3.82 times in 1995, and 4.80 times in 2000.

We don't yet have a comprehensive theory about the large disparity between the urban and rural elderly suicide rates. Some scholars believe that this disparity can

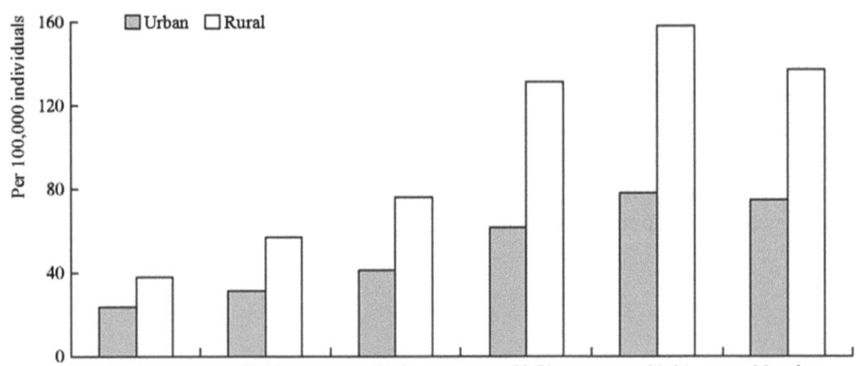


**Fig. 3** 2003 Elderly suicide rate: urban versus rural

be explained in part by the enormous differences between the cities and countryside. The economy remains relatively undeveloped in the countryside, and the lack of mental health services there hinders treatment of mental illnesses.[13]

Different Suicide Methods

The rural elderly generally use poison. City folk don't usually keep pesticides in their homes and need a doctor's prescription to get sleeping pills and other medications, so taking poison is not the method of choice for the urban elderly. Old people in cities live mainly in small housing units and tend to commit suicide by hanging or gas. In the countryside, especially in the western part of China, buildings of three stories or taller are very rare; but skyscrapers are common in the cities, so the urban elderly also are more likely to jump from buildings.

Different Motivations

In the countryside, the motivations for suicide tend to be finance-related. Poverty prevents the elderly from seeking treatment for their illnesses and creates discord within the family. In contrast, most of the urban elderly have pensions, having worked during their adult lives. The urban welfare system, though minimal, covers the urban elderly's basic needs. For these people, their financial situation is not the main factor, and their motivations for suicide have to do with poor familial relationships, loneliness, the empty nest syndrome, and the loss of spouse.

### 2.2.2 Elderly Suicide Versus Youth Suicide

Durkheim's study of nineteenth century Europe shows that suicide rate was directly proportional to age; elderly suicide rate was three to four times that of youth suicide rate. This is still the case with Western countries and the majority of other countries of the world today. But the situation is different in China where there are two suicide peak periods (elderly and youth), similar to Japan's situation. This is known as the Japanese, or East Asian, suicide model.

There are differences between the elderly and youth suicides. First, suicidal ideation tends to be stronger and methods more extreme with the elderly, so the elderly suicidal death rate tends to be higher. Second, the possible reasons of elderly suicide are related to the self, such as illnesses, poverty, and loneliness; with youthful suicide, the reasons tend to be socially directed, such as pressure from study, work, life, or emotional stress. Finally, in terms of telltale signs, the elderly tends to hide their suicidal thoughts and leave no telltale signs. They don't usually

[13]Song (2010a).

let other people know their intentions or seek help from others, and few of them leave a suicidal note. Young people tend to leave suicidal notes or tell other people about their intentions, actually as a way of seeking help.

#### 2.2.3 Elderly Suicide's Telltale Signs and Causes

There are telltale signs for elderly suicide in most cases, and the most effective way of preventing suicide is to recognize these signs. Tragedy can be prevented if family members can detect such signs in a timely way. These signs may manifest in the following ways: First, the elderly persons talk about death in conversations, saying things like "It'd be much better if I weren't here," "I can go now," or "If I go away, you have to take care of yourself." They would express a desire to see a deceased spouse or parent, give away things they treasure, or give burial instructions to a family member. Second, they have experienced a negative life event recently. Third, they have changes in their emotional states, becoming passive, pessimist, depressed, or emotionally unstable; sometimes they become anxious or sad for no reason and change to a state of calmness or happiness soon afterward, while at other times, they alternate between feeling happy and sad. Fourth, they exhibit stressed behavior such as self-inflicted injury or suicidal attempts. They begin to quietly hoard poison, pills, ropes, knives, etc. Moreover, more attention should be paid to them if they have mental illnesses such as depression or schizophrenia, which are important risk factors for suicide.

Zhai Dehua, a researcher at China Research Center on Aging, believes that factors of elderly suicide include the economic pressure brought to bear by illness, mental and bodily pain, strife in familial and social relationships, tragic life events (illness or death of a family member), lack of understanding of law or the concept of self-protection.[14]

## 3 Survey of Town S in Zunyi County, Guizhou

### *3.1 Target of Study*

Authors of this book chose Town S in Zunyi County of Guizhou Province as a target of our study, since we heard about the problem of suicide in this town earlier. Zunyi County, established in 1601 during the Ming Dynasty, has an area of 2487 km$^2$. A population of 1.135 million includes people from twenty ethnicities including the Han and the Miao. The northern and central parts of the county are the fluvial terrace of the Wujiang River and have one of the great dams of Guizhou. With an elevation ranging from 800 to 1300 m, the county has plenty of scenic and

[14]Zhang (2008a).

ecological resources. Forest covers 55.70% of the county, which has nine towns and one ethnic village. Town S is located on the banks of the south part of Zunyi County, having five villages, one resident community, and 23,150 residents according to the Fifth National Population Census.

The authors set the 60-and-over age group as the target of the study and obtained information through non-standardized interviews and literature review. The team began by gathering elderly death information in the villages around Town S from census data. Since there was missing or unverified data from relevant authorities, the team went to all the villages where abnormal deaths have occurred. By examining the household registrations, the team was able to obtain information on suicidal deaths; and the data obtained included the gender and age of the dead, the time and location of suicide, the method used, and the reason.

The team studied existing materials and used the qualitative method in its survey. The qualitative method views the researcher as a tool of study and analyzes social phenomena in totality. It uses induction to analyze data and form theories and interacts with the target of study to explain their behavior.[15]

The qualitative research method is not empty speculation or useless theoretical inference; it employs written narratives, demonstrates by induction, and presupposes constructivism. It believes that human predicaments are anchored in social conditions, relationships, and historical background. The researchers are well-versed in human psychology and the social processes which create psychological phenomena; they regard the individuals as participants in society and history, understand the social choices which the individuals make, and the complex relationships which shape them.[16]

In the course of the survey, the authors adopted the general interview guide approach and described elderly suicides of Town S from the point of view of the interviewees through non-standardized interviews. This is how the preliminary study was based.

The team adopted the multivariate detection method in the survey and used observation, research, and interviews to collect information and verified it by cross-reference. Moreover, it interviewed family members, relatives, and neighbors for their input and studied elderly suicide from their as well as the researchers' point of view. The multivariate detection method maximizes the objectivity of the survey.

The authors got a more comprehensive understanding of elderly suicide by interviews and by gathering census information and data provided by the local family planning office.

---

[15]Chen (2002).

[16]Maxwell (2007).

## *3.2 Basic Information*

The total population of Town S is 23,150, of whom 1579 are aged 60 or above. In this age group, 754 are male and 825 are female. Table 5 illustrates this.

### 3.2.1 Elderly Suicide Rate in Town S

Here, the elderly suicide rate is the ratio of elderly suicides to total elderly deaths. We can see the seriousness of elderly suicide by looking at this rate.

According to the local family planning office of Town S, there were 296 cases elderly death between 2004 and 2008. Table 6 shows the causes of death as illness, natural, and accidents, but does not show suicide. This is because most of the time the families do not want to report they have lost a loved one due to suicide and these deaths will be reported as caused by illness. Deaths by natural causes and accidents are by and large correct.

But, the authors looked into the household registrations of Town S and found that 68 of the 296 elderly deaths between 2004 and 2008 were due to suicide, representing 23% of the total. We can see from Table 7 that suicide is the No. 3 cause of elderly deaths in Town S.

**Table 5** Population details of Town S

| | | | |
|---|---|---|---|
| Total population | 23150 | 0–14 male | 3578 |
| Male | 12282 | 0–14 female | 3189 |
| Female | 10868 | 15–60 age group total | 14804 |
| No. of households | 6507 | 15–60 male | 7950 |
| Household population | 23108 | 15–60 female | 6854 |
| Household male | 12251 | 60 and over total | 1579 |
| Household female | 10857 | 60 and over male | 754 |
| 0–14 age group total | 6767 | 60 and over female | 825 |

**Table 6** Causes of elderly deaths, 2004–2008

| Cause | No. of deaths | Share (%) |
|---|---|---|
| Illness | 171 | 58 |
| Natural death | 110 | 37 |
| Accident | 15 | 5 |
| Total | 296 | 100 |

**Table 7** Project team's estimate of causes of elderly deaths, 2004–2008

| Cause | No. of deaths | Rate (%) |
|---|---|---|
| Suicide | 68 | 23 |
| Illness | 103 | 35 |
| Natural | 110 | 37 |
| Accident | 15 | 5 |
| Total | 296 | 100 |

**Table 8** Elderly suicide in Town S, 2004–2008

| Year | 2004 | 2005 | 2006 | 2007 | 2008 | Total |
|---|---|---|---|---|---|---|
| Suicidal deaths | 7 | 10 | 13 | 24 | 14 | 68 |
| Total deaths | 36 | 43 | 63 | 89 | 65 | 296 |
| Share (%) | 19 | 23 | 21 | 27 | 22 | 23 |

Table 8 shows that suicidal deaths climbed in 2007 and then dropped back in 2008. We have to find an explanation for this.

In the 1990s, in order to save precious arable land resources, a funeral reform was adopted in the countryside and cremation became mandatory. In the villages of Town S, full implementation of the new policy was preceded by an awareness-raising campaign that was carried out between April 1 and July 31, 2007, regarding the benefits and advantages of cremating the dead. Surprisingly, the number of elderly deaths shot up within that very period. Some villages had more than three elderly suicides, all involving people over the age of 70; in some families, both the patriarch and the matriarch killed themselves together. Such high suicide rate was unprecedented, and we will provide our analysis below.

### 3.2.2 Age Distribution

Rural elderly population here means people of age 60 and over. The authors divided this population into five age groups: 60–64, 65–69, 70–74, 75–79, and 80 and over. The survey found that the highest number of suicide cases happened in the 65–69 and 70–74 age groups, representing 34 and 37% of the total. respectively, as shown in Table 9.

### 3.2.3 Gender

There are 32 cases of male suicides and 36 cases of female suicides, representing a ratio of 0.89:1, with slightly more female cases than male cases.

**Table 9** Age distribution of elderly suicide, 2004–2008

| Age group | No. of elderly suicides | Share (%) | Age group | No. of elderly suicides | Share (%) |
|---|---|---|---|---|---|
| 60–64 | 14 | 21 | 75–79 | 3 | 4 |
| 65–69 | 23 | 34 | 80 and over | 3 | 4 |
| 70–74 | 25 | 37 | | | |

### 3.2.4 Methods

The main methods of suicide include poisoning, hanging, and drowning. The preferred method for both men and women is poisoning; women also take their lives by drowning, as shown in Table 10. These methods are somewhat mild, and except for a few cases of hanging, there are no cases involving the more extreme methods like jumping, self-immolation, explosion, or disembowelment. Taking poison is highly effective; practically all the households in the countryside have pesticides and rat poison which can be easily purchased. Moreover, healthcare is poor and facilities few in the countryside and town centers and cities are far away, so having taken poison, a person will most likely die. The elderly people who hanged themselves had problems with their legs or feet; since they had difficulty walking, the easiest way is hanging. Baima Village has a small reservoir for fish farming and the water level rises in April and May. Some of the elderly in that village, thus have chosen drowning during this period of the year.

### 3.2.5 Season, Time, and Location

As Table 11 shows, the elderly of Town S often choose the summer to commit suicide, and this is consistent with what the majority of researchers find in studies on suicide at the national level. Most elderly people commit suicide in their bedroom at night or during the day when no one is around. They have the time to do it calmly this way. This shows that they are strong-willed, desperate, incapacitated, or stubborn in the traditional belief that to die outside means that their bodies cannot enter the house again.

**Table 10** Methods of elderly suicide, 2004–2008 unit: person

| Method | Male | Female | Total |
|---|---|---|---|
| Poison | 17 | 19 | 36 |
| Hanging | 7 | 8 | 15 |
| Drowning | 8 | 9 | 17 |
| Other | 0 | 0 | 0 |

**Table 11** Season, time, and location of elderly suicide, 2004–2008

| Season | No. of cases | Time | No. of cases | Location | No. of cases |
|---|---|---|---|---|---|
| Spring | 22 | Day | 21 | Home | 48 |
| Summer | 29 | Night | 47 | Outside | 20 |
| Autumn | 11 | | | | |
| Winter | 6 | | | | |

# 4 Factors of Elderly Suicide

## *4.1 Characteristics*

### 4.1.1 Age

Generally speaking, the suicide rate is positively correlated to age. That is to say, it increases with age. Data from many countries shows that the 55–65 age group is the most prone to suicide, and the elderly male population has a higher suicide rate than the youth. In China, there is a pattern for elderly suicide in China. The first peak appears in the young, while there is a second one at the 70-and-over age group. The authors divided the elderly population of Town S into five age groups: 60–64, 65–69, 70–74, 75–79, and 80 and over. The two age groups with the highest suicide rates are 65–69 and 70–74, representing 33% (23 deaths) and 37% (25 deaths) of the total, respectively. In the ten typical cases selected, seniors in the 70-and-over age group account for 73%, while the remaining three cases are in the 65–69 age group.

### 4.1.2 Marital Status

It was first revealed by Durkheim that in the married elderly population, those who don't have children have a higher suicide rate than those who do, and this is true for both men and women. Japanese scholar Hiroshi Inamura found that in Japan, elderly males who are single have the highest suicide rate while elderly females who are separated from their spouse and childless have the highest suicide rate.[17] In China's countryside, the divorce rate is practically zero among the elderly. This is why those who are single or living alone due to spousal death are more prone to suicide. Spousal death is difficult to handle in one's golden years and it is seen in over half of elderly suicides. Some reports have shown that the first year of spousal death is a peak of elderly suicide, and, precisely for this reason, the newly widowed elderly population should be regarded as most prone to suicide. Another reason for elderly suicide is the death of a younger family member, especially a son.

### 4.1.3 Gender

Outside China, women of any age group have a lower suicide rate than men, and this is especially true in the elderly population. In China, this is also the case with the elderly in the countryside, but with one exception: The peak of suicide among women is not in the 45–55 age group but in the 74-and-over age group, as is the case with men.

[17]Inamura (1977).

But our study has found that the ratio between men and women in elderly suicide in Town S is 89:100. This means that the elderly suicide rate is higher with women than with men. There are several reasons for this: First, Town S is a typical town in Guizhou, where elderly women don't have much say or independence within the family. Their lives center around their husband or son(s). Second, elderly women in Town S are generally uneducated, and some could barely write their own names. They often have the feudal mindset which makes them think, "If God wants me to die, I won't have any choice but to die." Third, relative to men, women of the countryside are less strong psychologically; their emotions are more prone to the influence of the external world. Added to the mix is the traditional conflict between women and the mothers-in-law. The rush of migrant workers into the cities means that the husbands are not at home to mediate the disputes, and the possibility of conflict between the wife and the mother-in-law increases greatly. In the heat of the moment, the aggrieved party may very well take it to the extreme and kill herself. A main characteristic of suicide among rural women is that it is done out of impulse.

### 4.1.4 Health

Health, or the lack thereof, is an important factor of elderly suicide. The older one gets, the more prone he or she will be to illnesses, physical or mental. Physical illnesses which may lead to suicide include epilepsy, cancer, cardiovascular diseases, or the effect of a traffic accident; while mental illnesses which may lead to suicide include depression, Alzheimer's disease, emotional issues, or dementia. Many rural families and individuals are impoverished due to illnesses, which then lead to suicide. Some ill and impoverished elderly people, especially in the countryside, are afraid to become a burden to their children. They are more prone to suicide when they live alone or when their children are uncaring.

### 4.1.5 Economic Situation

Generally speaking, the economic situation is negatively correlated to the suicide rate. When the economic conditions are poor, the suicide rate is higher. The social security system in China is not good enough and there isn't much of an insurance system against old age. In the countryside, one's health deteriorates as one gets older. Sooner or later, the day will come when one can't work for his/her own livelihood and has to depend on one's children. In the study of Town S, the elderly suicide rate is higher among families which have financial difficulties. The elderly people wish to die sooner because they can no longer work and can only be a burden to their children. Each day they are alive depletes the family coffers. What a heart-breaking choice they are making!

## 4.2 How and When

### 4.2.1 How

The suicide methods are different depending on regions, nationalities, and beliefs. In the UK, elderly men tend to hang themselves while elderly women tend to take poison. In the US, due to the laxity in gun control, many elderly people use guns to take their own lives. In Hong Kong, where there are so many skyscrapers, jumping and inhaling gas indoors are the preferred methods of suicide. Things are somewhat different in China. The elderly choose poisoning, hanging, and leaping from buildings in the cities whereas in the countryside, pesticides and rat poison are used more often due to the separate system of control regarding the usage of pesticides, though hanging, drowning, and electrocution are not uncommon either. Few choose violent methods such as leaping from buildings, slitting, self-immolation, or explosion. The reasons for such choices may be convenience and the traditional belief that the corpse should be in one piece. In the countryside where healthcare is limited and antidotes and stomach pumping machines are often lacking, taking poison can be an effective method of committing suicide, which is not likely to cause much pain for themselves or burden to the loved ones, and will leave the corpse intact.[18]

The authors found that the elderly of Town S choose only three methods of suicide: poisoning, hanging, and drowning. The team has not found any violent ways of committing suicide. This reflects the fact that Town S is rather typical of rural China in choosing convenience and tradition over histrionics in committing suicide.

### 4.2.2 When

Some knowledge can be gleaned from the season and the time of day when one is more prone to committing suicide.

Emile Durkheim found that more people in the West commit suicide in the spring, with the number of cases moving upward from January to May.

In China, the high season for suicide is summer. People become irascible in the hot weather and family strife come to a boil. This is the case for the countryside as well. Having studied 268 rural suicide cases, Peng Gongde found that elderly suicide peak during July and August.

This is the time when farmers are at their busiest and need a large amount of cash flow. Picking this period to commit suicide reflects a large extent that the elderly is not getting the care they need at home during this period.[19]

---

[18]Rong (2010).

[19]Gongde (1997).

Of the 68 suicide cases of Town S, 22 were committed in the spring, 29 in the summer, 22 in the autumn, and 6 in the winter. This is consistent with the national data. Moreover, that the rural elderly won't consider the winter has a lot to do with the spring festival. This is the most important holiday in China, when all family members get together to celebrate the festival and worship the ancestors. The elderly has no time to think about committing suicide around this time.

Most of the elderly suicides happen in the dead of night or during daytime when nobody is around. Of the 68 suicide cases of Town S, 21 happened during the day and 47 during the night. This strong contrast regarding the time of suicide indicates that the elderly does not want other people to intervene when they take the action; they have made up their minds and given up all hopes for life. They just want death to free them from misery.

### 4.2.3 Where

Our survey finds that 48 of the suicide cases in Town S happened in the home and 20 happened outside the home. This shows that the rural elderly does not want to die outside. They commit suicide in their beds because they may be ill and have trouble with movement. Even when they decide to die outside, they won't go very far, choosing a reservoir or some places which have special meaning for them. There is a Chinese saying that "when leaves fall, they go back to the roots".

## *4.3 Other Factors of Rural Elderly Suicide*

In China, over 90% of the suicide cases happen in the countryside, and this is why we pay particular attention to the rural elderly population here. According to sociopsychologists, high population density leads to more complicated social relationships and more conflicts, and makes people more prone to frustration in their relationships or emotional life; and this leads to more suicides. But things are different in China in that suicide rate is much higher in the countryside than in the cities. Rural suicide rate has been rising since the 1980s. It was 15.40 per 100,000 individuals in 1980, and 29.10 per 100,000 individuals in 1991.[20] The rate gradually declined after the 21st century. It is an incontrovertible fact that rural life has improved over the years, so rural suicides may very well have non-economic factors behind them.

As suicide studies develop along the path of empirical sociology advocated by Emile Durkheim, it has found the impetus for new theories from explanatory sociology of which Max Weber is the originator. Human activities are conscious, intentional, interrelated, and full of social significance. As a result, to understand a

---

[20]He (1997).

social activity such as suicide, we need to go into the system of significance which the suicide has constructed and through which his or her inner thoughts are expressed by the very act of committing suicide. We have to consider the suicide's environment, social conditions, and his or her relationships with other people.[21] Why do the elderly have such an elevated suicide rate? What are the factors prompting them to take their own lives? We have to find out the hidden motivations to explain the phenomenon of suicide. Only by getting to the source can we effectively prevent elderly suicide.

The negative life events most associated with elderly suicide are difficult social relationships, financial trouble, illness, and other kinds of loss. Outside China, the relationship between social stratum and suicide has been amply studied and proven intimate. The lower the social status, the higher the suicide rate; the higher the social status, the lower the suicide rate. There has not been much study regarding this subject in China, and this is why it is necessary and practical to examine this and find out the social groups that are at high risk of suicide.

It must be pointed out here that it is unscientific to lump high rural elderly suicide rate under the effects of social transformation. We have to discover how the inner (psychological) and outer (social) factors interact to lead to elderly suicide.

### 4.3.1 Change in Rural Family Structure

As the reform and opening up deepens in China, the pace of industrialization and urbanization accelerates and rural social structure undergoes an acute transformation. The traditional culture and family structure have never been under such powerful assault. As William J. Goode once pointed out, during the modernization process, the husband-wife relationship constitutes the core of the family structure while the parent-child relationship weakens.[22] Rural families in China are undergoing exactly this kind of transformation.

#### More Empty Nests

As the government continues to implement the family planning policy and promote urbanization, able-bodied men and women leave the countryside to look for work in the cities, leaving many empty nests behind. The social problems facing the elderly bubble up to the surface. First, the sources of income in the countryside are limited. When young people leave to work in the cities, their income is by no means certain. This makes the empty nesters' financial situation highly problematic. The migrant population are sometimes barely able to support themselves in the cities, and they are seldom in a position to help the parents they left behind in the countryside.

[21]Zhang (2012a).

[22]Goode (1986).

Second, the migrant population's children are often left under the care of the grandparents who become responsible for the cost associated with raising them. This is a particularly heavy burden for the grandparents who have limited income sources in the first place. In addition, empty nesters would also have to do all the labor as well as daily trivialities at home. Third, the severe shortage of care services for the rural elderly means many of them are left to their own devices and experience poor quality of life. This is a huge challenge to the already weak social security system of China.

### Smaller Families

Traditionally, rural families in China have tended to be large. Even when family members do not dwell together, their residences are close enough so they could help one another. The children treated the elderly with respect and care which afforded the rural elderly some protection as they lived out their old age. But urbanization, modernization, and the national family planning policy have brought huge changes to the rural family structure. Families have become much smaller, often with only one or two children. In addition, because the living conditions have improved generally in the countryside, the children no longer wish to live with their parents. The families, nuclear or extended, have shrunk, and the traditional big and senior-centered families are basically a thing of the past. This has brought many difficulties to the rural elderly regarding their living arrangements, social care, and mental stability.

The traditional Chinese family is hierarchical and headed by a patriarch. The father and the husband dominate family relationships. Though the husband and wife (parents) are the heads of household, it is often the older generation (grandparents) who have the highest authority. In contrast, the modern family consists of individuals who have equal statuses. The older generation have gradually lost their superiority within the family while the younger generation has become the decision-makers. In a traditional rural family, the older generation had more agricultural experience which allowed them to retain their authority over the younger generation. In the modern era, science and technology have transformed agriculture and introduced new crops and new ways of producing and selling. The expertise of the older generation is no longer germane, and this has quietly transformed the relationships within the family. The older generation have seen their status reduced. Having lost their authority within the family, they experience an erosion of economic independence and social support, and a higher likelihood of living by themselves. Socially isolated, they may lose their will for living.

### Lower Status in the Family

When the income from cultivating the land can barely cover the cost of living of a rural family, the elderly of the family, who have no income, fall to a subordinate status. What little income the family has will be spent on the parents and the children, while very little of it will go to the care of the grandparents. Elderly care becomes a point of contention for the next generation, who try to shirk their responsibility as much as possible. The grandparents, invaded by a profound sense of inferiority, become embarrassed, sensitive, and jealous of their peers who are better off. They are often anxious and pessimistic. Some take refuge in superstitions or delusions to alleviate the mental and social pressure brought on by the family as well as the social transformation that is raging outside. The various forms of suppression they have to endure may cause them to commit suicide.

### 4.3.2 Rural Problems and the Rural-Urban Gap

The transition from an agricultural society to an industrial society is the general trend of modernization. Social transformation is a comprehensive and fundamental change in social structure and social life.

#### Rural Problems

As the Chinese society undergoes a transformation, a very important change in the rural society is that the basic unit of resource distribution has changed from the production team to the family, causing all the original social organizations to undergo different levels of decay and paralysis. The traditional rural society has been transformed in recent years by marketization, industrialization, and urbanization. People's mindsets and values have changed as well. Deep-seated social contradictions bubble up, and so does the problem of rural elderly suicide.

Before the reform and opening-up policy was launched, the vast rural population depended on the powerful people's communes, which had administrative and social functions, for their everyday needs. They did not concern themselves too much with the disparity between the cities and the countryside. The core of the people's communes was the production team which represented the government's administrative power. It distributed work and resources to the rural population, arbitrated disputes, and managed important life events such as birth, death, sickness, and retirement. The production team was the veritable lifeline of the rural population. When the household contract responsibility system was instituted, the family became the basic unit of production and audit. The production team morphed into the "villagers' committee" or the "villagers group." Its original function as the distributor of work and resources disappeared, and its duties as the arbitrator of disputes and social relationships were diluted. Apart from blood ties, the family was cut loose from all government organizations and had to bear all the risks relating to production and survival. The social barriers between the cities and the countryside disintegrated as people and ideas began to flow in this bifurcated system. Some parts of the countryside, especially in the coastal regions in East China, changed dramatically. Township enterprises rose spectacularly during industrialization as farmers went into the cities to look for work. People began to feel the wide gap between the cities and the countryside. Rural economic development lagged far behind that of the cities, and rural income rose at a snail's pace as farmers lost their land-based entitlements. The income gap between the cities and the countryside gaped to unprecedented levels. The average urban income was three times the average rural income in 2001, and even more remarkable in the more backward parts of China. If we put non-monetary factors into the equation, China has the highest income disparity in the world.[23] According to the data published by the National Statistics Bureau in August 2012, the average urban disposable income stood at RMB 21,810 in 2011 while the average rural disposable income was RMB 6977,[24] the former being 3.13 times the latter.

When we look at rural income, we see that it has two major sources: wages earned from work in the cities or township enterprises, most of which is used for house building and weddings and very little is for public infrastructure. There have been changes in the demand for agricultural products in recent years. The market has diversified and the trend is for products of better quality. The existing structure of agriculture has become unfit for what the market prefers. Even though the government tries to guide the farmers to upgrade their work, many rural families lack the technical know-how, funds, and experience to industrialize or push up the scale of their business. The result is high investment, low output, and difficult sales. Moreover, since agricultural work tends to be labor-intensive and unprofitable, many able-bodied men and women prefer to work in the cities. The people who stay behind tend to be less educated and have difficulty in absorbing new technology and business ideas. They would rather do traditional work than pursue more profits in areas such as animal by-products, aquatic products, vegetables, plant-based drinks, flowers, and medicinal products. If this trend continues, a vicious cycle will form and dash any hope of income growth.

### The "38-99-61" Phenomenon

"38" refers to March 8, International Women's Day; "99" to September 9 of the Chinese lunar calendar, the Double Ninth Day for revering the old; and "61" to June 1, Children's Day. The rural demographics exhibits this curious phenomenon: since many able-bodied people leave home to find work in the cities, those who remain in the countryside are called Troop 38-99-61, consisting of women, the elderly, and the young. The common thread running through these groups of people is that they all face problems of one kind or another. The case of the elderly is particularly poignant. With their children working elsewhere, they are now the heads of households and have to care for their grandchildren when they themselves

[23]Hu (2004).

[24]National Bureau of Statistics (2010).

need care. They are suddenly thrust with the myriad of daily chores when they should be enjoying retirement.

### 4.3.3 Filial Piety Truncated

In *Shuowen Jiezi*, a Chinese dictionary from the second century, the character *xiao* (filial piety) is defined as "Looking after one's parents. The character is a composite of two components: on top is the character for "old" and underneath that the character for "son". Together they signify the son supporting the parents." Zengzi says, according to the Book of Rites, that "[t]here are three levels to filial piety, which are, in descending order, displaying utmost reverence, protecting their honor and providing and caring for them." This means that the least a pious son is expected to do for his parents is to make sure the latter are well cared for. When Ziyou asks about filial piety, Confucius says: "Nowadays people think of filial piety as caring for their parents. But people care for their horses and dogs too. If this is all they do, what is the difference between parents and horses or dogs?" Confucius thinks that we should respect our elderly, trust our friends, and care for our young. Liyun in the Book of Rites states, "The old should live happily to the end; the strong should be put to work; the young should grow up properly; the quiet, the widowed, the solitary, the disabled, and the sick should all be cared for." The report to the 18th National Congress of the CPC states, "we should… ensure that all the people enjoy their rights to education, employment, medical and old-age care, and housing."[25]

In the traditional rural family, the parent–child relationship is backed by filial piety as the underlying mindset, paternalism in the government as a political basis, and the natural economy as the economic foundation. These together form a rigorous clan system that upholds filial piety as a traditional moral requirement and a philosophical and ethical consensus, against which, all people are subject to public scrutiny and judgment. It is the moral compass for the individual, the family, and the government. Filial piety has three parts: care for the old, respect for the old, and carry on with their pursuits.

Even though it is part of the traditional Chinese culture, filial piety is relevant today as a universal belief that the elderly should be cared for and respected with both their material and spiritual needs satisfied.

In the contemporary rural family, filial piety is still the dominant norm because there is a need for it both in the home and in society as a whole. On the one hand, to care for and respect the parents is an expression of the children's gratitude and of the symbolic permanence of the parents' wealth, knowledge, and life. On the other hand, if society has its share of responsibility in caring for the old, then filial piety is no longer a private matter but a social one. Confucius says, "I care for the elderly of my family and then extend this caring to the elderly of others." The

[25]Hu (2012).

intergenerational relationship ameliorates itself in a climate of respect and support, and this will no doubt help reduce elderly suicide.

But, as China transforms from a planned economy to a market economy, the rural elderly, who represent 75% of the elderly population, have ceased to be the magnet of their children's attention. The parents, who are rapidly growing old, feel neglected by their children whereas the children, lured by the excitement of the cities, question their parents' values and no longer see caring for them as their responsibility.

Confucianism, the reigning philosophy in China for two thousand years, calls for taking care of and honoring the elderly. But the traditional culture is under assault in the era of globalization and marketization. The folkloric belief in the spirits has always been historically connected with filial piety. Many people believe that our ancestors will protect us if we care for our parents and observe rituals to remember them after they die. If we don't, our ancestors won't rest in peace and may come back to haunt us.

But this kind of belief which has lasted thousands of years is rejected by many people today. In the conflict between tradition and modernity and between Eastern and Western cultures, many people have adopted values which prefer the new to the old, and they have lost a sense of balance regarding culture and ethics.

### 4.3.4 Deficient Rural Social Security System

Social security refers to provision from the government that all members of a society who are unable to provide for themselves due to old age, sickness, disability or other debilitating difficulties are entitled to that would allow their basic needs to be met. It is a system prescribed by law obligating the government to protect the people's basic right to survival. Simply put, social security is a set of measures which the government implements to protect the people from social risks; it is a duty emanating from the government's right to rule, a right of the people's to maintain basic human dignity, and a lubricant or safety net ensuring social harmony. Social security is the actions taken by a modern nation to protect the people from the threat of disease and other difficulties, and these actions may involve healthcare, social insurance, welfare, and other services which offer protection for basic social life.[26]

Article 45 of the Constitution of the People's Republic of China stipulates that Chinese citizens have the right to receive material help from the government in case of old age, sickness, or the loss of the ability to work. As such, social security as a basic entitlement is enshrined in the Constitution. The existing regulations regarding rural social security system include: Basic Program for County-level Rural Pension (Trial) issued by the Ministry of Civil Affairs in 1992; Opinions Regarding the Implementation of Rural Medical Aid promulgated jointly by the

[26]Guimin (2006).

Ministry of Civil Affairs, Ministry of Health, and Ministry of Finance in 2003; Guiding Opinions Regarding Further Work on Pilot Programs of New Rural Cooperative Medical Scheme issued by the Ministry of Health and other authorities and forwarded by the General Office of the State Council in 2004. But these regulations were rather basic and lacked consistency and authority; they were never fully implemented. Toward the end of the 1990s, five ministries including the Ministry of Agriculture forbade the collection of fees for retirement and healthcare regarding them a burden to the farmers. China does not have a complete social security system for the elderly yet, especially the rural elderly. A social security system will certainly mitigate the upward trend of rural elderly suicide. The county-level pension program of 1992 saw large-scale pilot programs launched on its basis in Shandong and other places. At the end of 2007, a basic system for subsistence was established in places where conditions are ripe and covered three million poor farmers. This was a big step forward.

Generally speaking, the rural social security system is less developed than the one in place in urban areas. China's national social security expenditure in 1990 was RMB 110.3 billion, of which 97.7 billion, or 88.6%, went to the cities and 12.6 billion went to the countryside. This means RMB 413 pcr capita for urban residents compared to RMB 14 per capita for rural residents, a gap of 30-fold. Between 1991 and 2001, urbanites spent 15% of their income on social security, reaching the level of developed countries in the 1970s. In contrast, this figure was 0.18% for the rural people, one-ninetieth of the urban figure.[27] At the same time, as the market economy develops, the demand for rural social security rises with the increase in social risk. A lack of government funds along with increased demand severely crimps the development of the rural social security system.[28]

There is a host of problems attending the rural social security system, and they hamper poverty alleviation and subsistence in the countryside. In its narrow definition, social security should include five insurances: retirement, healthcare, work-related injury, childbirth, and unemployment; and three protections: social assistance, welfare, and special care. It is, therefore, an eight-pronged system. If we compare the current rural social security system to this, we see the following problems: First, a serious lack of coverage. Though the first pilot programs were launched back in 1986, it has been on and off over the years and we are still in the initial stage today. The old rural cooperative medical insurance system is no longer viable while the new system is still in the incipient stage. Compensation for work-related injuries, and insurance for childbirth, and unemployment remain absent in rural areas. Second, the system of social assistance is not comprehensive. Viewed from the angle of demand, social assistance should include subsidies for disasters, basic living, employment, housing, retirement, education, healthcare, and legal matters. Rural social assistance is now limited to basic living subsidies and disaster relief. Healthcare assistance basically does not exist while education and

[27]Cuiyin and Jinfeng (2006).

[28]Zhang (2008b).

housing assistance is of limited scope. Disaster relief does not include help for work disruption or any kind of post-disaster assistance. Third, the lack of a welfare system. There are some senior centers and benefit offices in the vast countryside of China, but due to a lack of funds, they have shrunk tremendously. Apart from some prosperous pockets, these organizations are basically paralyzed.[29] The unsophisticated funds management system offers little protection against increased financial risks. As of the end of 2006, 31 provinces (autonomous regions and municipalities) and 2000 counties have started pension insurance at various levels of sophistication with 53.74 million participants and a combined fund of RMB 35.4 billion. There are 3.55 million pensioners drawing on their pensions. According to the existing model of fund management, RMB 35.4 billion need to be distributed to several thousand units on the county and city levels (even to some units on the township level). On September 1, 2009, The State Council's Guiding Opinions on the Pilot Program for the New Rural Pension Insurance was adopted and implemented in selected counties and county-level cities and prefectures. As of May 2010, 320 counties in 27 provinces and 4 municipalities participated in the pilot programs and 51.99 million people were covered by the pension insurance, representing 78% of the rural population above 16 years old, and 16.33 million qualified rural elderly started to draw on their pensions.[30] But pension funds face certain risks due to the lack of proper management. Moreover, the decentralized way of management makes it impossible to benefit from the economy of scale. Because the scope of the rural pension system is limited, it can only use the most basic methods (certificates of deposit, bonds) to increase value, and this is certainly a waste of resources.[31]

The current rural social security system does not yet provide adequate support for the elderly and has much room for improvement. Therefore, it is very difficult for work on a rural pension system, a cooperative medical insurance scheme, or a welfare system to get started.

On March 1, 2011, Director Zhang Kaidi of China Research Center on Aging said at a news conference that as of the end of 2010, partially and completely disabled elderly people in the countryside numbered 33 million, about 19% of the total elderly population. Office of the National Working Commission on Aging and China Research Center on Aging joined hands in 2010 to study the conditions of disabled elderly people. They found that there were 10.8 million completely disabled elderly people or 6.22% of the total elderly population. Based on the internationally adopted list of six everyday activities (eating, dressing, getting in and out of bed, going to the bathroom, walking indoors, and bathing), we define "light disability" as the inability to do one or two of the above activities, "medium disability" the inability to do three or four, and "serious disability" the inability to do five or six. As the Chinese population ages, there will be more disabled people. In 2015, the final year of the 12th Five-Year Plan period, the disabled population

[29]Cuiyin and Zuhui (2007).

[30]Song (2010b).

[31]Zhao (2008).

will reach forty million, or 19.5% of the total elderly population, 7 million more than the 2010 figure. Of the 40, 12.4 million, or 6.05%, will be completely disabled, an increase of 1.6 million from 2010.[32] A disabled person is someone who cannot take care of himself or herself and has to rely on the aid of another person. Long-term care involves providing the disabled person with everyday care, rehabilitation, spiritual consolation, social interaction, and hospice care. In 2007, 13.5 million disabled elderly people needed 5.65 million (a conservative estimate) institutional beds and the government could only provide 1.73 million. The lack of 3.92 million beds is a very acute problem.

Disability is a natural phenomenon of old age. While the lack of care for the elderly is a personal and familial tragedy, it becomes a social disaster when a preponderance of the elderly cannot get the care they need. The civility of an aging society is measured by the way it treats its disabled elderly.

There is not yet any legal stipulation in China regarding the relationship between social welfare level and economic development. It is very clear that the current standard of the rural social security system is low, and this has to do with the current conditions of China. The social security system may be able to feed the hungry, but it can't do too much for healthcare and education. It can't really lift people out of poverty, let alone pushing them into and keeping them in moderate prosperity.

Currently, the core of the rural social security system is social assistance, but the assistance's scope is very limited. The disadvantaged, mainly widowers and the widowed, and the childless elderly, may get their basic living needs met, but any other assistance has only symbolic significance. That is to say, it only happens out of moral considerations. Much of the vast countryside does not have social security institutions in place; and the local government sometimes collects a social security fee in the form of a welfare fund or cooperative medical fund, but this fund is so limited that it can only aid those who live alone and have nobody to support them. At the same time, the rural social security system lacks effective management and the farmers lack basic knowledge of and interest in the system. All this makes it difficult to implement the social security system, which is in danger of existing in form only.

The majority of the Chinese people, or 50.32% of the total population, live in the countryside; they number 674 million, including two-thirds of the elderly population. Population aging is especially acute in the countryside. Most of the rural population, especially in the vast western part of China, have no savings or social protection. The vast majority have no pension or health insurance, even though an incipient social security system has been implemented in some areas. The rural elderly depend on their children for their care and livelihood and are on track to become a huge social problem. Nobody knows if the traditional family ethics can continue to serve its social function of caring for the elderly. A serious imbalance exists between the rural and urban social security systems. A national social

[32]Zhang (2012b).

security system has taken shape in the cities, with a multitude of funding sources and coverage plans. Even though the idea of social security has taken roots in the cities, the main model of social security in the countryside is still the family. That is to say elderly care results principally from the interaction among family members. A rural social security system based on pension and medical insurance has been implemented in some limited areas, but it is far from a national system. This system is limited both in terms of funds and the number of people it covers. The implementation of the new rural cooperative medical insurance scheme solves some problems, but the scope is only regional, not national.

There are a myriad of problems in the rural social security system. First, the pension insurance is problematic and cannot effectively resolve retirement issues. The government issued a basic plan for that in 1992, but the scope was small and its effects negligent. The funding of this plan came from the participants and not from the government, which only offered policy support. The plan was effectively a mandatory pension savings plan in which the farmers had no incentive to join. It was self-help, not social help. The plan lacked management know-how and fared poorly financially. Second, the health insurance is far from comprehensive in scope and cannot meet the needs of the rural elderly. The rural cooperative medical insurance scheme of the 1960s had fulfilled some important functions but disintegrated with the planned economy. The new rural cooperative medical insurance scheme has limited coverage and many problems. It does not provide enough medical protection for the sick rural elderly.

### 4.3.5 Influence of Traditional Culture

Self-preservation is a natural instinct. How people feel about life and death has to do with their values and is intimately related to their culture, social environment, and family relationships. Some scholars think that how the elderly think about life and death reflects how happy, satisfied, and valued they feel.[33]

#### Life and Death Are Predestined

Confucianism believes that life and death are predestined and that life may be given up for a noble cause, such as justice or benevolence. If life and death are predestined, then it is a logical conclusion that one should attempt to be happy no matter what life brings. Confucius says, "One can't know about death if one doesn't know about life." This is the traditional Chinese way of looking at life and death. The elderly want to feel valued and respected at the time of death, even if death is predestined and natural. The Chinese culture casts aspersions on people who escape

[33]Zeng (1992).

death only to live ignobly. The elderly are therefore afraid to say that they fear dying or that they fear living too long because they can't be of service to anyone.

Abandonment

In September 2009, a large number of caves big enough for only one person were discovered amid the shrubs around Mt. Wudang, Hubei Province. They were called "death caves" because scholars believe that they were used to dispose of old people who had lost the ability to work. According to legend, when people got to be sixty years old or when they became disabled, their children would send them to these caves to die. We need more historical data to prove that such elderly abandonment was indeed an ancient custom, but we cannot excuse the cases of elder abuse and abandonment which exist today on the grounds that it was an ancient custom. We need to honor and respect the elderly as that is truly the culture of filial piety which has existed for thousands of years.

Some elderly people think that they are no better than a baby if they become disabled and lose their freedom and basic human dignity. To lose one's health, habitual social relationships, and economic ability is tantamount to losing one's right to life. When a negative event strikes, one can lose one's will to live. A healthy elderly person may hope for long life, but a disabled one may wish for a quick death. These opposite viewpoints may happen to the same person. This is true for Japan as well as China, and the only difference is in what people believe about the afterlife.

### 4.3.6 Influence of a Sudden Negative Event

As people age, their physiological functions decline along with their ability to deal with mental pressure. Frustrations and challenges of everyday life, especially sudden negative events, may trigger mental disorder or physical illnesses which in turn may cause suicide. These sudden negative events may include natural disasters, social disturbance, or a change in public policy. For example, due to psychological trauma, an elderly person may commit suicide after being rescued from an earthquake or a tsunami. Sometimes a person can be at higher risk of suicide when he is told to have cancer. In our study of Town S, the number of suicide cases increased from 13 in 2006 to 24 in 2007, an increase of 84.62%. After investigation, we found out that the reason was a change in the funeral law of Town S which mandated cremation.

How do we prevent suicides resulting from loneliness, poverty, and depression in an era of rapid population aging? Zhu Qingfang, researcher at CASS Institute of Sociology, believes that a new community-based service network which allows elderly people to live in their own homes is the caregiving model which meets elderly needs best. This new model includes daycare, home visits, and clinics, and it allows the elderly to receive care on an out-patient basis. It creates jobs, gives care to the poverty-stricken elderly, and keeps the elderly happy as they are not confined to a nursing home.[34] We can create a community-based care delivery system by pooling resources from the maternity subsidy system, the rural poverty alleviation program, the Five Guarantees system, and the rural cooperative medical insurance.

For China, the rejuvenation of the nation, the building of a harmonious socialist society, and the achievement of the goal of building a moderate prosperous society in all respects all need to be based on the stability of the family. China will become an aged society before it becomes wealthy enough. In facing the challenges of an aging society, we need to build an elderly care delivery system and come to a consensus on social values.

Only when the elderly population is fully valued and respected in society can we all have a promising future for ourselves.

## References

Chen, X. (2002). *Qualitative research in social science* (p. 15). Taipei: Wunan Publishing House.

Cuiyin, Y., & Jinfeng, G. (2006). Difficulties in the rural social security system. *Journal of Zhejiang University* (Social Sciences Edition), no. 3.

Cuiyin, Y., & Zuhui, H. (2007). Establish and perfect a rural social protection system. *Journal of Northwest A&F University* (Social Sciences Edition), no. 1.

Du, P. (2006). *Population aging and the attendant problems* (p. 2). Beijing: People's Publishing House.

Gongde, P. (1997). 268 case studies of elderly suicide. *Rural Public Health Management*, no. 8.

Gonghuan, Y., Huang, Z., & Aiping, C. (1997). Trend of accidental harm. *Chinese Epidemiology, 18*(3), 142–145.

Goode, W. J. (1986). *The family* (p. 11). (W. Zhangling, Trans.). Beijing: Social Sciences Academic Press.

Guimin, C. (2006). *Rural sociology* (p. 301). Beijing: Intellectual Property Publishing House.

He, Z. (1997). *The pathology of suicide* (p. 182). Beijing: China Traditional Chinese Medicine Press.

Hu, Y. (2004). Urban-rural income disparity in China. *Caijing, 2,* 22.

Hu, J. (2012). Fight for a moderately prosperous society with Chinese socialist characteristics. *People's Daily*, November 8, 2012.

Inamura, H. (1977). *Suicide: Treatment and prevention* (p. 26). Tokyo: University of Tokyo Press.

Liang, J., & Li, J. (2012). *Too many Chinese?* (p. 196). Beijing: Social Science Academic Press.

Maris, R. W., et al. (2000). *Review of suicidology*. New York: The Guilford Press.

Maxwell, J. A. (2007). *Qualitative research design: An interactive approach* (p. 9), (G. Zhu, Trans.). Chongqing: Chongqing University Press.

National Bureau of Statistics. (2010). *New script for the new challenge in the new era*. http://www.stats.gov.cn/tjfx/ztfx/sbdcj/t20120815_402827873.htm. Accessed October 5, 2010.

Qing, W. (2007). *Study of elderly suicidal thoughts and risk factors from Yuanjiang, Hunan* (Master's thesis). Zhongnan University.

Qingfang, Z. (2005). Indexed view of elderly poverty. *Chinese Cadres Tribune*, no. 8.

Rong, L. (2010). American crisis interventionist suggests more poison control. *Xiamen Evening News*, April 24, 2010.

[34]Qingfang (2005).

Song, Y. (2010). *Main features of countryside elderly suicide*. http://www.snzg.cn/article/2008/1113/article_12362.html. Accessed April 17, 2010.

Song, L. (2010). New rural pension system attracts 50 million adherents. *China Information News*, May 18, 2010.

Xiao, L. (2010). *The epidemic of suicide in the countryside*. http://www.mingong123.com/news/72/20089/6e9d4c749683e03d.html. Accessed April 15, 2010.

Yan, T. (2003). Study on elderly suicide during social transformation. *Population Research, 9*(5), 73–79.

Yang, G., Huang Z., & Chen, A. (1997). China's accidental injury level and trends. *Chinese Journal of Epidemiology, 18*(3), 142–145.

Zeng, J. (1992). How the Shanghainese see life and death. *Psychology*, no. 5.

Zhai, S. (1997). *Crisis intervention and suicide prevention*. Beijing: People's Medical Publishing House.

Zhang, C. (2005). Tender loving care for the elderly. *CPPCC Magazine*, October 12, 2005.

Zhang, C. (2008). *Anatomy of elderly suicide: What a warm and lonely soul needs*. http://www.pharmnet.com.cn/health/2005/11/05/155765.html. Accessed June 15, 2008.

Zhang, W. (2008). Rural social security system: Difficulties and solutions. *Economic Studies*, no. 11.

Zhang, X. (2010). *China's elderly population has reached 160 million people and 20% of total population*. http://www.ce.cn/xwzx/gnsz/gdxw/200910/23/t20091023_20256579.shtml. Accessed October 5, 2010.

Zhang, Y. (2012). "Killer tree" and "killer". http://blog.sina.com.cn/s/blog_676f7600100iltj.html. Accessed May 14, 2012.

Zhang, X. (2012). *China's disabled population reaches 33 million*. http://www.xeeee.net/Item/55120.aspx. Accessed February 5, 2012.

Zhao, Z. (2008). Building a comprehensive pension system. *Building a social security system* (Vol. 1, p. 1055). Beijing: Labor and Social Security Publishing House.

# Chapter 5
# Suicide Prevention: Theories and Possibilities

Suicide prevention and crisis intervention are closely related but not quite the same thing. B. E. Gilliland and R. K. James point out that it is impossible to separate the two.[1]

Suicide is an extreme and non-normative human behavior. Regardless of the reasons, it has consequences so devastating that we can hardly justify it. In his book *Suicide*, Emily Durkheim says that suicide is a social pathology and must be viewed as such even if it is based on positive moral considerations. According to Durkheim, we may have two different views regarding suicide: First, we recognize the fact of suicide and condemn it. Second, we limit it by making a series of possible and necessary changes.[2] The former does not seek to condemn the people who commit suicide but to denigrate the act of committing suicide as an unhealthy social phenomenon and denounce the social environment which facilitates it, including social customs and cultural values. This view involves a negative reflective attitude whose purpose is to build what Erich Fromm called a "sane society" and provide a *raison d'être* for healthy people. The latter view involves a proactive attitude which seeks to implement necessary measures to prevent or reduce suicide.

Suicide prevention treats suicides or potential suicides (including groups, of course) as target or object. The target of preventive work is logically the society, but more specifically, it is the forces within the society which facilitate the suicidal behavior. At first glance, Durkheim's first view seems to have little connection with suicide prevention, but effectuating factual and moral judgment in order to create better social and psychological consensus has to be an important aspect of suicide prevention. We can explore the ways of prevention by combining the social theories of Durkheim and the psychological analyses of Freud and take as our point of departure the dynamic relationship between the social and the individual.

---

[1]Gilliland and James (2000, p. 275).
[2]Durkheim (1996b, p. 342).



J. Li, *A Study on Suicide*,
https://doi.org/10.1007/978-981-13-9499-7_5

# 1 Theories of Suicide Prevention

## *1.1 Durkheim's View*

Emile Durkheim is cautiously optimistic about suicide prevention. He is cautious because he does not believe that suicide is a necessary evil in cultural evolution. He says the following: many people believe that suicide is not the fault of society since a good society may still have a high suicide rate. This belief seems plausible since suicide is on the rise as our society gets more affluent. If society causes suicides, then preventing suicide may thwart social development. Following this logic, the conclusion is that it is not necessary to try and prevent suicide because not doing this benefits social development. However, Durkheim surely does not accept this.

Durkheim believes that the above viewpoint might actually encourage suicide. He thinks that suicide is a necessary pathology accompanying cultural evolution, regardless of the motives and purposes.[3]

The act of suicide is an emotional expression of some members of society, reflecting a basic and prevalent atmosphere. An increase in suicide rate has to be viewed as a horrendous social anomaly. It is not horrendous to have a social anomaly. What is horrendous is that this kind of social anomaly can be regarded as normal if people get used to it. Suicide prevention is difficult because most people live in what they perceive as a normal world and they think that everything is as it should be and simply go about their lives without much reliance on or intrusion from society. They endure omnipresent social pressure, disorder, and injustice; and they compartmentalize and bend themselves to satisfy unreasonable social requirements. If they do this long enough, the resulting alienation becomes a ticking time bomb. The ensuing suicide may be anomic or egoistic. Durkheim believes that these two kinds of suicide merit more of our attention because they are more symptomatic of social ills. We must eradicate these social ills if we want to prevent these two kinds of suicide.[4]

This view can be gleaned from Durkheim's theories: A better society can provide a healthy atmosphere and sufficient protective power to its members (by groups) to stop their abnormal behavior. The responsibility for suicide prevention falls therefore on society. We may say that the possibility or effectiveness of suicide prevention depends on how determined a society is for social reform and how radical the changes are.

Durkheim mainly believes in two things with regard to suicide prevention: Suicide should be condemned and limited. To condemn suicide involves the determination for social change, and to limit, it involves the depth of social change. Durkheim believes that this condemnation has to be total and unswerving. We cannot "partially condone" suicide. Durkheim states, "Our resolve comes from taking direct action on pessimism. We must return to the normal state by limiting

---

[3]Ibid., 349.

[4]Ibid., 354.

pessimism until society on the whole is no longer under its sway and gains more resolve. Once people's mental state returns to normal, they will find a way to repel unhealthy tendencies."[5] Here, Durkheim articulates the first step of suicide prevention: a total and universal rejection of suicide, rendering ineffective suicide's negative influences. As an extreme and pessimistic state of mind, the thought of suicide may be hidden in the depth of the consciousness of every single person. We can control the impulse to commit suicide, to harm ourselves, or to negatively impact others only when our consciousness is sober, normative, and strong. To condemn suicide is a corrective, not moral, judgment against the harm that suicide causes. It is society which has to find a way to limit the spread of suicide. Durkheim believes that, as long as society has enough stability and cohesion, its members will have a sense of security and belongingness and they will thus be able to find a purpose in their thoughts and actions, and live.

As we can see, Durkheim takes a macroscopic approach to suicide prevention. In his view, society can either facilitate or curtail the incidence of suicide. Religions, family, and the state all have a useful role to play in suicide prevention. So have other collective entities, such as professional organizations, which can facilitate coordination and cooperation. Durkheim contends that social organizations can be a source of "meaning of life" for people, demarcating the scope of what people should or should not do. So long as we do not breach those boundaries and limits, suicide prevention would be possible.

In the last chapter of *Suicide*, Durkheim concludes, "If there are more suicides now than before, it is not because it has become more difficult to sustain ourselves or satisfy our legitimate needs; it is because we don't know where our legitimate needs end and we don't see the significance of our sustenance."[6]

Apparently, Durkheim believes that suicide prevention lies in knowing what to do and what not to do.

## 1.2 Freud's View

Freudian psychoanalysts believe that suicide is an expression of something inherent to human nature that impels us toward self-destructive acts. Freud believes that the death drive is as deep-seated as the desire for self-love or self-realization. When people suppress themselves too much, they can't find happiness or vent their pain, and they will then satisfy their instinctual desire through the destructive force of suicide.[7] From this view, Eros, which opposes the death drive, may well be at the service of the death drive and can transform or yield its place to death. Is suicide the most typical manifestation of how immense the power of the death drive is? If so,

---

[5] Ibid., 353.

[6] Ibid., 367–368.

[7] Freud (1999, pp. 54–55).

there is no need for suicide prevention. But in reality, the death drive does not always express itself in such an extreme form but may be softened or neutralized by Eros. Although the death drive may express itself internally as self-punishment or masochism, these pseudo-suicidal actions will be resisted by Eros which will continue its desire to live psychologically and create defense mechanisms through a compromise with reality. The death drive may therefore transform itself into Eros and drive people to love life. We may say that it is precisely because the death drive is omnipresent that suicide prevention becomes necessary and urgent. We know that suicide is self-destruction. As such, internal problems cannot be solved by the external environment. This is the biggest lesson we can learn from Freudian psychoanalysts, apart from Durkheim's theories. Sigmund Freud tells us that suicide prevention is the resistance to death drive, an attempt to find things within us (such as Eros) which can mitigate the explosiveness of the death drive and lead to the creation of a self-regulating system of balance.

American psychoanalyst Karl Augustus Menninger studied suicide prevention based on the Freudian theory of death drive. He believes that suicide is not the result of heredity, hidden desire, or maladjustment, but an act of long hidden and omnipresent self-destruction.[8] He divides suicides into three kinds: chronic (abstinence, alcohol dependency, neurosis), local (self-mutilation, deliberate accident), and organic (illness). These kinds of suicides are battles between life and death, whether directly or indirectly, and a compromise or affirmation between construction and destruction.

Menninger regards suicide as a failure in life, an inability to manage the life process constructively; the person who commits suicide insists on a wrong way of managing life. Menninger believes that the urge to commit suicide can be controlled, and the only way to prevent suicide is through continually strengthening Eros and reducing the desire for self-destruction.

Menninger believes that the best way to prevent suicide is to love more. If one learns to love oneself and others and to sublimate love into a devotion to others which transcends the self, one may come to experience the power and nobility of love through the beloved and gain much more will and space for life. In loving others, we experience the value of life and the happiness of living, so that we no longer need to prove the meaninglessness of living by committing suicide.

In the end, suicide is an instinctual response to the fear of death. But, if we fear death, it is not because death is fearful but because it is a declaration that the value, meaning, and strength of life are all false. When we are alive, we resist death by such socialized constructs as reputation, status, and wealth. One commits suicide because one senses that these constructs not only are futile but also brings more and more suppression and anxiety. Suicide is the last resort when one can't live anymore.

For American psychologist Ernest Becker, the fear of death is in reality a defense mechanism. The death drive does not lead to suicide; on the contrary, it provides

---

[8]Menninger (1990, p. 74).

the impetus for living and for confronting the risks which threaten life.[9] He quotes psychoanalyst G. Zilboorg, "There can be no drive for living if there is no continuous fear of death. The term 'defense mechanism' implies the effort at resisting disintegration."[10] We can see from this that the death drive and Eros are two sides of the same coin. Death is a destructive force which has already disintegrated. We fear it because we can no longer use our defense mechanisms to protect our lives. Becker believes that suicide happens when defense mechanisms lose their effectiveness to such an extent that death drive transcends Eros. But in reality, we can absorb the death drive and the fear of death into life's abundance and proactivity. As a result, to prevent suicide we need to reconstruct defense mechanisms, renew life's vitality, discover life's renewable resources, and replenish energies which are stronger and more decisive. Although Becker does not agree with Freud's death drive and believes that the fear of death will transcend the death drive's narrow aim, they actually share the same assumption regarding suicide prevention.

In my opinion, the common assumption is this: Suicide prevention is possible as long as we are able to live in the face of death. Suicide prevention negates death; to live is not to die. To live, even if abjectly, is the biggest thing all of us have to face. Our most basic instinct is to fight death ceaselessly in order to live.

## *1.3 Chinese Scholars on Suicide Prevention*

While psychiatry, either theoretically or methodologically, is largely "practical" insofar as it focuses exclusively on issues of application, its understanding of the underlying causal mechanisms is still quite limited. What the deployment of such catchphrase as "one suicide is too many" shows is that, what Michael Phillips and other scholars have done is to call attention to suicide prevention (a genuine and serious issue facing society) and to help us realize that we all have what Karen Homey calls the "neurotic personality" to varying degrees.

Wu Fei offered his thoughts on suicide studies and prevention. He believes that suicide in China has its unique aspects which cannot be explained by Western psychiatry or sociology but has to be viewed from the perspective of Chinese culture and society. In his book *Suicide is a Chinese Problem*, Wu argues that Western theories on suicide are influenced by the Christian culture and the negation of suicide is based on Christian values of life and human nature. Suicides in China, however, happen in a different social and cultural context. Western psychiatry assumes that suicides have mental problems, whereas in China we consider most suicides normal people. In Chinese parlance, suicides with mental problems are rare and rarely studied. Based on this understanding, Wu gave us his theories and explanations on the "Chinese Style of Suicide." He writes, "In the final analysis, the

---

[9]Becker (1988, p.33).

[10]Ibid., 33.

question of suicide has to be understood from two angles. First, how a modern problem such as suicide manifests in China? Second, how do we understand Chinese people's view of life and death in a modern context? Suicide in China is a reflection of China's modernity."[11] In short, Wu views suicide as a cultural phenomenon. He believes that behind the cases of suicide is Chinese people's view on life, and we have to discover the underlying conditions which have existed for a long time before we can understand why people commit suicide. As such, Wu has proposed the concept of "living one's days" (*guo rizi*), a very familiar phrase in the Chinese language, to explain the causes and prevention of suicide. "Living one's days" is a summary expression of the life process; it denotes the general conditions and the minute details of life in China.[12] People in China commit suicide because "they live their days badly"; they can find no reason or meaning to continue living, so they use death to demonstrate the absence of meaning in life. What lies underneath this seemingly simplistic explanation is the Chinese view on life. Confucius says, "One can't know about death if one doesn't know about life." To know about life is to "live one's days." If in living their days people encounter devastating conflicts, injustice, loss of face, or negative family event, their days may end any time. The only way to prevent suicide is to bring back the normal conditions of "living one's days." Wu talks about suicide prevention at the end of his book *Finding Meaning in Life*. He writes, "As for potential suicides, suicide prevention should mean more than preventing mental illness. We should help them live a happy and dignified life, otherwise our efforts would be in vain."[13] We can see from this that suicide prevention has to be built on love, care, and an affirmation of the right to live.

It is probably fair to say that the non-medical views on suicide prevention within China, apart from the pithy and original ones above, don't have many interesting things to say. (Surely, this may be because I have not read enough.) One exception is He Xuefeng, Director of China Rural Governance Research Center of Huazhong University of Science and Technology where many sociologists studying suicide congregate. Many young scholars studying suicide prevention, including Chen Bofeng, Liu Yanwu, and Yang Hua, have emerged in recent years under He's leadership. Based on his research on Liwei Village in northern Anhui, Chen Bofeng feels that rural suicide is often a twisted kind of face-saving gesture, and that to prevent suicide, efforts must be made to rebuild the personal values of farmers and reduce the reliance on social values. Simply put, the farmers must discover some kind of meaning to their lives that will allow them to live peacefully and remain calm in the face of other people's harsh judgment.[14] In his article "Suicide: Plight, Theory, Solution", Liu Yanwu delineates the status quo of research on suicide and the limitation of the analytical models. He feels Wu Fei's suicide study has not gone

[11]Wu (2007b, p. 117).

[12]Wu (2007a).

[13]Wu (2010, p. 263).

[14]Chen (2008).

beyond Durkheim's sociological approach, that his theory and methodology lack clarity and comprehensiveness, and that his research is at best one man's opinion. What is more important is the light Liu shed on the question of suicide prevention: We must take up all the possible approaches to suicide studies to avoid drawing the wrong conclusions concerning prevention. He feels that there are many variables to consider in suicide prevention, including gender, age, the rural–urban dichotomy, and region; and that there is no one-size-for-all solution. Liu concludes his book by stating that there are confusion and uncertainty in Durkheim's way of finding balance between the society and the individual. He suggests that we look more into the humanist approach of sociology represented by Max Weber. This approach regards suicide as a social act and emphasizes the social significance of suicide. In contrast, Durkheim regards suicide as a social fact and attempts to find a single solution for all.[15] In other words, the first step to preventing suicide is to create an ideal type as proposed by Weber, and this will involve the domain of legal sociology. Li Jianjun has studied how suicide has changed from a crime to a human right in the history of Western law. Taking this study as a point of departure, Liu Yanwu explains in his article "National Law, Common Law, and Rural Suicide" that, when national law is insufficient to prevent suicide, common law may be used to mete out an appropriate punishment for committing suicide. Where common law is powerless to do so, national law has to be used for crisis intervention which comprises two levels: the definition of the suicide's legal responsibility and the definition of the legal responsibility of those who are directly related to the suicide.[16] In other words, it has to be made clear to potential suicides that the act of suicide has repercussions against him and those around him. The idea that death means the end of all troubles is completely irresponsible and contrary to the rights and responsibilities that emanate naturally from life.

In summary, Chinese scholars have not reached a consensus on suicide prevention, and we cannot speak about implementation yet. But they have at least agreed on the following point: Suicide prevention is everyone's responsibility, but the government ought to take the leading role. The winners of suicide prevention will always be the individuals and society.

## 2 Conditions, Difficulties, and Approaches of Suicide Prevention

### 2.1 *Current Conditions and Difficulties*

The high rates of suicide have become a serious public health issue and a social problem.

---

[15]Liu (2010a).

[16]Liu (2010b).

As the series studies done by Michael Phillips et al. of Beijing Suicide Research and Prevention Center show, China registered a suicide rate of 23 per 100,000 individuals in 1999, equivalent to 287,000 deaths by suicide a year, and 2 million failed suicide attempts. This takes a huge economic toll on the country. As many as 1.7 million people suffer the emotional trauma of losing a friend or relative to suicide, and 162,000 minors lose a parent to suicide. According to Phillips, suicides in China differ significantly from those in other countries. Rural suicide rate is three to five times the urban rate and women's suicide rate is 25% higher than men's. Suicide is the fifth cause of death of the Chinese population and the leading cause of death in the 15–34 age group.[17] Some scholars such as He Zhaoxiong and Jing Jun questioned these figures.[18] Michael Phillips also said in an interview on September 8, 2009, that the death rate went down according to the new data of the Ministry of Health. He produced some data later: There are 195,600 suicides per year on average, and the ratio of suicide deaths to total harmful deaths went down from 34% in 1987–1988 to 20% in 2005–2006.[19] This book reflects this trend as well: In Chapter Three, we analyzed in detail rural suicides according to gender and age based on the data of the Ministry of Health for the year 2009. Even though this study by itself cannot accurately predict suicides, the number of suicides is declining, so is the ranking of suicide among causes of death in various age groups. Notwithstanding the difference in time, Phillips' findings show the enormity of the problem of suicide, which has become a serious public health issue and social problem. The government and the society have to be mobilized to pay more attention to suicide prevention. The media reports frequently on suicide cases, and this shows that our efforts at suicide prevention are far from sufficient.

As was previously said, suicide rates have been declining in various age groups and in larger margins. This reflects the increased attention the government, the academia, and volunteers have paid to suicide prevention in recent years (we won't comment on the validity of some of the government reports on this subject). As the Chinese society undergoes transformation, many social problems bubble to the surface, and we see the difficulties and challenges facing suicide prevention. Moreover, elderly suicide will become the subject of more studies as China ages. That China tops the world in terms of the absolute number of suicides has become a stigma, yet we are only at the initial stage of tackling suicide prevention. The world's experience in this area shows that the government has to get involved; otherwise, any effort would be limited in effectiveness.

A conference on China national suicide prevention program was convened jointly by China Center for Disease Control and Prevention and Beijing Suicide Research and Prevention Center on November 19 and 20, 2003, attracting mental health experts from China and abroad. This was still a nongovernmental effort despite the name of the conference. Based on the characteristics of suicides in

[17]Phillips (2004).

[18]He (2008).

[19]Jing et al. (2010).

China, the program proposed to improve the overall mental health conditions and endurance in the face of adversities of the general public, enhance social interaction, tell children how to handle emergency situations, and change the way movies and other media depicts mental illness and suicide. Given that pesticides play a prominent role in suicides in China, the program also called upon the Ministry of Agriculture to join the efforts to control the inappropriate use of pesticides, which should constitute an integral part of a national suicide control program. It seemed at the time that a national plan for suicide prevention was in the making, but unfortunately it hasn't materialized yet.

A 2005 report of *Nanfang Daily* stated that more chilling than the high suicide rate was society's indifference and the lack of suicide prevention work. For this report, the reporter interviewed Hu Shenzhi and Dr. Zhan who worked to prevent suicide in Guangzhou. They did not get paid for the work they did, but the pressure they felt did not come from a lack of funds but from social prejudice and the lack of government involvement. Both of them felt the important work of suicide prevention was completely ignored by the society and their work in this area was very limited in scope.[20] Another report of 2007 told about what had currently been done for suicide prevention. Beijing Suicide Research and Prevention Center was established in December 2002, and a hotline was put in place to help those thinking about suicide. This marked the start of suicide prevention in China with a scientific method. From that time on, a dozen or so suicide intervention centers opened across the country, utilizing hotlines, the Internet, and clinics to deliver their services. Suicide intervention work was met with many obstacles from the beginning because it involved a taboo subject. Zhang Chun of Nanjing Suicide Research and Prevention Center said that his organization celebrated the World Suicide Prevention Day on September 10 each year like the Spring Festival because that was the only day when he could talk about his work openly and make publicity and awareness-raising efforts. Shanghai psychiatrist Shan Huaihai made a proposal to the People's Congress in 2003 to build a suicide intervention center in his city, but he said he felt like a lone fighter to this day. Xu Kun, University Professor in Beijing, started a suicide intervention hotline for seniors at his own initiative, but it morphed gradually into a dating service. Chen Si volunteered to patrol the Yangtze River Bridge in Nanjing for potential suicides, but people questioned his motives constantly.[21]

We can see from the above that suicide intervention in China is limited to a small number of psychological help centers, volunteer organizations, and mental health clinics. There doesn't seem to be a national consensus regarding suicide prevention and the government is reluctant to get involved. When Zhang Chun was interviewed in 2010, he said that what perplexed him was not the scarcity of volunteers or the limited scope of his work but the lack of legal basis for suicide intervention. There is currently no law authorizing crisis intervention. As a result, mental health

[20]Lu and Cui (2005).

[21]Wen and Zeng (2007).

workers cannot count on the law to protect them in doing their work.[22] Prior to the World Suicide Prevention Day of 2011, Deputy Director Mao Yu of Beijing Municipal Health Bureau said during an interview, "Suicide has many possible causes including mental and physical illness, mental disorder, heredity, and domestic violence. Moreover, the raging social and cultural transformation plays a part too…In a society of many diverse cultures, government organizations have to cooperate to create different measures for the different cultures in order to prevent suicide."[23] But how will the organizations cooperate and who will implement the various measures? There are no answers yet.

The author made the suggestions about creating a suicide prevention mechanism with coordination between the police, the firefighters, and the medical team.[24]

Public security organizations at various levels should pay more attention to potential suicides. They should evaluate high-risk groups, predict potential incidents, establish a crisis management system, create a contingency plan, and gather relevant information through different channels. They should be prepared to tackle serious suicide attempts and to reduce the number of such occurrences. The police, firemen, and medical personnel should combine forces to create a single crisis prevention mechanism which unites their different functions. There should be a team of experts including psychologists and negotiators, life-saving equipment specialists, and a crisis prevention contingency plan. When necessary, different branches of the police should be mobilized to jointly deal with suicide-related emergencies.

Other countries have systems that we can emulate. For instance, "911" calls in the USA reach a central command center which uses the GPS system to quickly gather the forces needed from the closest positions for crisis prevention. These teams then coordinate perfectly to deliver highly efficient and effective interventions.

In creating a new system of social management, we should pay attention to the possibility of suicide cases leading to mass incidents. Land expropriation and housing demolition over the past years have resulted in suicide attempts. If badly managed, suicide attempts may create serious mass incidents.

On June 22, 2008, a female secondary school student drowned in Weng'an County of Guizhou. The relatives had questions about the cause of her death and rumors began to swirl around the county. On June 28, tens of thousands of people gathered in the street in the county seat and some of them attacked government buildings. In the end, over a hundred administrative offices in the county government building and 47 offices in the public security bureau building were destroyed, all the household registration files were burned. On June 17, 2009, a hotel cook in

[22]Chen (2010).

[23]Li (2012).

[24]Li (2007a, p. 286). Also, National Planning Bureau of Philosophy and Social Science (2007) *Results*, no. 14.

Shishou, Hubei, committed suicide and his families refused to accept suicide as the cause of death.

In this era of massive social transformation, any incident of suicide may provide the fuse for social unrest.

The problems with suicide prevention may be reduced to the following factors.

First, the lack of understanding: The government and society at large have never paid enough attention to suicide prevention and this subject has never reached the fever pitch of "creating a harmonious society" or "attaining moderate prosperity." We have to ask ourselves: Is it possible to create a harmonious society or attain moderate prosperity when people commit suicide in droves?

Second, the lack of government involvement: The efforts at suicide prevention are weak, poorly organized, and concentrated in a few nongovernmental organizations and the academia.

Third, the lack of coordinating mechanisms: Suicide prevention is a large-scale systematic undertaking requiring the cooperation among diverse disciplines and organizations and the mobilization of social resources for public health, social security, education, culture, public security, and law. This kind of a comprehensive system should ideally include a command center (such as a suicide predictive organization), government and educational organizations, the media, intervention team (including volunteers), psychologists, psychiatrists, families, school authorities, communities, intervention experts, public security organizations (such as the police), a steady budget (for personnel, equipment, and technology), and methods of intervention (psychological counseling and medical treatment).[25] But this system has not been established, and plans remain under discussion.

Fourth, unclear goal, plan, and policy: Nongovernmental organizations have their own views on suicide prevention and their own ways of delivering services. Their plans are not community-based and lack comprehensiveness, expertise, and operability. Goals are unscientific, unclear, and full of empty promises such as "we should reduce suicide rate by x percent in y years." Policies lack frameworks on the macro- and micro-levels and are not supported by scientific evidence.

Fifth, the lack of the right conditions: The conditions are not right in terms of personnel, materials, funds, and technology. There is no policy support or legal protection. A national monitoring system, restrictions on pesticides, and standards in media reporting are yet to be established.

## 2.2 *The National Approach*

The study of suicide, be it from the psychological, psychiatric, social, or cultural perspective, is ultimately about the causes and characteristics, prevention, policies,

---

[25]Mao (2010).

education, and last-minute help before the final act of suicide. Its ultimate goal is to foster healthy minds which value and love life.

Regrettably, there is no real progress in suicide prevention in the world, even in developed countries or those with high suicide rates. The reasons are threefold: First, suicide is a complicated social behavior with many factors which cannot be effectively controlled for the time being. Second, suicides are in the minority and do not receive the attention they deserve. General preventive measures lack focus, and it is not easy to identify high-risk groups to implement preventive measures. Third, preventive measures lack the binding force of law. Suicide prevention efforts come mainly from nongovernmental organizations and not from the government. Fourth, preventive measures leave much to be desired.[26] Moreover, the traditional view is that suicide is shocking and people who commit suicide have mental problems and therefore unworthy of pity or attention.

While it is true that suicide is a complex issue with many different explanations and that much ignorance and confusion attend its prevention, one thing is certain: Suicide is preventable, and the key issue is how to prevent it. We already have a World Suicide Prevention Day every year to remind the public that suicide is preventable.

The year 2010 saw the eighth anniversary of the World Suicide Prevention Day. The theme for that occasion was global unity. The WHO published a statement on that day: Not every suicide cases are preventable, but most are; national policy and local measures can reduce suicides.[27] The WHO made four recommendations for suicide prevention: Restrict access to tools of suicide, establish community-based prevention plans, set standards for media reporting, and offer training to frontline personnel.[28]

We need the might of the country to build a comprehensive suicide prevention system. The government ultimately has to be responsible for it. Suicide prevention is a huge and serious undertaking, and it is impossible to implement without strong government support. In 1986, Finland was the first developed country to implement a national suicide prevention plan and it was a success, lowering the suicide rate markedly. The Netherlands adopted a national policy in 1989 and created a suicide prevention committee under its National Health Board to implement the policy on the national, regional, and local levels. Based on the result of these actions, the UN adopted an article for setting and implementing a national suicide prevention policy, declaring that suicide is a national problem and prevention is an urgent matter. Japan created a Suicide Response Headquarters in September 2010. China was late in creating a system of suicide intervention. A conference on suicide prevention was convened in November 1992, and China Mental Health Association created a crisis intervention committee in 1994. China has thus taken the first step in suicide prevention.

---

[26]Xiao (2012b).

[27]Liu and Fan (2010).

[28]Ibid.

## 2.3 Legal Basis of Suicide Prevention

There are several issues from the legislative perspective: First, is suicide a human right and should it be allowed by law? The Western world has had this debate for a thousand years. Second, should aiding and abetting suicide be legal? Third, is it our duty to prevent others from committing suicide?

We have seen in Chapter One of this book how suicide has changed from a crime to a human right in the evolution of Western law.

In 2004, the second session of the 10th National People's Congress adopted the 33rd Amendment to the Constitution, and one paragraph in it stipulates that the government respects and protects human rights. Human rights are a measure of freedom which originates in human nature and which allows people to exist and develop. They can be categorized into individual rights (citizen's rights), collective rights (rights of social groups or races), and national rights (sovereignty). Human rights can also be divided by content into the right to life, political rights, and the rights to economic, cultural, and social development. The core of human rights concerns the individual.[29]

Theoretically, the right to life belongs to the individual. In terms of constitutionalist values, the right to life is supreme. Suicide can have no legal basis in a constitution because it is inconsistent with the system of values and rights of a modern constitution.

A constitution's aim in the modern era is to protect basic individual rights, including the right to life. Due to cultural, religious, and historical reasons, some countries declare that the right to life is relative and permits death sentence. But death sentence is incongruous with modern constitutional values which stipulate that the right to life is absolute. When life is stipulated as the precondition for human existence, it means that individual values have become social values, and whether to deprive someone of life is for society to decide.[30] As a subjective individual right, human right guards against the intrusion of national rights, but modern constitutionalism does not allow the individual to decide on the right to life. As an objective prioritization of values, human right is expressed as the collective pursuit of values and the individual has no right to end his or her life. As a result, human life is the most important social value and a basic component of society. What to do with one's life involves collective values, not just individual values. The individual does not have legal basis for suicide or euthanasia.[31]

Some scholars believe that the law ought to tackle suicide intervention in two ways. First, define the suicide's legal responsibility. The law should not talk about individual rights in an abstract way but in real terms. Even though some theorists such as David Hume suggest that suicide is a human right, history did not prove them right. Second, define the legal responsibility of the persons close to the

---

[29]Lin (2004).

[30]Han (2011).

[31]Ibid.

suicide. For those people directly involved with the suicide, are they liable for intentional homicide, negligent injury, or nothing at all?[32] In 1997, a person in New York State wanted to commit suicide. He was then sued, because a state law prohibits this act. The case went to the Supreme Court of New York State where the Chief Justice declared that the state law prohibiting aiding and abetting suicide does not violate the US Constitution and therefore conforms to the basic values of the Constitution.[33]

There was no mention of suicide in the national law; PRC Criminal Law, adopted in 1979, and the ensuing amendments do not define suicide. "Homicide is defined as committed by a third person and not the first person. No national law defines suicide as a human (or legal) right; the law is unclear and ambivalent about suicide."[34]

We have to take a serious look at suicide and provide the legal basis for suicide prevention.

## 3 Three Levels of Suicide Prevention

Borrowing from the theories and methods of public health and preventive medicine, we propose a three-level approach to suicide prevention. Primary prevention ameliorates the social environment and raises people's happiness level. Secondary prevention provides aid to sufferers teetering on the edge of life and death. Tertiary prevention prevents repeated attempts.

### *3.1 Primary Prevention: Change the Social Environment*

The aim of primary prevention is to control suicide by changing the social environment.

We are in an era of rapid social transformation where conflicts are conspicuous, personal interests diverse, and social problems acute. Based on global experiences in social development, the period where per capita income goes from USD1000 to USD3000 is usually full of turbulence. It is a period when the industrial structure and social interests undergo massive transformation, and a time of great opportunities and risks. Samuel P. Huntington believes that people's desires and expectations are high during this period; social problems and pressure rise because society is unable to satisfy people's rapidly rising needs, resulting in resentment and

[32]Liu (2010a).

[33]Han (2008, p. 134).

[34]Liu (2010a).

frustrations.[35] During this period in China, changes to social life were rapid, far-reaching, and profound; and social interests began to diversify along with the socioeconomic structure, resource distribution, and employment. Conflicting interest groups, values, behavior models, and expectations interacted with and reacted to one another; and the society was turbulent and unstable.

In creating a socialist market economy, we had to face the additional challenge of promoting equity and justice. China experienced huge changes over the past thirty years since the reform and opening-up policy was launched, along with high economic growth. The society as a whole benefitted from it and people's lives improved. But the Confucian ideas of equity and justice remained deep-rooted as the Chinese society underwent transformation. Differences in income, residence (urban–rural), regions (eastern–western), and employment widened; social problems such as unemployment, loss of rural land, unpaid income, over-qualification, lack of healthcare, insufficient education, and poor public security conditions all point to the fact that we have to do a better job at promoting equity and justice.

"Equity and justice are inherent socialist qualities and provide the foundation for social stability. They shine as brightly as the sun."[36] The key to realizing equity and justice is to implement policies which protect the interests of disadvantaged people. This is an important function of the government, the basis of CPC governance, and the guarantor of a harmonious socialist society.

People want a reduction in the social ills brought about by social transformation, such as the wide income gap, regional inequality, unequal educational opportunities, lack of health care, and corruption. This is in reality a call for equity and justice, and the government must strengthen and be innovative in social management, resolve social conflicts, and allow people to partake in the fruits of reform.

Moreover, the old method of suicide prevention is to micromanage the environment and keep tight control over the tools of suicide. As was said earlier, suicide caused by relationship problems is often impulsive; the thought of suicide diminishes once the impulse passes. Increasing protective measures by restricting access to tools of suicide can reduce the impulse to suicide and therefore reduce the number of suicides. Erwin Stengel was the first to propose controlling the environment to prevent suicide. He pointed out that changing to cleaner energy (such as natural gas which gives off less carbon-monoxide) could reduce suicide. Gas conversion was tried out in England and Wales, and Stengel's theory was proven true. The WHO published a report on controlling the environment to prevent suicide, suggesting a number of ways to control the environment, such as gun control, fuel purification, exhaust reduction, limited access to poison or medication, and less sensational media report on the subject. All these practical methods can effectively prevent suicide.[37] China's housing construction specifications can be adjusted to require a parapet on the roofs of buildings, a safety net around elevated

[35]Huntington (1988).

[36]Wen (2010b).

[37]Wasserman (2003b).

passageways, bridges, and subway tracks. Regulations may be adopted to necessitate proper packaging of dangerous products such as pesticides, sleeping pills, and other controlled substances. The packaging should include a telephone number for psychological counseling. Studies have shown that a potential suicide usually does not seek a different way of suicide when his intended method is disrupted.

Thoughts of suicide may be reduced if we take care to instill a positive view on life in young people, promote scientific thinking, tighten gun control, strengthen the management of poisons and controlled substances, and increase the delivery of mental health services.

### 3.1.1 Improve Social Security System and Create a Happy Environment

Happiness is a basic human value.

It has become a buzzword in recent years, and the pursuit of happiness is a fond topic of discussion by ordinary people as well as the chairman of the CPC. Durkheim states, "In a harmonious and lively society, the collective opinions and feelings are transmitted to each of its members. This interaction is akin to moral support, and people do not feel abandoned or forced to find their own way. They are led instead to a path where they share in the collective energy."[38] Durkheim also believes that social being and social environment determine suicide rate.

Many empirical and clinical studies have shown that people are less likely to consider suicide when they are satisfied with their environment. From the ecological viewpoint, the degree of satisfaction is a reflection of the mutual adaptability between the people and the environment. People can adapt to the environment when their interaction with the environment is good. Bad interaction with the environment implies that the environment does not adapt well to human actions, and if this situation persists for a long term, people lose their ability to adapt and become dissatisfied or frustrated. If there is no assistance, this vicious cycle will spiral downward. Suicide is the manifestation of the lack of mutual adaptability with the environment.

China's social security system includes social insurance, social benefits, social assistance, and special care. It is a safety net which protects people's interests and promotes social stability and development.

The report to the 17th CPC National Congress states that a comprehensive social security system covering all the people will be built based on social insurance, social benefits, and social assistance; its focus will be on basic pension, basic healthcare, and minimum living subsidy. It will be supplemented by charities and commercial insurance. The basic pension insurance system of enterprises and public institutions will be reformed, and efforts will be made to explore the building of the rural pension insurance system. The basic health insurance schemes for urban

[38]Kang (2002a).

employees and for urban residents and the new rural cooperative medical insurance scheme will be promoted.[39]

The goal of the social security system is to reduce social inequality and maintain social justice. Justice is the value and nature of the social security system.

The former premier, Wen Jiabao says, "Social security is a safety net for the society and a safety valve for the economy. Globally, social security has a history of 120 years. It has gone through many rounds of economic depression and shown its functions of balancing income distribution, alleviating social conflicts, and promoting economic development and social stability. During an economic crisis, social security can calm fear, stimulate consumption, and promote economic recovery. It is a benchmark for a modern society and the duty of a modern government…But by and large, our social security system is far from ideal. Its main problems are: urban-rural imbalance with severe backwardness in the countryside, low coverage, fund pooling at a low level, and insufficient funds. These problems are more acute with disadvantaged groups such as farmers, migrant workers, farmers without land, the urban unemployed, and urban and rural people with disabilities. For all these, we need to accelerate the pace of reform. Our goal is to have a basic social security system with wide coverage by 2020 so that everyone has their basic needs in life covered. This is the overall plan and deployment in terms of social security development for the present and the next period. This goal is relevant to the future of the Chinese nation, beneficial to every citizen, and a blessing for future generations. It bears special significance in the great cause of building socialism with Chinese characteristics."[40]

The former premier Wen Jiabao said in an online interview, "Our society must march forward and develop. We must resolve the huge problem of people's livelihood and let them live peacefully, comfortably, and have enough confidence for the future."[41] This is the standard of happiness.

The report to the 19th National Congress of the CPC states, "We will improve the public service system, ensure people's basic quality of life, and keep up with people's ever-growing needs for a better life. We will continue to promote social fairness and justice, develop effective social governance, and maintain public order. With this we should see that our people will always have a strong sense of fulfillment, happiness, and security.

We will develop a sustainable multi-tiered social security system that covers the entire population in both urban and rural areas, with clearly defined rights and responsibilities, and support that hits the right level. We will work to see that everyone has access to social security. We will improve the basic pension schemes for urban employees and for rural and non-working urban residents, and quickly bring pension schemes under national unified management. We will improve the unified systems of basic medical insurance and serious disease insurance for rural

---

[39]Hu (2007).

[40]Wen (2010a).

[41]Premier Wen Jiabao's interviewed with www.gov.cn and Xinhuanet on February 27, 2011.

and non-working urban residents, and improve unemployment insurance and work-related injury insurance. We will establish a unified national platform for social security public services. We will promote the coordinated development of the social assistance systems for urban and rural residents, and improve the subsistence allowances system. We must adhere to the fundamental national policy of gender equality, and protect the legitimate rights and interests of women and minors. We will improve our systems for social assistance, social welfare, charity, and entitled groups7 benefits and services. We will improve the system for supporting and caring for children, women, and elderly people left behind in rural areas- We will develop programs for people with disabilities and work to provide better rehabilitation services for them. We will move faster to put in place a housing system that ensures supply through multiple sources, provides housing support through multiple channels, and encourages both housing purchase and renting. This will make us better placed to meet the housing needs of all of our people.

### 3.1.2 Educate People, Especially the Young and Teach Them to Respect Life

Suicide is a complicated issue of sociology and mental health. It has social, economic, and cultural factors and causes. But these are external factors, and the fuse to suicide is ultimately psychological in nature. For this reason, mental health is a very important topic in suicide prevention.

Mental health implies self-control, mental balance, self-respect, self-love, self-confidence, and self-knowledge. It connotes sound psychological behavior and processes and leads to social adaptability.

The youths lack life experience and analytical skills. When the imperfections of the world are revealed to them during social transformation, they may come up with extreme thoughts, confusion, and pessimism regarding life and existence. To prevent such psychological crises, we must build young people's adaptability with the environment. Good education can lead them to think about the purpose of life and their function in society and to affirm the value of life. Meanwhile, they must understand the reality of a diverse world. Some imperfections will not go away, and they have to take them as they are, cultivate a positive outlook, make adjustments, combine idealism and realism, and interact with the environment in a healthy way. All these things will shield them from the threat of suicide.

Various studies have shown that the youth are a high-risk group for mental health issues, with 50% of them having such problems. They are more prone to mental problems, and their suicide and crime rates are on the rise. Many social organizations have established mental health education or consultation committees; they include Chinese Psychological Society, Chinese Association for Mental Health, the Chinese Society of Education, and many institutions of higher learning. Chinese Association for Mental Health has organized more than ten conferences on mental health education and counseling for college students. Since 2004, the Ministry of Education has conducted pilot programs in some higher education institutions to take mental health surveys of new entrants and establish mental health records. The Communist Youth League, the Ministry of Education, and the All-China Students' Federation jointly launched a mental health education website (www.psyhealth.cn). The Ministry of Education published *Opinions on Strengthening Mental Health Education for Primary and Secondary School Students* in August 1999, *Implementation Outline for Mental Health Education in Higher Education Institutions (Trial)* in April 2002, *Implementation Outline for Mental Health Education in Vocational Schools* in July 2004, and *Implementation Outline for Mental Health Education in Higher Education Institutions* in July 2018. These documents specified the content, tasks, principles, and methods of mental health education, as well as relevant team building. Students' mental health finally received extensive attention from society.

There are courses dedicated to mental health in primary and secondary schools to help students learn more about their own psychology and gain skills to analyze problems, respond to frustrations, and express their emotions. In developed countries such as the USA and the UK, elementary school students are required to take classes on life skills and emergency response. In universities and colleges, student tutors, counselors, and Communist Youth League officials should be trained regularly on the psychological characteristics, mental health, and counseling of college students, so that they can teach students about mental health and adjustment skills. There should be mental health counseling centers in schools at all levels to do crisis intervention and help students deal with mental health issues. Mental health forums and programs should be created by the media to raise the overall mental health level of the young.

To be mentally healthy, one must fight the feeling of inferiority. Avoidant personality disorder (AVPD) is quite common among young people. Those who suffer from AVPD often find themselves easily influenced or controlled by exterior events. Through suppression, they have less and less psychological room for their feelings and emotions and their minds become hostage to external events. When there is no room for psychological life, people commit suicide as a protest for their existence. Young scholar Shi Yong says, "What makes us feel small in this world are the unfair rules of the game, the fake self, the uncertain future, the influence of others, violence, and the fear of death."[42] These things create a big psychological trap into which many young people fall. To avoid this trap, one must become mentally stronger and gain more insights into life. As long as we can gain more understanding of the world and experience it more deeply, we can overcome the uncertainties of life and become stronger. To be mentally strong is to be self-sufficient psychologically, to view all the external excitement with a calm mind, and "not to feel happy about external things or sad about oneself." This calmness comes with practice, and it can only come from the mind, if not from any religion. In short, one must find one's true self, attain psychological self-sufficiency, and refuse to march to the rhythm of the external world. This is what Zhang Zai

[42] Shi (2011).

(1022–1077), a sage of the Song Dynasty, means when he says, "I have found my Way and don't need anything else."[43]

Death education began in the USA in the late 1950s and early 1960s and became part of regular education. It developed later into life-and-death education. Developed nations of the West followed suit and offered life education in primary and secondary schools. By the end of the twentieth century, it was taught universally in schools. Life education spread to China in the 1990s, but it remained on the theoretical level. Few studies have been devoted to delivering life education in class.[44]

"Life education is life-centered education. Life means the life of the students and the general public."[45] The purpose of life education is to spread the scientific knowledge of life and death to the general public, and the goal is to make society understand the value of life.

After the big earthquake of 2008 in Wenchuan, Sichuan, the government made May 12 a day of national mourning with flags flying at half-mast. This act shows respect for life and serves as a good example of life education.

Many studies of recent years show that young suicides (successful and unsuccessful) often have erroneous ideas or no knowledge of death. Schools at all levels have avoided the topic of death for a long time. Parents, teachers, and society at large don't know how to broach the subject with the children. When death occurs, most people are reticent as if it is something ineffable. Most children have no idea about death. Educators don't know how to explain death to students, let alone suicidal death. When schools have to deal with tragic events such as an accidental death or suicide, they often ignore students' feelings and the mental trauma brought about by the event. The response to many crisis situations is silence. Schools do what they have to do hastily, without giving students an opportunity to express their sorrow. After a suicide of a student, most schools don't allow a memorial ceremony or gathering, don't offer condolences, and don't explain what has happened. They view the absence of emotion as a sign of strength and praise those who don't take time off for mourning as diligent students or dutiful teachers. In reality, this way of dealing with death is dangerous. For those directly involved, the reaction to the tragedy is shock, and without proper guidance, negative emotions will hide deep but won't disappear, forming a wound that has a scar on the top but inflammation underneath. These negative emotions will continue to consume the hosts' energy for life, hamper psychological healing, and wreak havoc on relationships. In more serious cases, they cause long-term emotional trauma. In a traditional society, people dealt with a tragedy with religious or customary rituals or ceremonies. But in a modern society, people have fast-paced lives and weak relationships. So they don't have time to talk about death and mourning or don't know how to. This lack of communication or interaction sows the seeds of mental illness without our

[43]Tang and Chen (2005).

[44]Wang (2007b).

[45]Zheng (2011, p. 131).

knowing. To suppress pain will only prolong it, in the form of future illness such as depression or other adverse symptoms.[46]

Orbach and Glaubum studied Israeli children between the ages of 10 and 12 and found that those with suicidal tendencies thought that the major cause of death was suicide, that they could be brought back to life, or that there was an afterlife. This shows that children with suicidal tendencies have incorrect views about death. Other scholars have found that some children want to change the way they were brought up through the act of suicide ("I want to come back again to win the love that my parents give to my brother"), to bring back the harmony once existed in their family ("I want to come back and start over"), to escape an impossible situation ("I might as well be dead"), or to view death as reversible ("I can still live after I die.")[47] There was a study of primary school children in Nanjing. When asked about death, 60.30% of the students picked "When people die, they don't come back;" 27.62% picked "When people disappear from this world, they go to another world;" 10.67% picked "Death is sleeping and dreaming;" and 10.87% picked "You can come back after death."[48] In reality, young people, especially children, got erroneous understanding of death from our social culture, such as the mythological or supernatural stories in television, cinema, on the Internet, or from video games and novels. These stories exert great influence on children and fill them with romantic and false notions about death. They would commit suicide for love or for their idols. We can see from all this that an important cause of suicide is the misunderstanding of death. As a result, we have to promote life education to teach young people the correct notions of death, thereby preventing suicide.

Life education is a basic tool for preventing youth suicide. Some scholars also proposed death education as a basic and paramount tool for preventing suicide. This shows how important death education is for suicide prevention.

The goal of life education for young people is threefold: First, it imparts some basic knowledge about death. Second, it strengthens young people's ability to face the issue of death. Third, it invites young people to search for life's meaning and cultivates the right values of life, including respect for life. In short, the ultimate goal of life education is to instill the right knowledge of and appreciation for life; and it encourages people to cherish life. To love life is to love living and to search for meaning and value in life. Life education helps students know their own lives better, respect other people's lives, ponder life's meaning, discover the value of existence, and treat every life with kindness.

In addition to promoting life education, we should perform crisis intervention through mental health clinics and suicide hotlines, targeting high-risk groups and other people plagued by thoughts of suicide, to subdue their suicidal impulses and treat potential suicides medically.

---

[46]Zheng and Lai (2003).

[47]Zhang (1997).

[48]Wan et al. (2005).

### 3.1.3 Strict Control Over Tools of Suicide

Once a person has the idea of committing suicide, he or she has to plan for the act. There is a process of preparation. As a result, many scholars suggest controlling the tools of suicide to hold them back.[49]

#### Strengthen Management of Poisonous Substance

There are many successful cases overseas. For instance, suicide rate in the UK rose between 1962 and 1971, but deaths from suicide dropped during the same period. A main cause is that British households began to use purified gas which made suicide difficult. In China, since the launch of the reform and opening-up policy and especially with the adoption of the household contract responsibility system in the countryside, pesticides were sold openly in stores and almost all households had a stash of them. This led to an increase in suicide by poison, especially among rural women. We should educate rural people about the safekeeping of pesticides and advocate for less poisonous pesticides and natural gas. It is gratifying to see that the government banned the production and sale of industrial-strength rat poison in 2003.

#### Restrict Access to Controlled Substances

We should better manage the dispensation of sedatives and antidepressant drugs. Drugstores and pharmacies should not sell this kind of drugs without prescription. Prescribed dosage and frequency should be regulated, especially concerning medications for depression and schizophrenia which may cause the sufferer to contemplate suicide. Before benzodiazepines, doctors prescribed large amounts of short- or medium-acting barbiturates which caused intentional overdose. When Australia restricted the dosage of sleeping pills, suicide rate lowered somewhat. In recent years, there have been more cases of suicide by the ingestion of antidepression drugs and benzodiazepines. The 15th World Suicide Prevention Conference held in Brussels in 1989 saw discussions on the harmful effects of amitriptyline and other tricyclic antidepressants.[50]

#### Restrict Access to Sites of Suicide

Potential suicides often pick scenic or dangerous sites for their intended act, such as rivers, bridges, tall buildings, railroads, lakes. We should strengthen management of

[49]Xiao (2008).

[50]Zhai (1997b, p. 307).

these sites, create safety support teams, and put in protective barriers. A special police team on the Yangtze River Bridge in Nanjing has stopped many suicide attempts. Chen Si volunteered to patrol the bridge on weekends and stopped more than a hundred cases of suicide in three years. He earned the moniker “Gatekeeper of Life” from grateful Nanjing residents. The patrol team of the Golden Gate Bridge of San Francisco has rescued many people over the years. Kevin Hines climbed over the protective barrier on September 16, 2000, and jumped the 250-feet distance into the Bay. He was one of the only 26 survivors. It takes four seconds to fall into the water, at a speed of 120 mph. Kevin changed the position of his body in those four seconds and saved his own life. He said afterward, “I wouldn’t have jumped if there were pesky obstacles.” Pat Hines, Kevin’s father, said, “To have a bridge without anti-suicide barrier is like throwing a loaded gun into the room of a psychotic patient.”[51] The management organization of the Golden Gate Bridge allotted USD2 million in 2005 for protective work and planned to spend USD2 million more to build a barrier area.[52] The Niagara Falls between the USA and Canada was a prime spot for suicide. Intricate protective measures implemented over the past thirty years have greatly reduced suicide cases. In China, scenic Mount Huang, Mount Emei, Mount Tai, and Mount Hua are all prime spots for suicide. There should be more patrolling in these areas to discourage people from taking their own lives. We have to think of ways to disrupt the deadly rhythm of these tourist attractions. Mr. Tao Xingzhi erected a wooden arch at Nanjing’s Swallow Promontory to remind people to value life. It has proven effective.[53]

Restrict Access to Ammunition and Explosives

Gun control can effectively reduce suicide and many countries, including China, have strict gun laws. If legal possessors of guns (soldiers, policemen) show signs of contemplating suicide, there should be measures to take their weapons away. Moreover, civilian-use explosives should be monitored and controlled.

### 3.1.4 Encourage More Study of Suicide and Create Prevention Systems

Researchers in suicide prevention should combine forces with experts in sociology, anthropology, psychology, public health, preventive medicine, and psychiatry. Some developed countries have established research centers for suicide prevention, such as the National Institute of Mental Health in the USA. China established the first medical organization for suicide prevention—Beijing Suicide Research and

[51]Chen (2006).
[52]McKinley (2006).
[53]Zhai (1997c).

Prevention Center at the Huilongguan Hospital—in December 2002. But other countries and regions only have limited resources for suicide prevention. They are limited in personnel and funds which are poorly coordinated. The challenges facing China are insufficient knowledge, attention, and ineffective response (see Chapter One). As suicide becomes more frequent, suicide data is often missing in relevant annals such as China Statistical Yearbook or census surveys. If there is data, it is often incomplete. One example is suicides of college students. To ignore this data is to imply that these suicides did not happen.[54] There has to be a dedicated suicide study organization to fulfill the important function of lowering suicide rates. We need a system of prevention like the one established in 2003 to combat SARS.

We need to create a community-based service organization to effectively prevent and manage suicide. This organization can be independent or affiliated with a mental health or public health organization.

As was discussed before, many countries and regions have established dedicated suicide prevention organizations such as suicide prevention centers, crisis intervention centers, disaster-relief centers, or "lifelines". They are connected to the police via phone or the Internet for crisis intervention. Some examples are the Samaritan Befrienders Hong Kong, and "Teacher Zhang" and "Lifeline" of Taiwan. Even though there isn't sufficient evidence showing that these organizations have lowered suicide rates, they are certainly needed for giving timely support for people in crisis. There are similar organizations in large Chinese cities such as Beijing, Nanjing, Shanghai, Tianjin, Guangzhou, Changsha, Chongqing, and Hefei. It is highly significant to build such organizations and form networks for suicide prevention.

From the situation of the suicide research and prevention centers in big cities, we can hardly see what the future national strategy for suicide prevention is. The UN has drawn up a suicide prevention plan on the national level which gives detailed instructions on creating a public support model. These instructions have to do with creating an advocate organization (governmental or nongovernmental) for community action which uses forums and the media to involve the general public, enlists government support, drafts national strategy for suicide prevention, and coordinates between government and social resources.[55] We may glimpse the future of suicide prevention through the UN plan.

### 3.1.5 Adopt Mental Health Legislation

It is indisputable that relevant laws and regulations can help lower suicide rates. We will discuss the necessity of a mental health law below.

[54]Shi (2001).

[55]United Nations Program for Policy Coordination and Sustainable Development (2012).

As was discussed in Chapter Five, mental illness and suicide are closely linked. Mental health issues are a big challenge to public health and constitute a serious social problem.

Mental illness has the biggest share of government expenditure for illnesses, around 20%. According to WHO data, 5% of the Chinese population have psychological impediments, 13% have mental illness, and 80% of mental patients do not get proper care. A third of mental patients are aggressive, putting the safety of those around them in jeopardy. Only 2% of mental illness sufferers receive psychological counseling, and the figure is even less for those who have suicidal tendencies. China lags behind other countries in mental health legislation. Among the 160 member states of WHO, 75% have mental health law and half of them enacted such laws in the past ten years. Basically, all European nations have mental health law; such laws cover 87% of the population of the Americas, 95% of the population in Southeast Asia, and 59% in Africa and the Middle East. As of 2010, China, Laos, and Cambodia were the only countries in the Western Pacific region that did not have mental health law. China was the only major country without mental health law.[56]

What is cause for celebration is that on October 26, 2012, the Standing Committee of the 11th National People's Congress adopted the first Mental Health Law, to be implemented on May 1, 2013. This legislation took 27 years to pass.

China finally has a mental health law! The purpose of this law is to prevent and treat mental illness, promote mental health, protect mental illness sufferers' rights, ameliorate the mental health system, and maintain social stability.

The ultimate goal of the Mental Health Law is to benefit all Chinese people, including the disadvantaged groups.

How a society views its mental patients shows how civilized it is. Mental illness sufferers constitute a disadvantaged group because they are unable to fight for their rights. Should aggressive mental patients be treated as criminals? How should we view them? Do the family members or the society have any responsibility? How should the government help them? There were no precise answers to these questions before May 1, 2013. Mental health work was randomly and haphazardly done. It takes the government's involvement to protect the legal rights of the sufferers as well as the people who treat them.

Should the mental health law encompass all psychological impediments? There are three views from abroad. First, the mental health law in some twenty countries, such as the UK, India, and Pakistan, encompasses all psychological impediments. The law of the State of Indiana in the USA includes mental retardation, epilepsy, alcohol poisoning, nicotine, and narcotic dependency in the definition of mental illness. Second, in about ten countries such as Egypt, Japan, and Brazil, mental illness is defined as including mental retardation but not alcohol poisoning or narcotic dependency which is dealt with in other laws. Third, in a small number of

[56]Li and Bao (2007).

countries such as Denmark and Norway, separate laws exist for various mental illnesses.[57]

There is similarity in the different mental health laws around the world. In terms of public policy, these laws set the minimum standards for mental health resources, policy, and goals. In terms of administration, the laws create administrative organizations to plan and implement public policies concerning mental health. In terms of budget, the laws set fiscal policies and provide financial support for implementing public health plans. In terms of implementation, the laws provide the details of implementation, accountability, and evaluation. In terms of research and training, the laws provide plans for education and training for basic, clinical, and application research. In terms of service, the laws mandate service without prejudice. In terms of protecting members of society, the laws protect the rights, benefits, property, and integrity of mental illness sufferers and their families. In terms of medical treatment, the laws ensure the supply and quality of services in the realm of mental health and set policies for treatment. In terms of authority, to the extent permissible by law, the laws use administrative regulations, directives, and other orders to improve the current state of mental health.[58]

China created a law drafting team in 1985 to draft a mental health law. After twenty years of research and revisions, a Mental Health Law (Draft) seemed ready in September 2005, but it underwent further revisions until May 2009, when it was declared finished. It was approved by the State Council and the legislature in September 2011 but failed to be adopted a month later by the Standing Committee of the 11th National People's Congress.[59] The Mental Health Law was finally adopted on October 26, 2012. It has seven chapters and eighty-five articles detailing the principles of mental health work, the ways to manage and promote mental health and prevent mental illness, the diagnosis and treatment of mental illness, and the protection of mental patients' and mental health workers' legal rights.

Once the national Mental Health Law was adopted, local regulations were put in place quickly in cities such as Beijing, Shanghai, Hangzhou, Wuhan, Ningbo, and Wuxi. The treatment of mental illness became mandatory in Shanghai, Tianjin, Wuhan, Shijiazhuang, and Heilongjiang.[60]

There is more legislative work to be done in the area of restricting the production and sale of highly poisonous pesticides and managing controlled substances.

### 3.1.6 Training

In March 2000, a symposium on suicide prevention was organized jointly by Beijing Suicide Research and Prevention Center and the WHO. The two

[57] Li (2004).
[58] Cheng and Wang (1999).
[59] Wang (2011).
[60] Guan (2011).

organizations had agreed to collaborate on a long-term project about mental health, and this symposium was part of this collaboration. Attendees included Dr. Bertolote of WHO, Dr. Olsson of Sweden's National Suicide Prevention Center, and forty Chinese representatives from organizations such as the Ministry of Health, Beijing Municipal Health Bureau, Chinese Academy of Preventive Medicine, All-China Women's Federation, UNDP Small Grants Program, Institute for the Control of Agrochemicals under the Ministry of Agriculture, China Health Education Research Institute, and China Agricultural University. The goal of the symposium was "to provide public education, train healthcare personnel, and improve crisis support and suicide prevention in urban areas."[61]

Many studies show that persons attempting suicide often seek help first from healthcare organizations or hospitals. This is true for many developing countries. But healthcare personnel in China often lack the knowledge of suicide and mental illnesses such as depression and schizophrenia which can cause suicide. They are not ready for crisis intervention or psychological counseling. They prescribe physical, not mental, treatment for failed suicides, look down on the latter, and often cause even more suicide attempts. Many farmers commit suicide using organophosphorus pesticides, but healthcare personnel often have no knowledge of these deadly substances.[62] The Ministry of Health should take the lead in mandating proper training for healthcare personnel of various areas to respond to suicides and suicide attempts.

Moreover, there should be professionally trained mental health personnel in schools, including dedicated and supporting personnel who together form a stable team that cover all relevant specialties. Psychological counseling is underdeveloped in China. Many people who do counseling are not professionally trained, and they lack the knowledge and skills for crisis intervention. Some counselors are not even trained in psychology or psychiatry and lack understanding of why people commit suicide. It is therefore urgent that we give proper training to mental health workers at all levels if we are to do a better job in suicide prevention.

Concrete efforts must also be made to train school personnel related to suicide prevention in relevant knowledge and skills so that they can identify signs of depression and other mental illness, signs of self-harm or suicide, know how to evaluate a crisis and intervene properly. In 2003, the Professional Skill Assessment Center established some training centers for psychological counselors in some cities. They accept applications from people with degrees or work experience in psychology, education, and medicine. Upon finishing the training courses, the students receive Professional Qualification Certificates issued by the Department of Labor and Social Security. These certificates have three categories: psychological consultant, psychological counselor, and senior psychological counselor.

---

[61]From the report of the symposium on suicide prevention organized by the Ministry of Health/WHO, March 22–24, 2000. *Chinese Mental Health Journal*, no. 5.

[62]Xiao (2012a).

### 3.1.7 Check Media Reports to Avoid the Werther Effect

Rapid advances in information technology fuel the development of mass media. Sensational reports of suicides can easily be found on the Internet. These reports are numerous and detailed with pictures and videos to satisfy the curiosity of the general public. Reports of suicide attempts by celebrities (movie stars, politicians, teen idols) are often serialized and romanticized, inviting copycat reactions from potential suicides, especially among the younger generation. These are known, as was mentioned earlier in this book, as the Werther effect. In extreme cases, there are websites which teach people how to commit suicide successfully, and some may even offer help or broadcast the deadly act live.

There should be regulations to ensure that the media does not sensationalize suicide, much like those regulating pornography.

The media have the responsibility to respect life and do their share in suicide prevention.

Moreover, publications such as *Complete Suicide Manual* should be banned.

### 3.1.8 Suicide Prevention Targeted at High-Risk Groups

People with Mental Illness

People with mental illness are a high-risk group for suicide and the prime target for suicide prevention. Schizophrenia sufferers often don't reveal their suicidal intentions, need no stressful event to prompt their act, and show very strong determination to kill themselves. They are often driven to suicide by symptoms such as imperative auditory hallucination, persecutory delusion, or delusion of guilt. Some may also commit suicide due to depression or a negative event which people normally view as not serious.

Timely diagnosis of and proper treatment for mental illness can prevent suicide. B. Barraclough found a study of 100 successful suicide cases that 64% of the suicides suffer from depression, and the suicide rate among depression patients drops to 21% when they are treated with lithium carbonate. Prescott and Highly found that 67% of unsuccessful suicides had taken wrong medication, 65% of depression sufferers take benzodiazepines while only 32% take antidepressants. Unfortunately, negligence or ignorance on the part of family members can make medications prescribed for the patients the ones they take to commit suicide. To effectively prevent suicide among mental illness sufferers, proper medication must be used at the proper dosage and for full treatment courses. Apart from medications, psychological treatment and family and social intervention have to be strengthened in order to maintain long-term stability and relief for mental illness sufferers.[63] In

[63]Zhai (1997b).

England and Wales, the increased use of proper medications to combat mental illness in the 1980s has effectively lowered the number of suicides by drugs.[64]

All mental illness sufferers, whether they receive in-patient or out-patient care, should be evaluated for suicidal tendencies. Those with strong suicidal tendencies, especially when they are afflicted with serious depression, should be persuaded (or, when necessary and to the extent permissible by law, made) to seek in-patient care. Since there is strong prejudice against mental illness sufferers in China, families are reluctant to seek the help of doctors, even when the sufferers have attempted suicide. It is therefore important that medical personnel have ample interaction with the families to ensure patients get treatment they need. The suicide rate among college students is high in China, but the students usually would rather die than disclose their mental conditions. To the extent permissible by law, students with aggressive or suicidal tendencies should receive mandatory treatment. Apart from regular treatment, in-patient treatment for mental illness has safety requirements including the removal of potential suicide tools in the ward, restricting the use of controlled substances, assessment of suicide tendencies, management of visits or holidays (many suicides happen when the patients are on holiday). When the in-patient period ends, a suicide prevention plan has to be drawn up for the patient, including a schedule for follow-up visits, and support from family members must be secured. Outside China, the suicide rate among mental patients in communities is rising, so scholars suggest moving the focus of suicide prevention to communities.[65]

### Children from Single-Parent or Broken Families

Single-parent families result from divorce, death of a parent, abandonment, separation, or other reasons while broken families are those in which one or both parents are deceased or absent for at least six months. Broken families can also be caused by divorce, separation, or long-term conflict between the parents. Children living in such households lack maternal or paternal love and the communal feeling of being in a family. This lack gradually alters the children's psychology and may result in a feeling of inferiority, loneliness, rebelliousness, and violence. Some of them develop bad habits or mental impediments which may lead to antisocial behavior. Some studies show that children from single-parent or broken families are more prone to suicide attempts.

We should create some intervention mechanisms targeted at children with negative factors in their family backgrounds. Developed countries such as the USA have good experience in this regard. There should be mechanism to warn parents of the risks their children are exposed to when a people's court or any other authority works on divorce cases. District or sub-district offices or relevant social

---

[64]Xiao (2008).

[65]Ibid.

organization should communicate the above-mentioned risks to guardians of children. Schools and community organizations should work to protect children from single-parent or broken families from unnecessary social pressure. Other organizations such as school authorities and the Communist Youth League should also do their bit.

### Young Students

Young students are in the process of mental development, but they already face tremendous academic pressure from college entrance examinations, English aptitude tests, postgraduate entrance examination, and job hunting. Some of them, especially college students, face economic pressure as well, and this is a cause of the rising suicide rate among students, which has become a social problem. College students prefer to jump to their deaths, and the success rate is high, dealing a mind-shattering blow to the other students. That school buildings are getting higher is a red flag that something has to be done about the risks they engender. A survey should be conducted among new entrants to identify those with potential psychological impediments. Studies have shown that the prime reason for suicides among college students is the accumulated stress which is part of the growing-up process.[66] Stress can come from many sources such as the family, school, society, and cultural background. For example, high parental expectations create inordinate mental pressure, competition engenders anxiety and stress, unmet goals result in the feeling of inferiority and loss, poor grades promote anger and regret, economic difficulties beget worries and fear, and relationship issues generate loneliness and depression. If they are behind in learning, disciplined for incorrect behavior, or forced to quit school due to illness, the students become anxious, afraid, and depressed. Temporary failures and frustrations in love may provoke mental disorder and alienated sexual behavior. All these factors cause strong emotional pain which may lead to suicide attempts. Suicide caused by stress can be sudden, and there has to be effective crisis intervention.[67]

The Outline of the Mid- and Long-term National Educational Reform Program (2010–2020) states, "We should take students as the key player, make teachers the leader, give full play to the initiative of the students, and make the students' healthy growth the priority and ultimate purpose of education. We should care for every student, allow them the freedom to realize their potentials. We should respect the pattern of students' physical and mental development, and provide suitable education for everyone". "We should take health as the top priority, ensure sufficient time for physical education and extracurricular activities, provide higher-quality physical education, improve mental health education to build their mental health, physical strength, and will power. We should strengthen aesthetics education to

[66]Wang (1990).

[67]Ji (1999).

cultivate good aesthetic and cultural tastes."[68] The purpose of education is to promote all-round development of students and not to prime them for exams. We should reduce their workload and enrich their lives. We should devise activities appropriate for their age and development. The closed education of the past should be abandoned. All the academic methodologies should conform to the principles of education. Teachers need to be knowledgeable of mental health and create a learning environment in which the students are not at risk for suicide. Mental health has to be part of the curriculum, and they should be taught the skills to adjust their emotional state, relax, relieve stress, and anxiety and establish relationships of trust with others. They should be taught to love and value life and refuse the temptation to end it.

There should be mental health education in higher education institutions in which psychological counseling is available to those in need. Psychological counseling uses theories and methodologies of psychology to help students know and accept themselves and realize their potential.

In 2005, the Education Work Committee of the CPC Beijing Municipal Committee and the Municipal Education Commission published "Teaching Syllabus of Mental Health Education in Higher Education Institutions in Beijing", "Outline for Psychological Counseling for Higher Education Institutions in Beijing", and "Outline for Crisis Intervention for Higher Education Institutions in Beijing". These signify the first step in building a mental health educational system in institutions of higher learning in Beijing. This work is systematic, scientific, and standardizing.[69] It seeks to resolve the students' psychological confusion and facilitate their long-term development. The documents mandate that psychological counseling be done by properly trained professionals and specify the attendant requirements. They also propose five innovative systems of detection, monitoring, intervention, referral, and post-care in terms of suicide prevention. The Ministry of Education praised these documents as worthy of being promoted on the national level.[70] The guidelines have been implemented in Beijing for years and obtained good results.

### Disadvantaged Groups in Urban and Rural Areas

In the government work report to the 5th session of the 9th National People's Congress in 2002, then premier Zhu Rongji used the term "disadvantaged groups" for the first time. The disadvantaged groups are groups of people who find themselves at the lowest rung of the social ladder and on the margins of economic and political life. They can be disadvantaged in physical or social sense. The former is due to physical factors such as age or illness while the latter is due to social factors

[68]http://news.xinhuanet.com/2010-07/29/c_12389254.htm. Accessed: 29 July 2010.
[69]Cai (2005).
[70]Huang (2005).

such as unemployment or discrimination. In China, disadvantaged groups are formed mainly due to social reasons. They are weak in their ability to create wealth, uncompetitive in what they do, poor, unemployed, old, with disabilities, or victims of disasters. Since the reform and opening-up, fast growth has resulted in a wide income gap and the Gini coefficient is close to 0.5, far from the alarm level of 0.4. This means that there is huge income disparity between urban and rural areas, between eastern and western China, between the rich and the poor, and between those who have benefitted from the rapid growth and those who have not.

It is very important that we create a social security system which is consistent with the level of China's social development. The government has to find solutions to the social issues which matter the most to the Chinese people: education, employment, income distribution, social security, health care, and social management. The government must create a social security system which benefits the entire society and strive to realize the goals proposed at the 17th, the 18th, and the 19th CPC National Congress: There should be teachers in schools, paychecks for laborers, hospitals for the sick, retirement for the old, and housing for all.

We will develop a sustainable multi-tiered social security system that covers the entire population in both urban and rural areas, with clearly defined rights and responsibilities, and support that hits the right level; and make sure that more fruits of development are shared by all the people in a fair way.

## *3.2 Secondary Prevention: Help People in Distress*

Secondary prevention provides to people who are experiencing a psychological crisis, with strong suicidal ideation, and are the edge to attempting suicide early intervention, viable help, special care, medical treatment, and the removal of harmful environmental influence. Crisis intervention is an effective way of preventing suicide. It is closely related to suicide prevention but differs from it in concept. Studies have shown that if intervention is absent when a crisis happens, 12% of the crises will lead to suicide.[71]

### 3.2.1 Crisis Assessment

A crisis situation can manifest in a person's emotions (anxiety, stress, loss, fear, anger, shame), mindset (attention focused on sadness, extreme pain, confusion, inability to make decisions, fear of going crazy), behavior (inability to finish work, inability to act normally, isolation, broken relationships, refusal of help from others, action inconsistent with feeling, atypical behavior), and bodily discomfort (insomnia, dizziness, lack of appetite, digestive problems).

[71]Zhai (1997d).

Emotional disturbances may or may not result in a crisis. As a result, an assessment is always necessary. An untrained personnel often gives help without an assessment, and the result can be harmful to the sufferer. The goal of crisis assessment and intervention is to prevent suicide or the onset of mental illness. Crisis assessment is not rocket science, but it needs the cooperation between the frontline person (relatives, friends, doctors, volunteers), and the trained personnel (psychologists, psychiatrists, mental health workers). Crisis assessment has to be accurate and timely, and the key is to clarify the nature and possible consequences of the problem. Understanding the possible factors of the crisis can improve the precision and timeliness of the assessment.

Crisis assessment has to complete two tasks: First, determine whether there is danger to life; i.e., see whether suicide, physical assault, or killing is imminent. Second, determine whether the person is cognizant of the social environment and his or her normal social role. The first involves personal, familial, and social characteristics and has to be completed by a trained personnel. The second is more general and may include the following parts: Determine the source of crisis, which may be a dangerous event, temporary confusion, or sociocultural factors; track crisis development, determining whether the person in question is at the beginning of a crisis or in the emergency stage; identify crisis manifestation, which may involve the person's emotions, mindset, and behavior; find out whether a life event is perceived as a threat, loss, or challenge; and determine what the resources and the sociocultural environment involved are.[72]

We have to determine the person's emotional state, coping ability, the personal crisis encountered, and mobility to understand the past and present situation, the seriousness of the crisis (the person's subjective opinion and the worker's objective judgment), and the degree of danger (to the person or others), in order to formulate an action plan and ascertain viable resources for crisis response and support. A person in crisis has internal resources (personal, psychological) and external resources (environmental, such as friend or family). The internal resources may include reason and the tolerance for pain. If these resources are missing, the danger increases and external help and support become necessary.

### 3.2.2 Timely Crisis Intervention

Crisis intervention forms a part of psychotherapy in the broader sense. Generally speaking, it uses a simple method of psychotherapy to help a person manage a pressing problem, regain psychological balance, and overcome a crisis. The target of crisis intervention is not necessarily the sufferer in the traditional sense, although this is the case in many instances. The minimum goal of crisis intervention is to protect the party or parties involved and to prevent accidents (such as suicide), so it needs the support of the society.

---

[72]Ibid, 102.

The sufferer is emotionally unstable and feels weak and helpless at the beginning of a crisis. After a while, he or she becomes hesitant and amenable to outside influence. This is the reason why timely intervention can be effective once a crisis starts.

Crisis intervention is a psychological counseling and psychotherapeutic technique which mobilizes the sufferer's potentials to regain mental balance he or she possessed before the crisis; it has become the mainstay of clinical counseling. If a person in crisis can get appropriate and effective therapeutic intervention, the crisis can be prevented from developing, and the person can learn some new coping skills and reestablish mental balance, sometimes to a level higher than the pre-crisis one. We may therefore say that a crisis is both a turning point and an opportunity. It teaches the person that suicide does not solve any problem. Most suicide attempts happen because a predicament in life cannot be resolved, but once a solution can be found, the suicide will be averted.

Crisis intervention is temporary care and support given to a person in crisis or imminent danger (such as suicide) so that he or she may regain mental balance. It is a method of psychotherapy developed from brief psychotherapy. Its goal is to find a solution to a problem and does not involve personality correction or shaping. It is also called listening therapy because the therapist has to listen to the sufferer.[73] The method of intervention includes the telephone, the Internet (message and video), face-to-face assistance, letter counseling, and familial and social intervention.

The intervener has to prepare contingency plans for various possibilities during the intervention. For instance, he may have to decide on the spot that the sufferer needs to go to a hospital for medical treatment. If the sufferer feels that he or she has gained nothing from psychological counseling, the frustration may fuel her depression.

### 3.2.3 Creating a Social Support Network for the People in Distress

Through suicide prevention education, we can promote healthy interaction between people and their environment and cultivate a positive attitude when facing stress and frustration. To create a social support network, we need the cooperation of schools, employers, communities, sub-district committees, and villagers' committees. In its totality, suicide prevention may include pre-crisis education, guidance for the sufferer, and post-crisis guidance.[74]

We are all born with a social background and grow up within the safety net of interpersonal relationships. When experiencing a stressful life event, we need help from people around us (friends, teachers, schoolmates, relatives, coworkers, communities) to navigate the crisis. Studies have shown that this social support network is of invaluable help to people in distress. It is important for socialization and crisis

---

[73] Ibid., 10.

[74] US Department of Health and Human Services (1992).

intervention, even when the distress has reached the point of suicide attempt. The social support network is often in crisis along with the sufferer, making familial and social intervention necessary. Sometimes a crisis comes from the family, such as when a family member is prone to violence or has mental illness or previous suicide attempts. This kind of family lacks harmony and cohesion. Whether the social support network is in crisis or not, it is the most natural, direct, and effective support the sufferer can have.

The individual, family, and society form an organic and reciprocal whole. When this whole has problems which evolve into a crisis, the best solution may be to restore each part's natural function, and familial and social intervention can help mitigate the crisis. We can use education to raise awareness regarding the nature of suicide prevention, the importance of mental health, and the mental stress caused by poverty, unemployment, divorce, and death of a loved one. Helping the sufferer rebuild social support network and restore the intimacy and harmony of interpersonal relationships goes a long way in defusing the crisis for the sufferer. This can be done by reducing the sufferer's isolation, developing satisfactory relationships with other people, restoring healthy relationships with family members, and alleviating anxiety caused by a sudden negative event such as robbery, kidnapping, or a natural disaster.

### 3.2.4 Timely Closing the Exit

We have discussed this topic in the primary prevention section. Closing the exit means restricting the access to tools of suicide.[75] This includes gun control, restricted use of explosives, detoxification of gas and car exhaust, poison control (for rat poison, pesticides, psychotropics, and toxic chemicals), and safety mechanisms in buildings, bridges, railroad tracks, highway buffer belts, wharfs, and high voltage sites. Any obstacle or intervention from anyone that happens to be around can prevent suicide sometimes. This is especially true for impulsive suicide attempts. There is some debate over whether closing the exit should be considered primary prevention. Jose Bertolote of the WHO and British psychiatrist M. Gelder think so, whereas American psychiatrist David Lester thinks it should be considered secondary prevention. M. Gelder feels that primary prevention is difficult but can be done in three ways: reduced access to suicide tools, encouraging aid to people with emotional problems, and improved education on mental health.

[75]Zhai (1997e).

## 3.3 Tertiary Prevention: Prevent Repeated Attempts

Repeats in suicide attempt are quite common. The goal of tertiary prevention is to give sympathetic support to those who have attempted suicide in the hope that they won't try it again. We have to distinguish between failed suicides attempt and self-harm. People who have attempted suicides are more likely to try again. Studies have shown that more attempts are often made within one or two years of the previous one.[76]

There are studies which show that the risk factor of failed suicides to die from suicide is 1%, 100 times that of normal people. About 3–10% of those who have tried to take poison will eventually die from suicide. Risk factors for repeated attempts are multiple, so the prevention models have to be multiple as well.[77] Eddleston and Phillips believe that instances of self-harm in the countryside will be reduced if we can lower the instances of mental illness and increase the sufferers' coping ability and social support.[78] Past history of suicide is an important risk factor of suicide. Western studies have shown that mental illness is a leading cause of suicide; about 90% of failed suicides have been diagnosed as having mental problems.[79]

In 2003, the WHO implemented a failed suicide intervention project in 14 countries; the goal was to systematically investigate the risk factors which influence suicide and to evaluate the effectiveness of suicide intervention by simple contact methods such as telephone or face-to-face counseling. The findings for five countries of different cultural backgrounds and development levels show that intervention lowered the suicide death rate during the 18 months after the suicide attempt but did not lower the rate of suicide attempts.[80]

### 3.3.1 Post-crisis Intervention

It is not easy to prevent repeated intentional self-harm after attempted suicide. Depending on the purpose of a suicide (e.g., to protest, to win sympathy, to cause shock, to gain advantage, or just to end life), guidance or therapy should be provided as a way for the victims to properly express their feelings or needs, so as to prevent the risk of them taking their own lives. In addition, counseling and psychological treatments are important to the improvement in their mental health. When patients with personality disorders (such as borderline personality disorder) show signs of struggling in coping with challenges or hardships, crisis intervention should be promptly employed to boost their ability to restore psychological balance.

[76]Tejedor et al. (1999).

[77]Li and Qin (2008).

[78]Eddleston and Philips (2004).

[79]Mann (2002).

[80]Xu et al. (2012).

Post-crisis intervention is targeted at two groups of people: the failed suicides and the people close to them who are at high risk of suicide attempts. The fact that these two groups of people are at higher risk of suicide is often ignored. For the failed suicides, the goal of post-crisis intervention is to prevent the crisis from happening again. For those who are close to the failed suicides, the goal of post-crisis intervention is to prevent possible copycat reaction and to help heal their psychological wound. This intervention involves timely treatment and active and long-term follow-up, so it can be called "consolidation therapy." For the failed suicides, there are physical and psychological wounds to be healed; the key is to understand their motives for suicide, evaluate their risk of repeated attempts, and show them that the society cares about them. The interveners, friends, and relatives have to be more attentive, protective, calm, and non-judgmental. For the people close to the failed suicides, social resources such as the community, hospital, and school should combine forces to give them psychological counseling and sympathetic support so that they may regain their sense of psychological balance.[81]

Most crises can be resolved through intervention in a matter of days or weeks. The sufferers should be weaned off social support in a timely way lest they become dependent on it; they should be encouraged to resolve future problems using the skills they have gained through the social support system and reduce the likelihood of the crisis happening again. At the same time, there should be follow-up visits to provide aid and support as needed.

### 3.3.2 Treatment

For the failed suicides, we can minimize their chances of repeated attempts by treating the accompanying mental illnesses such as depression and schizophrenia. Failed suicides are often afflicted with personality disorders, neuroses, and sexual deviation; we can give them medical treatment, psychological counseling, and attentive monitoring. We should create a model of psychological intervention for the failed suicides. If they don't live in the big cities, it is unlikely that they would receive the kind of treatment they need. It is more realistic to mandate period visits by social workers, psychological counselors, or doctors to provide psychological service and evaluate risk factors for repeated attempts.

### 3.3.3 Evaluate Repeated Attempts' Factors

It is very important to evaluate failed suicides' environment; an adverse environment can be conducive to repeated attempts. An evaluation may reveal the sources of stress, the micro-level negative factors (family and other interpersonal relationships), and the macro-level negative factors (social and cultural transformation). We

[81]Yao (2005, p. 75).

have to conduct more research in criminal psychology and deviant behavior, because if people cannot satisfy their needs through normal channels, they may resort to anomic or egoistic suicides as described by Durkheim or other unreasonable social behavior. We have to look at failed suicides from a larger context and help them socialize more satisfactorily, such as ensuring that young people have education, job training, and employment opportunities. This will surely help prevent suicide and create better models for thoughts, emotions, and behavior. Moreover, research can raise the effectiveness and pertinence of suicide prevention.

Durkheim writes at the end of his book *Suicide*, "A study of suicide involves more than the specific issues it discusses."[82] The reason he gives is that the abnormal development of suicide is intimately related to the prevalent ills of the contemporary society; both share the same causes. As a result, to prevent suicide means to eliminate social ills. But he also believes that "there is no reason to artificially recreate a superficial social phenomenon that is already in the past or to create a wholly new and historically unseen social phenomenon. What we need to do is to find seeds for a new life from past phenomena and help them germinate, grow, and bear fruit."[83] Durkheim believes that suicide will not cause the collective death of a society and that prevention only involves a few simple reforms in the existing society. He believes that prevention lies in the soil of the society; we will grow and blossom if we can find sustenance in the soil that is our social environment. But Freud's psychoanalysis tells us that the society is also our biggest problem because it creates a fake self within us and forces us to play by unfair rules; we seek psychological balance in vain and the resulting suppression, anxiety, and neuroses distort our personality. If Durkheim wants to prevent suicide by creating the new from the old in the society, then Freud wants to do the same thing in the psyche. We have tried to describe in this book what this means.

We have to emphasize again here: Suicide prevention in China comes back to the healthy relationship between the individual and the society. A healthy society is composed of healthy individuals, and conversely, healthy individuals live by default in a healthy society. But to build a healthy society, we need a government which knows what to do and what not to do. When put in this organic context consisting of the individual, the society, and the government, we see the long and tortuous road of suicide prevention in front of us.

---

[82]Durkheim (1996c, p. 372).

[83]Ibid.

# 4 From Isolated Suicide Prevention to Integrated Suicide Prevention

Effective suicide prevention not only helps with the reduction of individual tragedies and alleviation of public health problems, but serves as an approach to defuse social tensions in a time of social transformation. Despite the fact that there has been a fall in China's suicide rate, China is still at a preliminary stage to curb suicides by using isolated suicide prevention and control model. It is hoped that an "integrated suicide prevention and control model" with Chinese characteristics that involves diverse social participants would be established in the future.

## *4.1 A Suicide Prevention Method to Cope with Social Tensions*

Suicide prevention, in a nutshell, deals with the prevention and control of suicides.

Cases from real life warn that we should attach a great importance to managing potential secondary risks derived from suicidal actions. Effective suicide prevention is able to decrease these tragedies, and it is also essential to prevent and mitigate our social tensions over the course of China's social transformation. The 19th CPC National Congress pointed out that it is paramount to improve mechanisms preventing and defusing social tensions, to improve the system of public psychological services and cultivate self-esteem, self-confidence, rationality, composure, and optimism among our people, so as to promote the construction of a harmonious socialist society. With that being said, we can see that suicide prevention is crucial to the goal of building a mechanism for preventing and defusing social tensions, as well as enhancing public psychological services.

## *4.2 The Current "Isolated Suicide Prevention"*

The 2005 World Suicide Prevention Day was themed "Prevention of Suicide is Everybody's Business", and the theme of 2017 was "Take a minute, Change a Life". We notice that both themes focus on individuals. Life is precious, one suicide is too many, and it is everyone's business to prevent suicide. However, what we can do is still far from what we hope for.

Earlier in November 2003, Beijing Suicide Research and Prevention Center and several other organizations held a seminar themed "China National Suicide Prevention Initiative", where it gathered experts from both China and other countries. The seminar proposed the "National Suicide Prevention Initiative", which is also the biggest achievement of the seminar. The initiative made the following appeals: 1) to improve the overall mental health of the society; 2) to enhance the connections among people; 3) to train the children, teenagers, as well as their custodians and school faculty, with necessary skills in dealing with emergencies; 4) to control the media broadcasting and movies related to suicides and mental diseases. Given that drinking pesticides is the main way to commit a suicide in rural areas, it is suggested that the Ministry of Agriculture take the lead in the legislation of controlling the production, selling and use of such substances, and make it a national-level approach upon the matter. In fact, the initiative turned out to be solely a folk plan, the real "National Suicide Prevention Initiative" is yet to be born.

Yet, statistics from *China Health Statistics Yearbook* released by China's Ministry of Health show that over the course from 2003-2018 suicide rate among different ages sharply declined in both urban areas and rural areas. It is an achievement made by the joint effort from the government, citizens, scholars, relevant departments (include volunteers), who have taken pains to study the matter. Xiao Shuiyuan noted that, "There are many factors contributing to the dip in suicides, to wit, China's economic growth, improvement in mental health services, governments' preventative mesures, and the rising educational level."[84]

But that various non-mainstream sources of statistics and media's myriads of reports on the matter of suicide prevail is also warning us that China needs to do more. Many problems begin to emerge as China is deepening its economic and social transformation. As China is inevitably coming to an aging era, there is an urgent need to dive into the research and practice on the current suicidal situation of the old and causes of suicide, as well as suicide prevention. The fact that China tops the number of suicides across the globe is grieving the country.

There has not been a unified effort when it comes to suicide prevention, and suicide prevention practices are only seen in a few psychological counseling centers, institutions and hospitals organized by volunteers. "National Efforts" have not yet been able to involve in suicide prevention on an overall sense, not to mention leading it.

## 4.3 From Isolated Suicide Prevention to Integrated Suicide Prevention

Earlier on September 10th, 2008, the WHO put forward that suicide prevention should embark on global thinking, nationwide planning and reginal action, which focuses on a close collaboration among different departments and organizations as well as a need of specific yet different prevention measures. It is in accordance with the strategic thinking raised in the 19th CPC National Congress Report—"to integrate multiple channels and involve everyone to manage the country's public affairs, establishing a social governance model based on collaboration,

[84]Zhang Le. Stunning Decrease in China's Suicide Rates [EB/OL]. Xinhua Net. http://news.xinhuanet.com/society/2011-05/14/c_121416339.htm. 2015-5-10.

How the integrated suicide prevention system works

| Development of a suicide | Specific suicide prevention |
|---|---|
| Factors causing depressions | Improvement in educational, employment, social welfare and housing policy; addressing issues concerning child abuse, child nursing and caring; media guidance on avoiding drug abuse; public education; facilitating school mental health (coping strategies, social support, anti-bullying); facilitating mental health at work; controlling excessive alcohol drinking, combating illicit drugs; proper treatment for those with physical diseases and the disabled. |
| Depressive disorders and others | Close attention to suicidal groups; prompt evaluation; diagnosis, treatment and effective training |
| Suicidal inclination | A good preliminary risk management; include safety into daily assessment |
| Suicidal plans | Caring for people with suicidal inclinations during primary and intermediate treatment |
| Access of tools and approaches | Exert control over suicidal tools and approaches |
| Committing a suicide | Effective interference; evaluation and follow up with unsuccessfully attempted suicides |
| After suicide | Reflect on media policies held accountable and learn from experiences |

participation, responsibility and common interests." The incisive statement in the 19th CPC National Congress Report about strengthening and developing new approaches for social governance suggests that we should adopt an integrated suicide model based on collaboration, participation, responsibility and common interests.

The Integrated Suicide Prevention aims at reducing mental disorders and improving the overall mental health of all people, so as to draft a holistic suicide prevention plan and establish a thorough system of suicidal data collection and risks monitoring. It is a mechanism that integrates macro social policies, mass media, governments, communities, medical institutions, the education system and social organizations for better providing potential suicidal individuals with necessary knowledge about suicide prevention, psychotherapy and counseling, as well as effective training, comforting and reassuring services. The Integrated Suicide Prevention differs from the isolated one as it takes coordinate controls in every step that could possibly lead to a potential suicide, and the purpose of that is to build a protective and preventative network against suicides.

To conduct effective and coordinate measures against every step towards a suicide, a unified suicide prevention mechanism is required, as the integrated suicide prevention model involves a series of fundamental public issues.

China is working toward this pattern in dealing with suicides. On April 16th, 2018, the Ministry of Emergency Management of China has been officially founded. It integrated 13 existing departments and organizations. Apart from the target

| Fundamental public issues classified in the integrated suicide prevention model |
|---|
| Public education |
| Media reports held accountable |
| School courses |
| Prompt treatment to depressive orders and other mental disorders |
| Close attention to alcohol and drug abusers |
| Close attention to people with physical diseases and the disabled |
| Increase the opportunity of access to mental health services |
| Improvement in suicide attempt evaluation |
| Interference after a suicide |
| Interference in suicidal risks |
| Policies on employment and unemployment |
| Training of professional personnel on public health |
| Limit the access to tools that could possibly lead to suicides |

to streamline government organs, more importantly, it is an effort to establish an authoritative, efficient oversight system with complete coverage under the Party's unified command, thus improving social security, stability, and modernization of China's social governance. We will take full advantage of different sectors to forge a unified command and dispatching system as well as a cross-department responding mechanism so as to eliminate information isolation that causes departments staying aloof and shifting responsibilities. It is indeed a whole set of management system of risk control, caution and emergency treatment, and it is truly a blessed message addressing suicides in China.

## Epilogue

This book first came into being in 2012, which is 6–7 years from now. Therefore, some of the statistics and cases appear to be outdated. In recent years, China has enjoyed a steady economic growth, rapid development in social undertakings, and improved social security.

Undoubtedly, China still has a long way to go to prevent and control suicide. Yet we should also note that the suicide rate in China has fallen dramatically, indicating that we have achieved remarkable results through our continuous efforts over the past three decades.

We have every reason to believe that, under the guidance of "Healthy China" strategy, the whole society would work together to facilitate suicide prevention and to take on an integrated suicide prevention method based on China's own reality.

# References


Becker, E. (1988). *The denial of death* (p. 33) (H. Lin, Trans.). Guiyang: Guizhou People's Publishing House.

Cai, C. (2005). Mental health educational system in institutions of higher learning of Beijing. *Guangming Daily* (6th ed.), February 2, 2005.

Chen, J. L. (Ed., Trans.). (2006). Deadly beauty, *The Economist*, June 8, 2006.

Chen B. (2008). Rural suicide under changing values. *China Rural Study* (Vol. 6). Fuzhou: Fujian Education Press.

Chen, Q. (2010). China's deplorable suicide intervention system. *Yangcheng Evening News*, September 12, 2010.

Cheng, W., & Wang, J. (1999). Mental health legislation in Japan. *Medicine and Philosophy, 5,* 32.

Durkheim (1996). *Le suicide* (p. 342) (Y. Feng, Trans.). Beijing: The Commercial Press.

Durkheim, E. (1996). *Le suicide* (p. 372). (Y. Feng, Trans.). Beijing: The Commercial Press.

Eddleston, M., & Philips, M. R. (2004). Self-poisoning with pesticides. *BMJ, 328,* 42–44.

Freud, S. (1999). *The future of an illusion* (pp. 54–55) (S. Yang, Trans.). Beijing: Huaxia Publishing House.

Gilliland, B. E., & James, R. K. (2000). *Crisis intervention strategies* (p. 275) (S. Xiao, et al. Trans.). Beijing: China Light Industry Press.

Guan, H. (2011). Challenges to mental health legislation. *Chinese Social Sciences Today*, January 20, 2011.

Han, D. (2008). *Spirit of the constitution* (p. 134). Beijing: Law Press China.

Han, D. (2011). Euthanasia's constitutional limit. *Tsinghua University Law Journal*, no. 5.

He, Z. (2008). Suicide rate too high? No!. *Academic Forum*, no. 2.

Hu, J. (2007). Report to the 17th CPC National Congress. *People's Daily*, October 15, 2007.

Huang, W. (2005). Cultivating healthy-minded university students. *China Education Daily* (4th ed.). January 21, 2005.

Huntington, S. P. (1988). *Political order in changing societies* (p. 51) (S. Li, & Y. Yang, Trans.). Beijing: Huaxia Publishing House.

Ji, H. (1999). Psychological survey and crisis intervention in normal universities. Journal of *Beijing Normal University (Social Sciences Edition)* (pp. 26–33), no. 1.

Jing, J. et al. (2010). How rural women affect suicide rate. *Journal of China Agricultural University (Sociology Edition)*, no. 4.

Kang, Q. (2002). An analysis of suicide among women in rural areas in china. *Journal of Jishou University (Social Sciences Edition)*, no. 1.

Li, Z. (2004). Mental hea0lth legislation. *Journal of Clinical Psychosomatic Diseases* (p. 305), no. 4.

Li, J. (2007a). *Suicide of young people* (p. 286). Beijing: China Social Sciences Press.

Li, W. (2012). *Disadvantaged groups at high risk of suicide*. http://www.cnr.cn/china/ygxw/201109/t20110909_508484799.shtml. Accessed on January 12, 2012.

Li, C., & Bao, X. (2007). China needs mental health law fast. *China Science Dailly*, December 20, 2007.

Li, H., & Qin, X. (2008). Risk factors and prevention of suicide repeated attempts. *International Psychiatry*, no. 2.

Lin, Z. (2004). What are human rights? *Study Times*, March 25, 2004.

Liu, Y. (2010). National law, common law, and rural suicide. *Journal of Yunnan University (Law Edition)*, Vol. 5.

Liu, Y. (2010). Suicide: Plight, theory, solution. *Journal of China Agricultural University (Sociology Edition)*, Vol. 3.

Liu, J., & Fan, Y. (2010). WHO: Most suicides are preventable. *Guangming Daily* (4th ed.), September 11, 2010.

Lu, Y., & Cui, C. (2005). Suicide intervention: Vision and difficulty. *Nanfang Daily*, October 7, 2005.
Mann, J. J. (2002). A current perspective of suicide and attempted suicide. *Annals of Internal Medicine, 136*(4), 302–311.
Mao, R. (2010). Creating an official suicide intervention system. *Central China Normal University Journal of Postgraduates*, no. 3, p. 16.
McKinley, J. (2006). San Francisco strives again to prevent suicide on golden gate bridge. *The New York Times*, August 11, 2006.
Menninger, K. (1990). *Man against himself* (p. 74) (C. Feng, Trans.). Guiyang: Guizhou People's Publishing House.
Phillips, M. (2004). How to deal with suicide. *Chinese Journal of Epidemiology*, no. 4.
Shi, H. (2001). *Suicides of college students*. (Master's dissertation, Wuhan University of Technology).
Shi, Y. (2011). *Tough world begets strong mind* (pp. 38–39). Beijing: Industry Printing Press.
Tang, Y., & Chen, G. (2005). Zhang Zai's ethics. *Studies in Ethics*, no. 5.
Tejedor, M. C., et al. (1999). Attempted suicide: Repetition and survival-findings of a follow-up study. *Acta Psychiatry Scand, 100*(3), 205–211.
United Nations Program for Policy Coordination and Sustainable Development. (2012). Suicide prevention—Instructions for national strategy creation and implementation. http://news.sina.com.cn/c/2011-09-06/152223115689.shtml. Accessed: 14 March, 2012.
US Department of Health and Human Services. (1992). Youth suicide prevention programs: A resource guide, Washington D.C., U.S.A.
Wan, S. et al. (2005). What 1068 Nanjing schoolchildren think about death. *Journal of Nanjing Party Institute of CPC and Nanjing Administration Institute*, no. 2.
Wang, X. (1990). *Psychosomatic medicine* (p. 916). Beijing: Chinese Medicine Science and Technology Press.
Wang, X. (2007). Life education and its implications. *Elementary and secondary schooling abroad*, no. 1.
Wang, P. (2011). New hope for mental health legislation. *The People's Congress of China*, no. 21.
Wasserman, D. (2003). *Suicide: An unnecessary death* (pp. 284–285) (M. Li, Trans.). Beijing: China Light Industry Publishing House.
Wen, J. (2010). A few problems regarding social and economic development, *Qiushi*, no. 7.
Wen, J. (2010). In *Speech at a press conference of the 3rd session of the 11th National People's Congress*. March 14, 2010.
Wen, J., & Zeng, Z. (2007). Suicide intervention. *New Generation Investigation*, no. 8.
Wu, F. (2007). On "living one's days". *Sociological Studies*, no. 6.
Wu, F. (2007b). *Suicide as a Chinese problem* (p. 117). Beijing: SDX Joint Publishing Company.
Wu, F. (2010). *Finding meaning in life* (p. 263). Beijing: China Renmin University Press.
Xiao, S. (2008). *Psychological studies on suicide*. http://hncic.virtualave.net/suibook/chapter4.htm . Accessed March 16, 2008.
Xiao, S. (2012). *A psychological study on suicide*. http://hncic.virtualave.net/suibook/chapter4.htm . Accessed March 15, 2012.
Xiao, S. (2012). *Psychological studies on suicide*. http://hncic.virtualave.net/suibook/chapter4.htm . Accessed March 15, 2012.
Xu, D. et al. (2012). Effect of socio-psychological intervention on suicides. *Chinese Mental Health Journal*, no. 1.
Yao, Y. (2005). Crisis intervention for youth suicides. *Chinese Education Journal* (p. 75), no. 8.
Zhai, S. (1997a). *Crisis intervention and suicide prevention* (p. 307). Beijing: People's Medical Publishing House.
Zhai, S. (1997b). *Crisis intervention and suicide prevention* (p. 308). Beijing: People's Medical Publishing House.
Zhai, S. (1997c). *Crisis intervention and suicide prevention* (p. 102). Beijing: People's Medical Publishing House.

Zhai, S. (1997d). *Crisis intervention and suicide prevention* (p. 306). Beijing: People's Medical Publishing House.
Zhang, S. (1997). Life-and-death education and suicidal children. *Educational Research, 5,* 33–40.

# Uncited References

Bai, Z. (1983). *Diseases of the Western Society* (H. Zhang, Trans.). Beijing: SDX Joint Publishing Company.
Becker, E. (1998). *The denial of death* (H. Lin, Trans.). Guiyang: Guizhou People's Press.
Benedict, R. (1946). *The chrysanthemum and the sword: Patterns of Japanese culture* (Z. Sun, et al., Trans. 1987). Hangzhou: Zhejiang People's Press.
Chen, Q., & Li, X., et al. (2002). Research on Lahu customs, religion, and suicide in Zhanmapo Village of Lancang, Yunnan. *Chinese Mental Health Journal*, no.4.
Cheng, Q. (2007). Dialogue between Taoism and Islam on life and death. *Journal of Tibet Nationalities Institute*, no. 2.
Da, D. (2001). Suicide studies over the past fifty years. *Medicine and Society,* no. 4.
Dahuan, T. (2011). *Migration of the century: Shift towards mega-cities that will determine China's fate*. Beijing: China Development Press.
Dai, K. (1999). *Contemporary emerging religions*. Beijing: Oriental Press.
Department of Social Statistics, National Bureau of Statistics. (1987). *China's social statistics*. Beijing: China Statistics Press.
Du, P. (2006). *Population aging and the attendant problems*. Beijing: People's Publishing House.
Durkheim, E. (1996). *Le suicide*, (Y. Feng, Trans.). Beijing: The Commercial Press.
Durkheim, É. (1998). *Suicide: A study in sociology* (X. Zhong, & L. Ma, Q. Lin, Trans.). Hangzhou: Zhejiang People's Press.
Fan, Z. (1997). Legal treatment of indifference, negligence, and cowardice. *China Legal Science*, no.4.
Fang, J. (2010). Stream of suicides by students in mainland China. *Lianhe Zaobao.*
Ferguson, H. (2003). *The end of happiness* (Z. Xu, Trans.). Beijing: China Renmin University Press.
Frued, S. (1999). *Die zukunft einer illusion* (S. Yang, Trans.). Beijing: Huaxia Publishing House.
Fu, C. (1994). *The dignity of death and the dignity of life*. Taipei: Cheng Chung Book Co., Ltd.
Fuse, T. (1992). *Suicide and culture* (L. Ma, Trans.). Beijing: Culture and Art Publishing House.
Gu, X. (2007). *Death by Naxi people for love*. Beijing: Writer's Publishing House.
Guan, M. et al. (1995). Relationship between the Mongolian, Han and Hui cultures and suicide. *Hebei Mental Health,* no. 4.
Guo, Q., & Wang, Z., Tatsumi, T. (1993). A comparative study of suicide in nine Asian countries and regions. *Journal of International Psychiatry,* no. 4.
Hai, B. (2007). *Buddha on death*. Xi'an: Shaanxi People's Press.
He, Z. (1997). *The pathology of suicide*. Beijing: China Traditional Chinese Medicine Press.
He, Q. (1998). *The trap of modernity: Economic and social issues in contemporary China*. Beijing: China Today Press.
He, S. (2003). *Social formations at a time of transformation in contemporary China*. Shanghai: Xuelin Publishing.
He, J., Jiang, Y., Xia, B., et al. (2002). Study on the impact of comprehensive intervention on rural suicides. *Chinese Mental Health Journal, 16*(2), 100.
Hu, Y. (2002). Sociological reflections on depression. *Journal of Xinyang Normal University* 2001, no. 4.
Hu, Q., et al. (1999). *Social psychology issues faced by university students today, and countermeasures*. Nanchang: Jiangxi People's Press.
Huang, Z. (Ed.). (2008). *Rural China studies* (Vol. 6). Fuzhou: Fujian Education Press.

Huang, P., et al. (1997). *In pursuit of survival: A study of contemporary rural migrant population in China*. Kunming: Yunnan People's Press.
Huo, T. (2010). *Out of death*. Beijing: China Renmin University Press.
Ji, J., & Zhao, J. (2007). *Suicide prevention and crisis intervention*. Shanghai: East China Normal University Press.
Kang, Q. (2002). Analysis of rural female suicides. *Jishou University Journal (Social Sciences Edition)*, no. 3.
Kasahara, R. (1988). *Ambitions of the warlords* (L. Hu, Trans.). Beijing: PLA Publishing House.
Lei, B., & Liu, H. (1995). *Brief history of Lahu literature*. Kunming: Nationalities Publishing House of Yunnan.
Li, F. (1988). A survey of 4,868 college students with neurasthenia in the Lanzhou area. *Chinese Mental Health Journal*, no. 5.
Li, J. (1991). Waste of life by the new generation: Youth suicide in Japan. *Contemporary Youth Research*, no. 3.
Li, J. (1995). Historical and cultural factors of Japanese suicide. *Sociological studies*, no.6.
Li, H. (2001a). *An interview on violence: A record of psychological harm on school campuses, and countermeasures*. Beijing: China Writers Publishing House.
Li, J. (2001b). *A socio-cultural study on suicide*. Guizhou: Guizhou People's Press.
Li, J. (2001c). *Women of Japan: Japanese women and the "Great East Asia War"*. Guizhou: Guizhou People's Press.
Li, J. (2002). A comparative study of suicide among young females in China and Japan. *Journal of China Youth University for Political Sciences*, no. 6.
Li, J. (2007). Suicide: From crime to right in Western legal history. *Political Science and Law*, no.2.
Li, H., & He, L. (2002). Survey report on suicide among Chinese. *Life week*, December 13, 2002.
Li, X., & Michael, P. (2001). Causes of death for those of reproductive age and who died from suicide in China in 1998. *Chinese Journal of Public Health*, *17*(7).
Li, B., & Zuo, G., (2010). The disorder model: An examination of the reasons for suicide among China's rural women. *Journal of Shijiazhuang University*, no. (1).
Liang, J., & Li, J. (2012). *Too many Chinese?*. Beijing: Social Sciences Academic Press China.
Liu, H. (1995). A comparative study on suicidal deaths among urban and rural women in China. *Chinese Journal of Behavioral Medical Science*, 4(2).
Liu, K. (2001). Case study on child suicide. *Journal of Clinical Psychiatry*, no. 6.
Liu, B. (2004). An analysis on the reasons behind the high suicide rate among rural women. *Journal of China Agricultural University (Social Sciences Edition)*. no. 4.
Liu, Y. (2009). Building rural social organization mechanisms towards social Self-Governance. *Southeast Academic Research*, Vol. 1.
Liu, H., & Li, X. (1996). The current state of research into suicide, and trends. *Foreign Medicien (Psychiatry Volume)*, *23*(2).
Liu, X., & Su, L. (2002). The impact of video games on the behavior of children. *Chinese Mental Health Journal*, *16*(1).
Liu, L., & Xiao, S. (2002). A follow-up study of individuals who have attempted suicide. *Chinese Mental Health Journal*. *16*(4).
Liu, Y., & Xiao, S. (2007). The impact of media reports of suicide incidents on suicide behavior in the community (an overview). *Chinese Mental Health Journal*, no. 5.
Liu, X., Huang, Y., & Li, L. (2000). A case-control study of personality disorders in college students. *Chinese Mental Health Journal*, *14*(2).
Lü, Z. (2005). 1,200 entrepreneurs commit suicide in two decades in China. *Corporate Culture and Management*, no. 6.
Mao, J. (2005). *The last myths: Suicide by poets*. Yinchuan: Ningxia People's Press.
Ministry of Health. (2004–2010). *China Health Statistical Yearbook (2004–2010)*. Beijing: Union Medical College Press.
Minois, G. (2003). *Histoire du suicide* (J. Li, & Q. Lin, Trans.). Beijing: Economic Daily Press.

Pan, S. (2004). Systematic cultural explanation of death caves in the Hanshui river basin. *Journal of Yunyang Teachers' College*, no. 5.
Pan, L., &Wang, Z. (2005). Literature review on suicide studies in China. *Chinese Journal of Behavioral Medical Science*, no. 7.
Peng, G. (1997). 268 case studies of elderly suicide. *Rural Public Health Management*, no. 8.
Philip, M. (2004). Current status of suicide in China and direction of future work. *Chinese Journal of Epidemiology*, no.4.
Qi, S. (1999). Genetic research on suicide by depression patients. *Journal of Clinical Psychiatry*, no.3.
Qian, M., et al. (1996). A study on the relationship between youth personality and parenting methods. *Chinese Mental Health Journal, 10*(2).
Shang, H. (1998). *Chinese and Japanese: A comparative study of social groups, way of behavior, and cultural psychology*. Beijing: Peking University Press.
Song, L. (1996). Migration of China's rural labor force and countermeasures. *Sociological Studies*, no.2.
Song, A. (1998). Study on the correlation between characteristics of and social support for infertile women. *Medicine and Society, 11*(3), 25.
Song, X. (2001). *Report on the reform and development of China's Rural social security system*. Beijing: China Renmin University Press.
The First Historical Archives of China. (2008). *Collection of social archives of emperor Jiajing's reign of the Qing Dynasty* (Vol. 1–3). Tianjin: Tianjin Antique Book Company.
Vago, S. (2007). *Social change* (X. Wang, et al., Trans.). Beijing: Peking University Press.
Wang, J. (Ed.). (2006). *Report on women development in China* (No. 1). Beijing: Social Sciences Academic Press.
Wang, W. (2006b). *Depression, suicide, and crisis intervention*. Chongqing: Chongqing Press.
Wang, F. (2007b). *The culture of funerals: A comprehensive interpretation of death culture*. Changsha: Hunan People's Press.
Wasserman, D. (Ed.). (2003). *Suicide: An unnecessary death* (M. Li et al., Trans.). Beijing: China Light Industry Press.
Wen, Z. (1998). *Transcending death: Prevention and control of suicidal behavior*. Shanghai: Shanghai Medical University Press.
Wu, Z. (1999). The confusion regarding sexual issues that senior high students face today. *Contemporary Youth Research (sic.)*, no. 4.
Xi, Y. (2005). Suicide for love by the Naxi people and socio-psychological analysis. *Journal of Yunnan Minzu University (Philosophy and Social Sciences Edition),* no. 3.
Xie, L. (Ed.). (1999). *Report on suicides among rural women in China*. Guiyang: Guizhou People's Press.
Xin, Z., & Chi, L. (2008). *Youth in the midst of social change*. Beijing: Beijing Normal University Press.
Xu, Z. (1995). Suicide among Hong Kong youth and prevention. *Journal of Clinical Neurology, 5* (2).
Xu, X. (2000). A sociological analysis on drug abuse among youth and the prevention and control of such abuse. *Youth Studies*, no. 3.
Xu, Y. (2001). A study of the psychological health and family environment factors of high school students with suicide ideation. *China Journal of School Health, 22*(5).
Xu, X. (2002). Characteristics and problems of Chinese suicide studies. *Society,* no.6.
Xu, Y., & Gao, H. (1999). A study of youth suicide and home environment factors. *Chinese Journal of Public Health, 15*(12).
Yan, M. (2008). A preliminary analysis on the social causes of the high suicide rate among rural women in China. *Journal of Tianzhong, 23*(6).
Yang, F. (1999). *Road of soul*. Shenzhen: Haitian Publishing House.
Yang, X. (2000). An evaluation of the impact of the Internet on Chinese youth. *Youth Studies*, no. 4.

Yang, R. (2002). Semantic and functional characteristics of *sha* in ancient Chinese. *Journal of Chinese Language History,* no. 2.

Yang, G., Huang, Z., & Chen, A. (2004). Trends and geographical distribution of suicide in the Chinese population. *Chinese Journal of Epidemiology, 25*(4).

Yang, C., & Huang, Z. (2007). Building and improving rural social security system in China: An approach based on urban-rural coordination. *Journal of Northwest A&F University (Social Sciences Edition),* no. 1.

Yang, H., & Li, Z. (2002). A preliminary analysis of the "ten Internet harms" to youth psychology. *Youth Work Forum,* no. 1.

Yang, Q., & Wang, W. (2009). Study on collective suicide by Hui'an women in the Republic of China period. *Fujian Tribune,* no. 7.

Yang, Y., & Wang, L., et al. (2010). Update on the study on tryptophan hydroxylase and depression and suicide behavior. *Chinese Journal of Public Health, 26*(3).

Yang, G., Huang, Z., & Chen, A. (1997). Levels of accidental harm among Chinese populations, and trends. *Chinese Journal of Epidemiology, 18*(3).

Yao, J., & Feng, Z. (2002). Suicide in Yunnan Province. *Journal of Clinical Psychiatry,* no. 4.

Ye, Y. (2006). A few interpretations relating to traditional attitudes about women. *Journal of the Fuqing Branch of Fujian Normal University,* no. 6.

Yin, D. (2002). United with a practical mind, we promote mental health on all fronts in the new century: Report of the 3rd National Conference on Mental Health Work. *Chinese Mental Health Journal, 16*(1).

Yu, D. (1997). *The door between life and death* (p. 187). Beijing: New World Press.

Yu, Z., et al. (2001). *Reflections on issues related to the education of the youth.* Hohhot: Inner Mongolia People's Press.

Yue, D., et al. (1993). Methods of parental upbringing: the preliminary draft of the EMBU and the applications of the EMBU with patients with neurosis. *China Mental Health Journal, 7*(3).

Yue, X. (1999). A comparative analysis of idol worship and learning from one's models among youth. *Youth Studies,* no. 7.

Zeng, G., & Cai, Y. (2001). Guard against growing psychological indifference and pay attention to psychological issues among youth. *Guangming Daily.*

Zeng, G., & Fu, C., et al. (2006). Survey on anxiety and depression among patients with cardia-cerebrovascular diseases. *Chinese Journal of Public Health,* no. 9.

Zhai, S. (1997). Bridge suicides. *Journal of Clinical Psychological Medicine, 7*(2).

Zhai, S. (2001). Social factors and suicide. *Medicine and Society* no. 6.

Zhang, W. et al. (1998). An epidemiological survey of mental illness in seven regions of China. *Chinese Journal of Psychiatry, 31*(2).

Zhang, C. (Ed.). (2001). *History of human suicide.* Changchun: The Time Literature and Art Press.

Zhang, D. (2002). On emerging religions in Japan and their response to social changes. *Japanese Studies,* no. 5.

Zhang, Y. (2002). Evolution of suicide studies in sociology. *Sociological Studies,* no. 4.

Zhang, Y. (2004). Supply of and funding for public health services in rural areas. *China Rural Survey,* no. 10.

Zhang, X. (2007). *Death and economy.* Guiyang: Guizhou People's Press.

Zhang, W. (2008). Fiscal deficiencies in rural social security system building and countermeasures. *Economic Research Guide,* no. 11.

Zhang, G., & Hou, G. (2003). Serotonin and molecular genetics of depression and suicide. *Foreign Medicine (Psychiatry Volume),* no. 2.

Zhang, L., & Liu, M. (Eds.). (2004). *A study of domestic violence in China.* Beijing: China Social Science Press.

Zheng, X. (2011). *Life and death: The Chinese wisdom* (p. 131). Beijing: Peking University Press.

Zheng, Y., & Lai, X. (2003). *More student suicides.* http://www.people.com.cn/GB/jiaoyu/1055/1998514.html.

MIX
Papier aus verantwortungsvollen Quellen
Paper from responsible sources
FSC® C105338

If you have any concerns about our products,
you can contact us on
**ProductSafety@springernature.com**

In case Publisher is established outside the EU,
the EU authorized representative is:
**Springer Nature Customer Service Center GmbH**
**Europaplatz 3, 69115 Heidelberg, Germany**

Printed by Libri Plureos GmbH
in Hamburg, Germany